Ultrasonics
Physics and applications

Online at: https://doi.org/10.1088/978-0-7503-4936-9

USE

Ultrasonics
Physics and applications

Edited by
Mami Matsukawa
Faculty of Science and Engineering, Doshisha University, Kyotanabe, Kyoto, Japan

Pak-Kon Choi
Department of Physics, Meiji University, Tama-ku, Kawasaki, Japan

Kentaro Nakamura
Institute of Innovative Research, Tokyo Institute of Technology, Midori-ku, Yokohama, Japan

Hirotsugu Ogi
Graduate School of Engineering, Osaka University, Suita, Osaka, Japan

Hideyuki Hasegawa
Faculty of Engineering, Academic Assembly, University of Toyama, Toyama, Japan

IOP Publishing, Bristol, UK

© IOP Publishing Ltd 2022

All rights reserved. No part of this publication may be reproduced, stored in a retrieval system or transmitted in any form or by any means, electronic, mechanical, photocopying, recording or otherwise, without the prior permission of the publisher, or as expressly permitted by law or under terms agreed with the appropriate rights organization. Multiple copying is permitted in accordance with the terms of licences issued by the Copyright Licensing Agency, the Copyright Clearance Centre and other reproduction rights organizations.

Permission to make use of IOP Publishing content other than as set out above may be sought at permissions@ioppublishing.org.

Mami Matsukawa, Pak-Kon Choi, Kentaro Nakamura, Hirotsugu Ogi and Hideyuki Hasegawa have asserted their right to be identified as the editors of this work in accordance with sections 77 and 78 of the Copyright, Designs and Patents Act 1988.

Multimedia content is available for this book from https://doi.org/10.1088/978-0-7503-4936-9.

ISBN   978-0-7503-4936-9 (ebook)
ISBN   978-0-7503-4934-5 (print)
ISBN   978-0-7503-4937-6 (myPrint)
ISBN   978-0-7503-4935-2 (mobi)

DOI   10.1088/978-0-7503-4936-9

Version: 20221101

IOP ebooks

British Library Cataloguing-in-Publication Data: A catalogue record for this book is available from the British Library.

Published by IOP Publishing, wholly owned by The Institute of Physics, London

IOP Publishing, No.2 The Distillery, Glassfields, Avon Street, Bristol, BS2 0GR, UK

US Office: IOP Publishing, Inc., 190 North Independence Mall West, Suite 601, Philadelphia, PA 19106, USA

Contents

Preface	x
Preface from the Institute for Ultrasonic Electronics	xi
Editor biographies	xii
Contributor biographies	xiv

Part I Basic physics and measurements

1 Ultrasound propagation — 1-1
Pak-Kon Choi

1.1	Ultrasound propagation in gases and liquids	1-1
	1.1.1 Frequency of ultrasound	1-2
	1.1.2 Adiabaticity of sound propagation	1-2
	1.1.3 Wave equation	1-3
	1.1.4 Sound velocity	1-5
	1.1.5 Plane waves	1-7
1.2	Ultrasound propagation in solids	1-8
	1.2.1 Elastic properties of solids	1-8
	1.2.2 Wave equation in solids	1-10
1.3	Absorption and velocity dispersion in fluids	1-12
	1.3.1 Ultrasound absorption	1-12
	1.3.2 The relaxation phenomenon	1-14
	1.3.3 Molecular vibrational relaxation	1-16
	1.3.4 Examples of the relaxation phenomenon in fluids	1-18
1.4	Sound radiation	1-22
	1.4.1 Sound field produced by a circular piston source	1-23
	1.4.2 Simulation of a sound field	1-26
1.5	Measurement of ultrasound fields by optical methods	1-28
	1.5.1 Schlieren method	1-28
	1.5.2 Photoelasticity imaging method	1-29
	1.5.3 Shadowgraphy method	1-31
	1.5.4 Luminescence due to acoustic cavitation	1-31
	References	1-32

2	**Wave propagation in/on liquids and spectroscopy of viscoelasticity and surface tension**	**2-1**
	Keiji Sakai	
2.1	Introduction	2-1
	2.1.1 Viscoelastic properties of, and wave propagation in liquids	2-1
	2.1.2 Dynamics of liquid surface properties	2-6
2.2	Recent progress in the light-scattering approach to viscoelasticity	2-7
	2.2.1 Accurate Brillouin scattering experiment based on an optical heterodyne technique	2-7
	2.2.2 Thermal phonon resonance	2-9
	2.2.3 Determination of shear, orientational, and coupling viscosities in liquids	2-11
2.3	Recent progress in the experimental approach to the dynamic surface phenomena of liquids	2-14
	2.3.1 Ripplon spectroscopy	2-14
	2.3.2 Manipulation and observation of micro liquid particles	2-19
2.4	Introduction to recent progress in rheometry	2-23
	2.4.1 The electromagnetic spinning (EMS) rheometer system	2-23
	2.4.2 Measurement of viscoelasticity using the EMS system equipped with quadruple electromagnets	2-25
	2.4.3 Examination of the quantum standard for viscosity	2-26
	References	2-30
3	**Optical measurements of ultrasonic fields in air/water and ultrasonic vibration in solids**	**3-1**
	Kentaro Nakamura	
3.1	Measurement of ultrasonic fields in air/water	3-1
	3.1.1 Problems arising in ultrasonic field measurement	3-1
	3.1.2 Probe sensors using optical fibers	3-2
	3.1.3 Imaging of ultrasonic fields using optical methods	3-14
	3.1.4 Super directivity in the detection of ultrasonic waves	3-18
3.2	Vibration measurement at ultrasonic frequencies	3-20
	3.2.1 Out-of-plane vibration	3-20
	3.2.2 In-plane vibration	3-25
	3.2.3 Fringe-counting method for high-amplitude vibration	3-26
	3.2.4 Sagnac interferometer for very-high-frequency vibration	3-28
3.3	Conclusions and outlook	3-29
	References	3-30

4 Picosecond laser ultrasonics   4-1
Osamu Matsuda and Oliver B Wright

4.1	Introduction	4-1
4.2	Basics of picosecond laser ultrasonics	4-2
	4.2.1 Overview	4-2
	4.2.2 Basic experimental setup	4-4
	4.2.3 Interferometric setup	4-5
	4.2.4 One-dimensional model	4-8
4.3	Extensions of picosecond laser ultrasonics	4-11
	4.3.1 Time-resolved Brillouin-scattering measurements assisted by metallic gratings	4-11
	4.3.2 Generation and detection of shear acoustic waves assisted by metallic gratings	4-19
4.4	Summary	4-25
	References	4-25

Part II   Industrial applications

5 Ball surface acoustic wave sensor and its application to trace gas analysis   5-1
Kazushi Yamanaka, Takamitsu Iwaya and Shingo Akao

5.1	Introduction	5-1
5.2	SAWs on a sphere	5-2
5.3	Principles of the ball SAW sensor	5-5
5.4	Hydrogen gas sensors	5-8
5.5	Trace moisture analyzer	5-12
	5.5.1 Ball SAW TMA using phase signal for temperature compensation	5-12
	5.5.2 Ball SAW TMA using amplitude signal for various background gases	5-14
5.6	Micro gas chromatography	5-18
	5.6.1 Concept and problems of gas chromatography	5-18
	5.6.2 Sensitive film used in the ball SAW gas chromatograph	5-20
	5.6.3 Palm-sized ball SAW gas chromatograph as an example of micro GC	5-21
	5.6.4 Analysis of the aroma components of sake — a crystal sommelier	5-24
5.7	Conclusions	5-26
	References	5-26

6	**Phase adjuster in a thermoacoustic system**	6-1
	Shin-ichi Sakamoto and Yoshiaki Watanabe	
6.1	Introduction	6-1
6.2	Thermoacoustic phenomenon leading to steady oscillation	6-3
	6.2.1 Loop-tube-type thermoacoustic cooling system	6-3
	6.2.2 Mechanism of thermoacoustic cooling	6-5
	6.2.3 Variation of resonant wavelength and cooling capacity	6-6
	6.2.4 Resonant frequency before stable self-excited oscillation: changes in cooling capacity and resonant wavelength observed in the boundary layer	6-8
	6.2.5 Resonant frequency under conditions of stable self-excited oscillation: influence of total length of, and pressure in the tube	6-11
6.3	Progression to phase adjuster	6-14
6.4	Beyond the PA	6-19
6.5	Conclusions	6-20
	References	6-20

Part III Biological and medical applications

7	**Ultrasonic characterization of bone**	7-1
	Mami Matsukawa	
7.1	Why should we study bone using ultrasound?	7-1
7.2	Ultrasonic wave properties in bone tissues	7-3
	7.2.1 Conventional ultrasonic characterization in the megahertz range	7-3
	7.2.2 Microscopic bone evaluation by Brillouin scattering	7-7
	7.2.3 Piezoelectricity in bone in the megahertz range	7-11
7.3	Ultrasonic characterization of cancellous bone	7-17
	7.3.1 Two-wave phenomenon and clinical application	7-17
7.4	Conclusions	7-25
	References	7-25

8	**Acceleration and control of protein aggregation**	8-1
	Hirotsugu Ogi	
8.1	Introduction	8-1
8.2	Mechanism of acceleration of protein aggregation	8-4
8.3	Nonlinear components as indicators for the aggregation reaction	8-13
8.4	Supersaturation: a new concept for protein aggregation phenomenon	8-18

8.5	Multichannel ultrasonication system for amyloid assay: HANABI	8-22
8.6	Summary and future prospects	8-25
	References	8-26

9 High-frame-rate medical ultrasonic imaging — 9-1
Hideyuki Hasegawa

9.1	Introduction	9-1
9.2	High-frame-rate ultrasonic imaging	9-2
9.3	Motion estimators	9-7
	9.3.1 Autocorrelation method	9-7
	9.3.2 Vector Doppler method	9-8
	9.3.3 Block-matching method	9-9
	9.3.4 Spectrum-based motion estimator	9-10
9.4	Applications of high-frame-rate ultrasonic imaging	9-13
	9.4.1 Strain or strain-rate imaging	9-13
	9.4.2 Measurement of propagation of mechanical waves in tissue	9-20
	9.4.3 Blood-flow imaging	9-26
	References	9-35

10 High-intensity focused ultrasound — 10-1
Shin Yoshizawa and Shin-ichiro Umemura

10.1	Introduction	10-1
10.2	HIFU devices	10-3
10.3	Measurement and visualization of HIFU fields	10-5
10.4	Cavitation	10-7
10.5	Ultrasound image guidance	10-9
10.6	Concluding remarks	10-12
	References	10-13

Preface

After initial studies by Langevin in the early 20th century, research areas related to ultrasonics have been expanding tremendously. Ultrasonics has recently become an interdisciplinary scientific field, because it is always discussed in conjunction with other studies, such as optics, mechanics, biology, chemistry, ecology, medicine, etc. This also confirms the wide applicability and flexibility of ultrasonic techniques for practical use in this age of diverse and innovative technological evolution.

It is very interesting that young scientists (students, engineers, and researchers) sometimes envision the development of a new technique and then knock on the doors of ultrasonics laboratories. One probable reason for this is that sound is a fundamental and important physical phenomenon that is learned about in high schools and universities, which makes them familiar with ultrasound even though it is beyond the audible range for humans. The other reason is very practical. Ultrasonic systems are comparatively inexpensive and safe, and can often be integrated into other facilities. Thus, we find a lot of ultrasonic techniques and studies in various scientific areas. Unfortunately, it may be difficult for young engineers to realize all their visions using ultrasound technology. Many aspects and limitations of ultrasound techniques have to be considered from the physical points of view.

This e-book will introduce some perspectives on ultrasonics for young scientists (and of course senior scientists) and how they commenced and developed. Each chapter reviews recent progress in ultrasonics, the details of which have been presented in the annual symposiums on Ultrasonic Electronics (USE) (https://use-jp.org/) since 1980. They have been partly published as papers in the Special Issue on Ultrasonic Electronics of the *Japanese Journal of Applied Physics*, which is a journal of IOP publishing. This book is divided into three parts: basic physics and measurements, industrial applications, and biological and medical applications. It is recommended to start with chapter 1, 'Ultrasound propagation', where the basic physics of ultrasound propagation is thoroughly introduced. Readers can then read any chapters they are interested in, and enjoy the recent and interesting topics of ultrasonics. Moreover, it is recommended to try reading chapters which seem to fall into different categories. In reading several chapters of this book, you may find a common feature among various ultrasound techniques and will gradually enjoy the interdisciplinary science of 'Ultrasonics'.

We would be delighted if this book would help to open a new window on the interesting world of ultrasonics.

The editors

Preface from the Institute for Ultrasonic Electronics

Since the first Symposium on Ultrasonic Electronics (USE) was held in Tokyo, Japan in 1980, it has been conducted every year at different meeting venues. Since the first meeting, the number of participants has continuously increased; today, more than 300 presentations are given in each symposium, and the total number of presentations given during the past 42 meetings has exceeded 8000. A feature of USE is that some presentations are published and archived as papers in the Special Issue on Ultrasonic Electronics of the *Japanese Journal of Applied Physics*, which is a journal of IOP publishing. A total of more than 3000 papers have been published to date. The special issues are now valuable resources that document the history of the development of ultrasonic research. The USE covers diverse research fields, such as physical acoustics, measurement technology, electronic devices, power ultrasonics and sonochemistry, marine and environmental acoustics, and medical and biological ultrasonics, and includes all current ultrasonic research. In 2014, the Institute for Ultrasonic Electronics (IUSE), a specified non-profit organization, was established to cooperate in the smooth operation of USE and support the further development of ultrasonic science. As part of its activities, the publication of this e-book aims to present the current basic knowledge and fruits of ultrasonic science, not only to experts but also to the wide spectrum of related researchers and students. We hope that everyone reading this e-book enjoys the latest advances in the world of ultrasonic science and technology.

Keiji Sakai
Representative Director
Institute for Ultrasonic Electronics

Editor biographies

Mami Matsukawa, Editor-in-chief

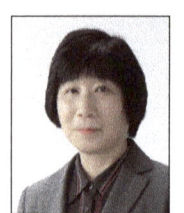

Mami Matsukawa is a professor at Doshisha University, Japan. She received her PhD from Doshisha University. Her research interests include bone ultrasound, Brillouin scattering, and pulse-wave analysis.

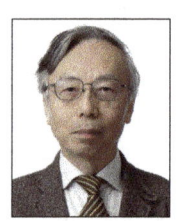

Pak-Kon Choi

Pak-Kon Choi is a professor emeritus in physics at Meiji University, Japan. He received his PhD from the University of Tokyo in 1979. His research interests include ultrasonic spectroscopy and acoustic cavitation. He is a co-author of *Sonochemistry and the Acoustic Bubble* (Elsevier, 2015, https://doi.org/10.1016/C2013-0-18886-1).

Kentaro Nakamura

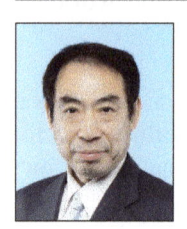

Kentaro Nakamura is a professor at the Institute of Innovative Research, Tokyo Institute of Technology, Japan. He received his DEng from Tokyo Institute of Technology in 1992. His research is focused on high-power ultrasonic applications including ultrasonic actuators as well as optical measurements of ultrasonic fields and vibration.

Hirotsugu Ogi

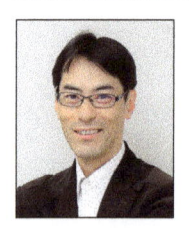

Hirotsugu Ogi is a professor at the Graduate School of Engineering, Osaka University. He received his PhD degree from Osaka University in 1997. His research areas are condensed matter physics using ultrasound and protein research using sonochemistry.

Hideyuki Hasegawa

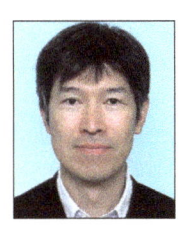

Hideyuki Hasegawa is a full professor at the Faculty of Engineering, University of Toyama, Toyama, Japan. He received his BE degree in electrical engineering and ME and PhD degrees in electronic engineering from Tohoku University, Japan, in 1996, 1998, and 2001, respectively. His research interests include ultrasound beamforming and functional ultrasound imaging.

Contributor biographies

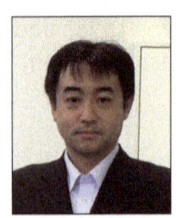

Shingo Akao

Shingo Akao is chief executive officer of Ball Wave Inc. He received his PhD from Tohoku University in 2009. His research interests include surface acoustic wave sensors and measurement system integration. He is a co-author of papers published in *Measurement Science and Technologies* (2019).

Takamitsu Iwaya

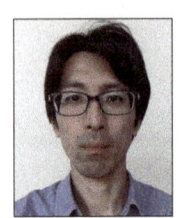

Takamitsu Iwaya is a researcher for Ball Wave Inc., Japan. He received his MEng from Tohoku University in 2012. His research interests include surface acoustic wave sensors. He has authored papers in *Measurement Science and Technologies* (2019) and the *Japanese Journal of Applied Physics* (2012).

Osamu Matsuda

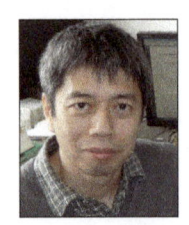

Osamu Matsuda is a professor at Hokkaido University, Japan. He received his PhD from Osaka University. His research interests include picosecond laser ultrasonics and time-resolved acoustic wave imaging.

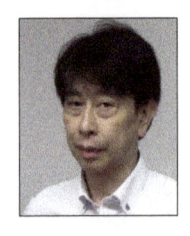

Keiji Sakai

Keiji Sakai is a professor at the University of Tokyo, Japan. He received his PhD from the University of Tokyo in 1991. His research interests include physical acoustics and rheology measurement.

Shin-ichi Sakamoto

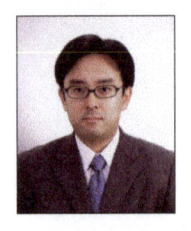

Shin-ichi Sakamoto is an associate professor at the University of Shiga Prefecture. He received his PhD from Doshisha University. His research interests include thermoacoustic systems, medical ultrasound, energy conversion, and time-series analysis.

Shin-ichiro Umemura

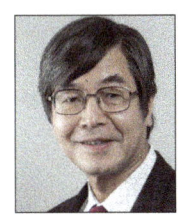

Shin-ichiro Umemura is a professor emeritus of biomedical as well as electrical engineering at Tohoku University, Japan. He received his PhD from the University of Tokyo in 1980. His research interests focus on ultrasonics for both medical imaging and therapy.

Yoshiaki Watanabe

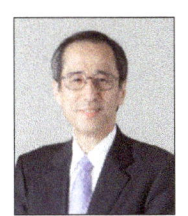

Yoshiaki Watanabe is a professor emeritus of engineering at Doshisha University, Japan. He received his PhD from Doshisha University in 1981. His research interests include ultrasonic electronics and nonlinear acoustics. Recently, he has become interested in the field of thermo-acoustics.

Oliver B Wright

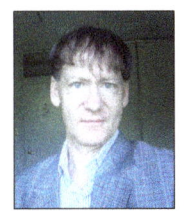

Oliver B Wright is a professor at Hokkaido University, Japan. He received his PhD in physics from Cambridge University. His current research interests include picosecond laser ultrasonics, acoustic wave imaging, and acoustic metamaterials.

Kazushi Yamanaka

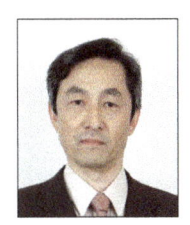

Kazushi Yamanaka is chief scientific officer of Ball Wave Inc. and a professor emeritus at Tohoku University. He received his PhD from Tohoku University in 1987. His research interests include acoustic wave sensors and ultrasonic nondestructive evaluation. He is a co-author of *Acoustic Scanning Probe Microscopy* (Springer, 2013).

Shin Yoshizawa

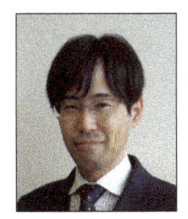

Shin Yoshizawa is a professor in the Department of Communication Engineering at Tohoku University, Japan. He received his PhD from the University of Tokyo in 2006. His research interests are therapeutic ultrasound, ultrasound imaging, and acoustic cavitation.

Part I

Basic physics and measurements

IOP Publishing

Ultrasonics
Physics and applications
Mami Matsukawa, Pak-Kon Choi, Kentaro Nakamura, Hirotsugu Ogi and Hideyuki Hasegawa

Chapter 1

Ultrasound propagation

Pak-Kon Choi

This chapter describes the fundamentals of ultrasound, as an introduction to the subsequent chapters. After a definition of ultrasound, the wave equation and sound velocity relevant to fluids are derived. For solids, the wave equation and elastic properties lead to the propagation of shear waves as well as longitudinal waves. The relaxation phenomenon, which is a key mechanism of sound absorption in fluids, is explained using examples. A theoretical treatment and a simulation of the sound field are provided for a circular piston source and a concave source. Finally, the optical methods used to measure sound fields are briefly described.

1.1 Ultrasound propagation in gases and liquids

We consider the generation of sound by an oscillating body in a fluid medium. When the body mechanically oscillates, disturbances consisting of compression and expansion transfer to the neighboring particles and then to successive particles. This produces a local density change, resulting in a local pressure change, as shown in figure 1.1. When we refer to particles, we imagine them as small volumes, each of which contains so many molecules that the effects of thermal agitation can be averaged out. The alternating compressions and expansions that travel into the medium at a specific velocity are sound waves. The pressure change p specified by time t and position (x, y, z) in Cartesian coordinates differs from the total pressure P by the amount

$$p(t, x, y, z) = P - P_0, \qquad (1.1)$$

where P_0 is the static pressure in the absence of sound waves, and $p(t, x, y, z)$ is called the *sound pressure*.

The displacement of particles is described by a vector $\boldsymbol{u}$ with components ξ, η, and ζ. To specify the oscillations, the velocity of the particles is used rather than the displacement, which is given by

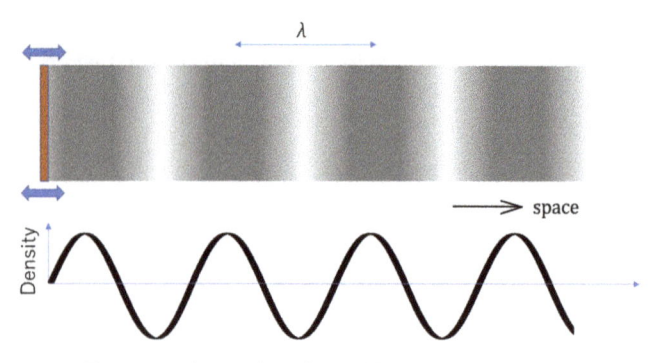

Figure 1.1. Generation of sound by an oscillating body.

$$\dot{u} = \frac{\partial u}{\partial t}. \tag{1.2}$$

This is referred to as the *particle velocity*, and it should be distinguished from the velocity at which the sound waves propagate as a whole. It is customary to use the sound pressure $p(t, x, y, z)$ as a variable that describes sound-wave propagation, because it is a measurable quantity.

1.1.1 Frequency of ultrasound

The frequency of audible sound ranges from 20 Hz to 20 kHz. Sound that has a frequency above this range is called *ultrasound*, although the boundary of the frequency is ambiguous. Sound that has a frequency of more than 1 GHz is sometimes called *hypersound*.

A low-frequency limit does not exist for sound waves, but a high-frequency limit (cut-off frequency) does exist. If we consider sound propagation in a perfect crystal, a possible waveform at the highest frequency is such that adjacent particles (atoms, ions, or molecules in this case) oscillate with exactly opposite phases; that is, the particle distance is equal to half the wavelength. The numerical value of the high-frequency limit can be estimated using values of 5000 m s^{-1} for the wave velocity and 0.3 nm for the particle distance, resulting in a value of 10 THz.

1.1.2 Adiabaticity of sound propagation

In adiabatic processes, the compression and expansion of a fluid volume causes a temperature change. We consider the applicability of the adiabatic condition to sound propagation. For longitudinal waves with wavelength λ in a fluid medium (as shown in figure 1.1), higher-temperature and lower-temperature regions are alternately produced at intervals of a half-wavelength, $\lambda/2$. The time T_{th} required for thermal conduction with thermal diffusivity D over the distance L, which is $\lambda/2$ in this case, is given by

$$T_{th} \approx \frac{L^2}{D} \approx \frac{\lambda^2}{4D}. \tag{1.3}$$

The period of sound τ is expressed by

$$\tau = \frac{\lambda}{v}, \tag{1.4}$$

where v is the sound velocity. If $T_{th} \gg \tau$, thermal conduction during the sound can be neglected, which implies an adiabatic process. Using equations (1.3) and (1.4), the adiabatic condition leads to

$$\lambda \gg \frac{4D}{v}, \text{ or } f \ll \frac{v^2}{4D}, \tag{1.5}$$

where f is the frequency of sound. When the frequency exceeds $v^2/4D$, the adiabatic condition cannot be applied. We can evaluate the boundary value of the limiting frequency in water, which is approximately 4×10^{12} Hz using $D = 1.4 \times 10^{-7}$ m^2 s^{-1}. The wavelength corresponding to this frequency is on the order of the molecular size. For propagation in a gas, the adiabatic condition breaks down if the wavelength is comparable to the mean free path of the molecules. This estimation indicates that the adiabatic condition can be safely applied to the ultrasound frequencies that we usually employ.

1.1.3 Wave equation

The propagation of sound waves is governed by the wave equation. Figure 1.2 shows a cubic volume element with small dimensions of Δx, Δy, and Δz imagined to be in a fluid medium. Applying sound pressure p, which is a scalar function of position $\mathbf{r}$ and time t, produces a displacement $\mathbf{u}(\xi, \eta, \zeta)$ which changes the length Δx to $\Delta x + (\partial \xi/\partial x)\Delta x$, with corresponding changes in Δy and Δz. Therefore, the element volume $\Delta V = \Delta x \Delta y \Delta z$ should change to

$$\Delta V' = \left(1 + \frac{\partial \xi}{\partial x}\right)\Delta x \left(1 + \frac{\partial \eta}{\partial y}\right)\Delta y \left(1 + \frac{\partial \zeta}{\partial z}\right)\Delta z \approx \left(1 + \frac{\partial \xi}{\partial x} + \frac{\partial \eta}{\partial y} + \frac{\partial \zeta}{\partial z}\right)\Delta x \Delta y \Delta z \tag{1.6}$$

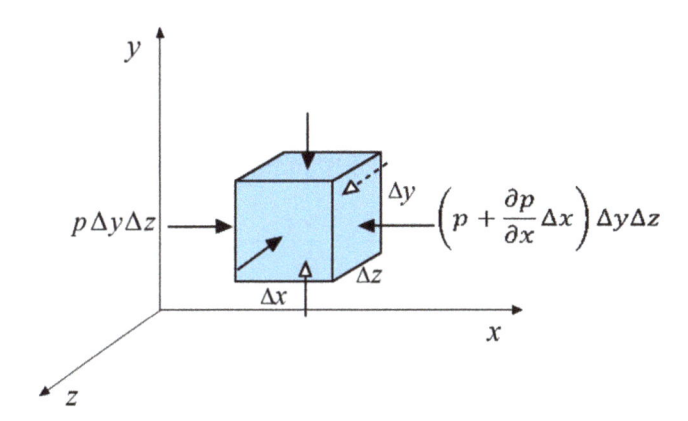

Figure 1.2. Forces acting on a cubic volume element in a fluid medium.

under the assumption of a very small displacement. The volume strain, or dilatation, is given by

$$\delta = \frac{\Delta V' - \Delta V}{\Delta V} = \frac{\partial \xi}{\partial x} + \frac{\partial \eta}{\partial y} + \frac{\partial \zeta}{\partial z} = \text{div } \boldsymbol{u}. \tag{1.7}$$

To relate the sound pressure to the volume strain, we define the bulk modulus (or volume modulus) K or adiabatic compressibility β, which is the inverse of K:

$$K = \frac{1}{\beta} = -V\left(\frac{dP}{dV}\right), \tag{1.8}$$

where V is the bulk volume. This leads to

$$p = -K\delta = -K \text{ div } \boldsymbol{u}, \tag{1.9}$$

which expresses Hooke's law in a fluid.

We consider the equations of motion for the volume element shown in figure 1.2. Forces are acting on its six faces, and their directions are perpendicular to each face. The forces in the x direction are $p\Delta y\Delta z$ and $-\left(p + \frac{\partial p}{\partial x}\Delta x\right)\Delta y\Delta z$. The net force in the x direction is then

$$\Delta F_x = -\frac{\partial p}{\partial x}\Delta x \Delta y \Delta z. \tag{1.10}$$

Similar relations hold for the y and z directions, and the net vector force on the volume element is

$$\Delta \boldsymbol{F} = -\nabla p \; \Delta x \Delta y \Delta z. \tag{1.11}$$

Since the mass of the volume element is $\rho_0 \Delta x \Delta y \Delta z$, where ρ_0 is the density of the fluid, Newton's second law requires that

$$\Delta \boldsymbol{F} = -\nabla p \; \Delta x \Delta y \Delta z = \rho_0 \Delta x \Delta y \Delta z \frac{\partial^2 \boldsymbol{u}}{\partial t^2}. \tag{1.12}$$

Dividing by $\Delta x \Delta y \Delta z$ gives

$$-\nabla p = \rho_0 \frac{\partial^2 \boldsymbol{u}}{\partial t^2}. \tag{1.13}$$

Taking the divergence of equation (1.13) and using equation (1.9) gives

$$\nabla^2 p = \Delta p = \frac{1}{v^2}\frac{\partial^2 p}{\partial t^2}, \text{ or } \left(\frac{\partial^2 p}{\partial x^2} + \frac{\partial^2 p}{\partial y^2} + \frac{\partial^2 p}{\partial z^2}\right) = \frac{1}{v^2}\frac{\partial^2 p}{\partial t^2}. \tag{1.14}$$

Here,

$$v = \sqrt{\frac{K}{\rho_0}} \tag{1.15}$$

is the wave velocity of the fluid. Equation (1.14) is referred to as the 'wave equation,' and the same form of equation holds for acoustic quantities such as the components of particle velocity or density variation.

1.1.4 Sound velocity

The wave velocity of sound depends on thermodynamic parameters such as the bulk modulus (compressibility), density, and ambient pressure and temperature, as shown in equation (1.15). The sound velocity is independent of frequency, except in the frequency region where the relaxation phenomenon occurs. Under intense ultrasound conditions, the sound velocity depends on the amplitude of the particle velocity, which is a nonlinear regime. The sound velocities in gases and liquids will be treated separately.

For most gases, the equation of state is adequately approximated by that of an ideal gas:

$$PV = nRT, \qquad (1.16)$$

where n is the number of moles, $R = 8.314$ J mol^{-1} K^{-1} is the gas constant, and T is the absolute temperature. The compression or expansion associated with sound propagation obeys the adiabatic equation given by

$$PV^\gamma = \text{constant}, \qquad (1.17)$$

where γ is the ratio of the specific heats at constant pressure and constant volume. Using equations (1.8), (1.15), and (1.17), the sound velocity in gases can be derived as

$$v_g = \sqrt{\frac{\gamma P}{\rho_0}}, \qquad (1.18)$$

which is rewritten using equation (1.16) to

$$v_g = \sqrt{\frac{\gamma RT}{M}}, \qquad (1.19)$$

where M is the molecular weight per mole. We can estimate the sound velocity in air at temperatures around room temperature from equation (1.19) using the values $\gamma = 1.402$ and $M = 2.897 \times 10^{-3}$ kg mole^{-1} (averaged) as

$$v_{\text{air}} \approx 331.5 + 0.6 t_C \text{ m s}^{-1}, \qquad (1.20)$$

where t_C is the temperature in degrees Celsius. Bhatia [1] discussed the deviation from the ideal gas behavior and the pressure dependence of the sound velocity.

In liquids, where molecular interactions have great variety, the equation of state is very complicated, and no exact expression for the sound velocity has been derived. Only semi-empirical equations are known [1]. Sound velocities and densities measured for typical liquids at 20 °C are listed in table 1.1.

Table 1.1. Sound velocities and densities in liquids at 20 °C.

Material	Sound velocity (ms^{-1})	Density (kgm^{-3})
Water	1482.3	998
Methyl alcohol	1121	791
Ethyl alcohol	1182	789
Glycerol	1923	1261
Ethylene glycol	1666	1113
Acetone	1190	791
Chloroform	1001	1487
Carbon tetrachloride	938	1594
Cyclohexane	1284	779
Benzene	1326	878

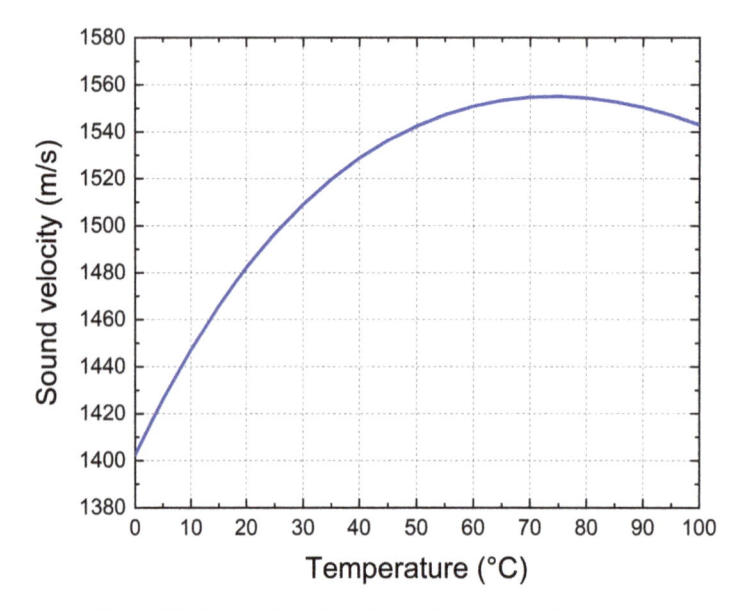

Figure 1.3. Temperature dependence of sound velocity in water.

We now discuss sound velocity in water, which has specific acoustic properties. Figure 1.3 shows the temperature dependence of the sound velocity measured at a frequency of 5 MHz in water [2]. The sound velocity exhibits a maximum at approximately 74 °C. This is attributed to the association between water molecules. Water has an ice-like structure consisting of a hydrogen-bond network, whose structure has a large compressibility compared with that of free molecules. As the temperature increases, the structure proportionally breaks and the number of free molecules increases, indicating a decrease in compressibility, i.e. an increase in velocity. At higher temperatures, near the boiling point, where molecular associations are scarce, the velocity decreases with increasing temperature. The negative temperature coefficient of velocity is typical for nonassociated liquids. The velocity of sound in water peaks at 74 °C.

1.1.5 Plane waves

The simplest case of sound waves is that of plane waves propagating in the direction of one coordinate, for example, the x-axis. In this case, the wave equation (1.14) can be rewritten as

$$\frac{\partial^2 p}{\partial x^2} = \frac{1}{v^2}\frac{\partial^2 p}{\partial t^2}. \quad (1.21)$$

The general solution of the above equation is

$$p(x, t) = f(x - vt) + g(x + vt), \quad (1.22)$$

where f and g denote arbitrary functions with existing second derivatives, $f(x-vt)$ describes a pressure disturbance propagating at a speed v toward an increasing value of x, while $g(x+vt)$ describes propagation toward a decreasing value of x. If we consider a harmonic function, plane waves traveling in the positive x direction can be written as

$$p(x, t) = p_0 e^{i(\omega t - kx)}, \quad (1.23)$$

where p_0 is the pressure amplitude, ω is the angular frequency, and

$$k = \frac{\omega}{v} = \frac{2\pi}{\lambda} \quad (1.24)$$

is the wave number.

We introduce the characteristic acoustic impedance (Z_0), which is the ratio of the acoustic pressure (input) and the particle velocity (output), a concept analogous to electric impedance. Using equations (1.13) and (1.23), the particle velocity can be obtained as follows:

$$\dot{u} = \frac{kp_0}{\omega \rho_0} e^{i(\omega t - kx)} = \frac{p_0}{v \rho_0} e^{i(\omega t - kx)}. \quad (1.25)$$

The ratio of the acoustic pressure and particle velocity is readily obtained from equations (1.23) and (1.25), as follows:

$$Z_0 = \frac{p}{\dot{u}} = \rho_0 v. \quad (1.26)$$

For plane waves, the value of Z_0 depends only on the material constants, i.e. density and sound velocity. This parameter plays an important role in reflection and refraction at the boundaries of different media. No reflection of sound waves occurs when two media have the same characteristic acoustic impedance.

Sound waves transport the energy contained in the medium through which they propagate. The energy content per unit volume is called the *energy density*. The energy flow is characterized by the *sound intensity I*, which is defined as the energy passing per second through an imaginary window of unit area perpendicular to the direction in which the sound waves propagate:

$$I = \overline{p\,\dot{u}} = \frac{p_0^2}{2Z_0}, \tag{1.27}$$

where the overbar denotes a time average.

For more details about the fundamentals of ultrasound, refer to Edmonds [3], Kuttruff [4], and Cheeke [5].

1.2 Ultrasound propagation in solids

1.2.1 Elastic properties of solids

Solid bodies try to maintain not only their volumes but also their shapes. This results in a variety of possible wave types in solids. Shear (transverse) waves as well as longitudinal waves can propagate in solids. The situation is very complicated in anisotropic solids, in which elastic properties depend on the material orientation. We confine the discussion to isotropic solids in the following. Figure 1.4 shows the forces acting on three faces of a small cube embedded in a solid in the directions x_1, x_2, and x_3. Stresses are denoted by T_{ij} ($i, j = 1, 2, 3$), where the first subscript indicates the orientation of the faces on which it is acting, and the second subscript indicates the direction of the force. The stresses T_{ii} acting on the faces in figure 1.4 are normal (tensile) stresses, and the stresses T_{ij} ($i \neq j$) are shear (tangential) stresses. Similar stresses act on the other faces of the cube. Nine elastic stress components form a second-rank stress tensor.

The elastic constants c_{ijkl} (a fourth-rank tensor) are defined as

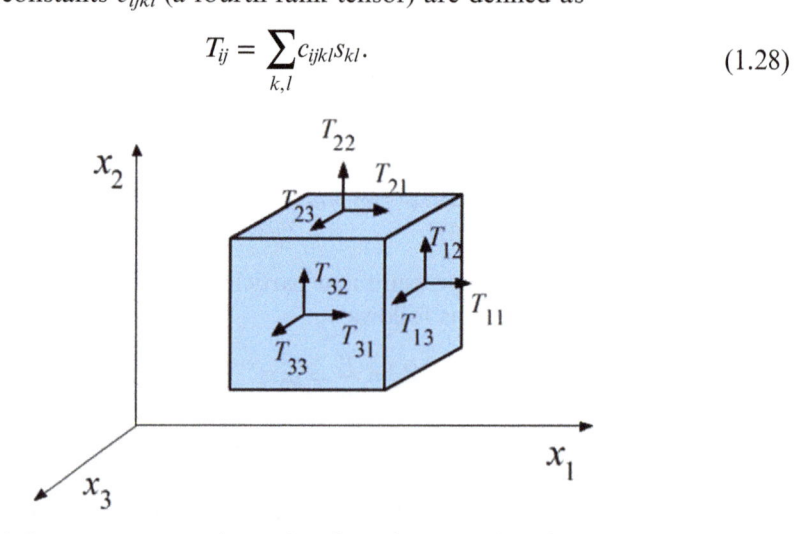

$$T_{ij} = \sum_{k,l} c_{ijkl} S_{kl}. \tag{1.28}$$

Figure 1.4. Stress components acting on three faces of a small cube embedded in a solid.

Here, s_{kl} is the strain given by

$$s_{kl} = \frac{1}{2}\left(\frac{\partial u_l}{\partial x_k} + \frac{\partial u_k}{\partial x_l}\right), \tag{1.29}$$

where u_k denotes displacement in the x_k direction. The strain components also form a strain tensor. Here, s_{kk} denotes the strain produced in the same direction as the displacement, that is, the extension per unit length in the k direction. The number of independent components of the elastic constant is reduced to 21 for crystals, due to symmetry rules. The indices of T_{ij}, s_{kl}, and c_{ijkl} are often reduced using the rules $11 \to 1$, $22 \to 2$, $33 \to 3$, $(23, 32) \to 4$, $(13, 31) \to 5$, $(12, 21) \to 6$, where ij and kl associate as pairs. The elastic constant tensor for isotropic solids is expressed as

$$c = \begin{pmatrix} c_{11} & c_{12} & c_{12} & 0 & 0 & 0 \\ c_{12} & c_{11} & c_{12} & 0 & 0 & 0 \\ c_{12} & c_{12} & c_{11} & 0 & 0 & 0 \\ 0 & 0 & 0 & c_{44} & 0 & 0 \\ 0 & 0 & 0 & 0 & c_{44} & 0 \\ 0 & 0 & 0 & 0 & 0 & c_{44} \end{pmatrix} \tag{1.30}$$

$$c_{11} = c_{12} + 2c_{44}. \tag{1.31}$$

The stress–strain relation for isotropic solids is expressed as

$$T_i = c_{12} \mathrm{div}\, \boldsymbol{u} + 2c_{44} s_i \text{ for } i = 1, 2, 3$$

$$T_i = c_{44} s_i \text{ for } i = 4, 5, 6. \tag{1.32}$$

Only two components are independent constants. The Lamé constants λ and μ are frequently used, and are represented by $c_{12} = \lambda$ and $c_{44} = \mu$.

$$c_{11} = M, \; c_{44} = G \tag{1.33}$$

are the longitudinal modulus and shear modulus (or rigidity), respectively. Each modulus is relevant to ultrasonic longitudinal-wave and shear-wave propagation, in which the wavelength is much smaller than the size of the medium. The bulk modulus K, defined by equation (1.8), is derived as follows:

$$K = c_{12} + \frac{2}{3} c_{44} \tag{1.34}$$

using the following relation:

$$-\mathrm{d}p = \frac{1}{3}(T_1 + T_2 + T_3). \tag{1.35}$$

We then obtain the relation connecting the three moduli:

$$M = K + \frac{4}{3} G. \tag{1.36}$$

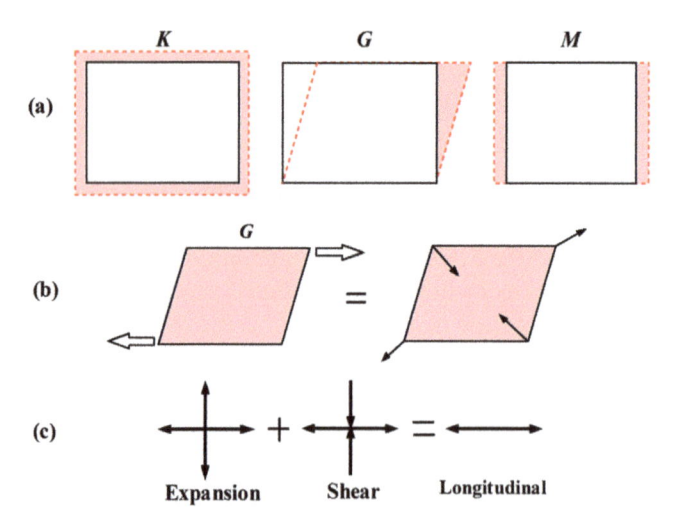

Figure 1.5. (a) Deformations for bulk, shear, and longitudinal moduli. (b) Shear deformation. (c) The combination of expansion and shear deformation results in longitudinal deformation.

The deformations appropriate for moduli K, G, and M are illustrated in figure 1.5(a). The reason that the longitudinal modulus M contains shear deformation is illustrated in figure 1.5(b) and (c). The shear deformation is realized by a couple of forces acting on a solid body, and the forces are divided into four, as shown in figure 1.5(b). Figure 1.5(c) explains that the combination of expansion (or compression) and shear deformation causes longitudinal deformation.

1.2.2 Wave equation in solids

Following a procedure similar to that used in the derivation for fluids, we can obtain Newton's second law for solids as follows:

$$\rho_0 \frac{\partial^2 u_i}{\partial t^2} = \sum_{j=1}^{3} \frac{\partial T_{ji}}{\partial x_j}. \tag{1.37}$$

Substituting equation (1.32) into equation (1.37) gives

$$\rho_0 \frac{\partial^2 \boldsymbol{u}}{\partial t^2} = (c_{12} + c_{44}) \text{grad div} \boldsymbol{u} + c_{44} \nabla^2 \boldsymbol{u}. \tag{1.38}$$

This is called the wave equation, which holds for isotropic solids. For further analysis, we make use of Helmholtz's theorem, which states that any vector field can be expressed as the sum of a solenoidal field whose divergence is zero and an irrotational field whose rotation is zero. This suggests that

$$\boldsymbol{u} = \boldsymbol{u}_l + \boldsymbol{u}_s. \tag{1.39}$$

For irrotational waves, rot $\mathbf{u}_l = 0$, and for solenoidal waves, div $\mathbf{u}_s = 0$. The wave equation (1.38) then becomes

$$\frac{\partial^2 \mathbf{u}_l}{\partial t^2} = \frac{(c_{12} + 2c_{44})}{\rho_0} \nabla^2 \mathbf{u}_l = \frac{M}{\rho_0} \nabla^2 \mathbf{u}_l \qquad (1.40)$$

$$\frac{\partial^2 \mathbf{u}_s}{\partial t^2} = \frac{c_{44}}{\rho_0} \nabla^2 \mathbf{u}_s = \frac{G}{\rho_0} \nabla^2 \mathbf{u}_s. \qquad (1.41)$$

If we assume that plane waves propagate in the x direction, the displacement is given by

$$\mathbf{u} = u_0 \mathbf{a}\, e^{i(\omega t - \mathbf{k}\cdot\mathbf{x})}, \qquad (1.42)$$

where $\mathbf{a}$ is the unit vector along the displacement, ω is the angular frequency, and $\mathbf{k}$ is the wave number vector. Inserting equation (1.42) into equation (1.40) and assigning rot $\mathbf{u}_l = 0$ leads to

$$\frac{\omega}{k} = v_l = \sqrt{\frac{M}{\rho_0}}, \text{ and } \mathbf{k} \| \mathbf{a}. \qquad (1.43)$$

The wave type whose k vector is parallel to the displacement vector is the longitudinal wave, and its velocity is given by v_l. Inserting equation (1.42) into (1.41) and assigning div $\mathbf{u}_s = 0$ leads to

$$\frac{\omega}{k} = v_s = \sqrt{\frac{G}{\rho_0}}, \text{ and } \mathbf{k} \perp \mathbf{a}. \qquad (1.44)$$

The wave type whose k vector is perpendicular to the displacement vector is the shear wave, and its velocity is given by v_s.

Another type of elastic wave can propagate along the free surface of solid body that fills a half-space. It is referred to as a Rayleigh wave, which is well known in seismology. The particle motion is localized beneath the surface and forms elliptical orbits that are a particular combination of longitudinal and shear-wave components. Over 90% of the Rayleigh wave energy is restricted a depth of less than one wavelength. The velocity of the Rayleigh wave v_R for isotropic solids can be obtained as follows:

$$v_R = \frac{0.87 + 1.12\sigma}{1 + \sigma}, \qquad (1.45)$$

where σ is Poisson's ratio, given by

$$\sigma = -\frac{s_2}{s_1} = \frac{c_{12}}{2(c_{12} + c_{44})} = \frac{3K - 2G}{6K + 2G}. \qquad (1.46)$$

Poisson's ratio denotes the negative ratio of the lateral extension to the axial extension when a rod-shaped material is subjected to elongation. As values of σ in

Table 1.2. Longitudinal and shear sound velocities in commonly used solid materials, along with their densities.

Material	Longitudinal velocity (ms^{-1})	Shear velocity (ms^{-1})	Density (kgm^{-3})
Fused quartz	5968	3764	2200
Pyrex glass	5640	3280	2320
Sapphire (z)	11100	6040	4000
Aluminum	6420	3040	2700
Brass (70Cu, 30Zn)	4700	2110	8600
Gold	3240	1200	2790
Copper	5010	2270	5010
Stainless steel (347)	5790	3100	7910
Polyethylene	1950	540	900
Poly(methyl methacrylate) (PMMA)	2720	1460	1180

the range $0 < \sigma < 0.5$ are allowed, the Rayleigh wave velocity varies from $0.87v_s$ to $0.96v_s$. The Rayleigh wave has been widely applied in the field of signal processing in sensors, delay lines, electrical filters known as SAW (surface acoustic wave) filters, etc. Chapter 5 describes a novel application of Rayleigh waves in sensors for trace gas analysis. Various wave types can propagate in solid materials, depending on their boundaries: Lamb waves in thin plates, Love waves in layered substrates, etc [5].

The values of the sound velocity and density for some typical solids are listed in table 1.2. The commonly used materials listed in table 1.2 can be treated as isotropic solids because they are polycrystalline or amorphous. In the case of crystalline materials, the velocities depend on the crystal axis along which the sound waves propagate [6].

1.3 Absorption and velocity dispersion in fluids

1.3.1 Ultrasound absorption

Thus far, we have disregarded the absorption of sound. However, each type of sound propagation is subject to inevitable losses. The losses of sound energy are caused by a variety of mechanisms related to the internal structure of the medium. Measurements of sound absorption over a broad frequency range allow the physical and chemical properties of matter and the interaction between its components to be investigated. This research field is referred to as ultrasonic spectroscopy. We define the term *absorption* to mean the energy losses caused by processes inherent to materials, such as viscosity and the relaxation phenomenon. The term *attenuation* is sometimes used when one wants to include energy losses due to sound diffraction and scattering in addition to absorption.

To take absorption into account in plane harmonic waves, we introduce a complex wave number

$$k^* = k - i\alpha, \quad (1.47)$$

where α is the absorption coefficient per unit length. Substituting equation (1.47) into equation (1.23) yields

$$p(x, t) = p_0 e^{-\alpha x} e^{i(\omega t - kx)}, \quad (1.48)$$

which expresses exponential decay with distance. The units of α are Np m^{-1} (Np = nepers). A decibel-scale representation is also used. The two units are related by

$$\alpha \text{ [dB m}^{-1}] = 20 \log_{10} e \, \alpha \text{ [Np m}^{-1}] = 8.686 \, \alpha \text{ [Np m}^{-1}]. \quad (1.49)$$

Using the complex wave number, the complex velocity v^* can be written as

$$\frac{1}{v^*} = \frac{k^*}{\omega} = \frac{k}{\omega} - i\frac{\alpha}{\omega}. \quad (1.50)$$

The complex longitudinal modulus is then

$$M^* = M' + iM'' = \rho_0 v^{*2}, \quad (1.51)$$

where M' and M'' are the storage modulus and the loss modulus, respectively. Comparing the real and imaginary parts of both sides of equation (1.51), we obtain

$$M' = \rho_0 v^2 \frac{1 - \left(\frac{\alpha v}{\omega}\right)^2}{\left\{1 + \left(\frac{\alpha v}{\omega}\right)^2\right\}^2}, \quad M'' = \rho_0 v^2 \frac{2\frac{\alpha v}{\omega}}{\left\{1 + \left(\frac{\alpha v}{\omega}\right)^2\right\}^2}. \quad (1.52)$$

Under the assumption that $(\alpha v/\omega) = (\alpha \lambda/2\pi) \ll 1$ or small absorption, equation (1.52) reduces to

$$M' = \rho_0 v^2, \quad M'' = \frac{2\rho_0 v^3}{\omega}\alpha, \quad (1.53)$$

so that the velocity and absorption are expressed as

$$v = \sqrt{\frac{M'}{\rho_0}}, \quad \alpha = \frac{\omega}{2\rho_0 v^3} M'' \quad (1.54)$$

The complex expressions for the bulk modulus K and the shear modulus G are

$$K^* = K' + K'' = K + i\omega\eta_v$$

$$G^* = G' + G'' = G + i\omega\eta, \quad (1.55)$$

where η_v and η are the volume viscosity and the shear viscosity, respectively. Using equations (1.36), (1.54), and (1.55), the longitudinal-wave velocity and absorption are given by

$$v_l = \sqrt{\frac{K + \frac{4}{3}G}{\rho_0}}, \quad \alpha_l = \frac{\omega^2}{2\rho_0 v_l^3}\left(\eta_v + \frac{4}{3}\eta\right). \tag{1.56}$$

K is much larger than G, except for very viscous liquids, so that the longitudinal velocity is governed by the bulk modulus. However, the absorption is governed by the viscosity. The volume viscosity originates from the relaxation phenomenon (molecular relaxation, structural relaxation, etc) which is discussed in the following. The volume viscosity dominates the shear viscosity in most liquids, with the exception of viscous liquids.

Heat conduction is another mechanism that contributes to absorption. In section 1.1.2, we showed that the temperature change that occurs during ultrasound propagation is adiabatic. In reality, it is inevitable that heat flows from the compressed warmer element to the expanded cooler element. Because heat conduction is an irreversible process, this effect causes absorption of the wave, depending on the frequency. The absorption due to heat conduction is given by

$$\alpha_h = \frac{\omega^2}{2\rho_0 v_l^3}\frac{(\gamma - 1)\kappa}{C_v}, \tag{1.57}$$

where κ is the thermal conductivity and C_v is the heat capacity at constant volume. The total absorption coefficient is given by

$$\alpha = \alpha_l + \alpha_h = \frac{\omega^2}{2\rho_0 v_l^3}\left\{\eta_v + \frac{4}{3}\eta + \frac{(\gamma - 1)\kappa}{C_v}\right\}. \tag{1.58}$$

The absorption due to the shear viscosity and thermal conductivity alone, i.e. the latter two terms in equation (1.58), is usually called *classical absorption*. The magnitude of the ultrasonic absorption in monatomic gases and liquids can be satisfactorily explained by these effects. However, the absorption measured in other fluids significantly exceeds classical absorption. The excess absorption is attributed to the volume viscosity, which originates primarily from the relaxation phenomenon.

1.3.2 The relaxation phenomenon

Ultrasound absorption arising from the relaxation phenomenon is the process of irreversible energy exchange between the external and internal degrees of freedom [7, 8]. The physical quantities representing the external degrees of freedom are strain, pressure, or temperature, and they are denoted by x_i. The internal degrees of freedom are, for example, the rotational or vibrational degrees of freedom of molecules, or the degree of chemically reactive species. Let the parameter representing the internal energy or internal reaction be denoted by ξ.

If external energy is applied to a system in thermal equilibrium, the energy is distributed among the internal degrees of freedom, causing a change in ξ from an equilibrium value of $\bar{\xi}$ toward a new equilibrium. The time dependence of ξ is represented by

$$\frac{d\xi}{dt} = -\frac{\xi - \bar{\xi}}{\tau}, \tag{1.59}$$

where τ is a constant that characterizes the time required for the energy redistribution to attain thermal equilibrium, which is called the *relaxation time*. Equation (1.59) indicates that it takes a finite time for the internal energy to follow an external energy change. In the case of sound waves, a periodic external energy with angular frequency ω is applied. The input to the system is the strain x_1, which has a time dependence of $e^{i\omega t}$. This strain causes ξ to have a similar time dependence, with the result that ξ acquires a phase lag, according to equation (1.59). Consequently, the output of the system, stress x_2, for example, has a phase lag with respect to the input (figure 1.6). If the frequency is sufficiently low that $\omega\tau \ll 1$ holds, the variations in external energy are so slow that the internal energy can follow immediately, and no phase lag occurs. Conversely, if the frequency is sufficiently high that $\omega\tau \gg 1$ holds, the internal energy cannot follow the variations in the external energy. The internal degrees of freedom effectively uncouple from the external energy change. In the intermediate frequency range, i.e. $\omega\tau \sim 1$, the energy exchange is only partial, and has a certain phase lag. The ultrasound absorption per wavelength reaches a maximum at $\omega = 1/\tau$.

The longitudinal modulus M is represented by $(\partial x_2/\partial x_1)$. The above consideration gives a frequency dependence of M:

$$M^*(i\omega) = M_0 + (M_\infty - M_0)\frac{i\omega\tau}{1 + i\omega\tau}, \tag{1.60}$$

where M_0 and M_∞ are the longitudinal moduli at the low- and high-frequency limits, respectively. The real and imaginary parts of M are as follows:

$$M'(\omega) = M_0 + (M_\infty - M_0)\frac{\omega^2\tau^2}{1 + \omega^2\tau^2} \tag{1.61}$$

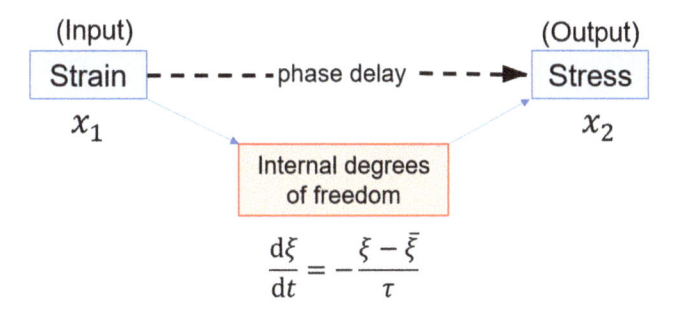

Figure 1.6. Energy exchange between a physical quantity and internal degrees of freedom.

$$M''(\omega) = (M_\infty - M_0)\frac{\omega\tau}{1 + \omega^2\tau^2}. \tag{1.62}$$

Substituting equations (1.61) and (1.62) into equation (1.53) yields the velocity dispersion and absorption change as a function of frequency. In the next section, we describe a typical example of the relaxation phenomenon, molecular vibration, as an internal degree of freedom.

1.3.3 Molecular vibrational relaxation

We assume a two-state model of vibration–translation energy transfer, as shown in figure 1.7. Level A represents a ground state with only translational energy. Level B represents a vibrationally excited state. Although polyatomic molecules have many vibrational levels, the two-state model is appropriate in most cases. Level B can represent many vibrational levels because vibration–vibration energy transfer among vibrational levels is much faster than vibration–translation energy transfer. The forward and backward rate constants are denoted by k_f and k_b, respectively. The numbers of particles occupying levels A and B are n_A and n_B, respectively, and their sum is constant:

$$n_A + n_B = N \tag{1.63}$$

The rate of decrease in n_B is obtained using equation (1.63):

$$-\frac{dn_B}{dt} = k_b n_B - k_f n_A$$

$$= (k_b + k_f)\left(n_B - \frac{N}{1 + k_b/k_f}\right)$$

$$= (k_b + k_f)(n_B - n_B^e), \tag{1.64}$$

where n_B^e is the value at thermal equilibrium, where the decreasing rate of n_B is zero. Using the relaxation time τ, defined as

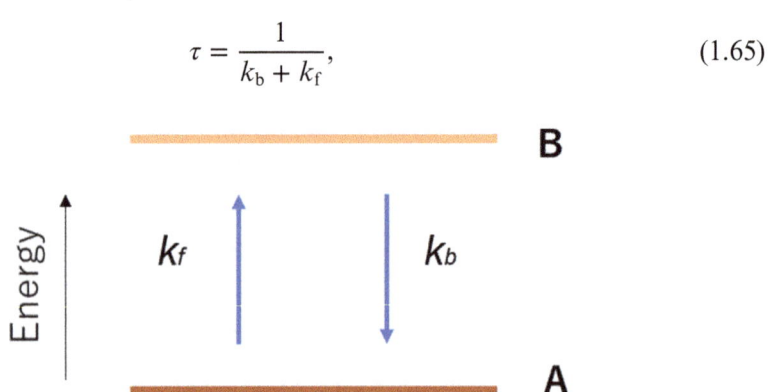

$$\tau = \frac{1}{k_b + k_f}, \tag{1.65}$$

Figure 1.7. Two-state model of vibration–translation energy transfer.

equation (1.64) can be rewritten as

$$-\frac{dn_B}{dt} = \frac{n_B - n_B^e}{\tau}, \quad (1.66)$$

which corresponds to equation (1.59). Ultrasound produces harmonic changes in the local temperature, which results in

$$n_B^e = A e^{i\omega t}, \; A = \text{constant}. \quad (1.67)$$

Because the value of n_B following n_B^e has a similar time dependence, equations (1.66) and (1.67) lead to

$$n_B = \frac{n_B^e}{1 + i\omega\tau} = \frac{A e^{i\omega t}}{1 + i\omega\tau}. \quad (1.68)$$

The heat capacity arising from this reaction is proportional to n_B, and equals some constant C_i at frequencies $\omega \ll 1/\tau$; it equals zero at frequencies $\omega \gg 1/\tau$. At intermediate frequencies, the total heat capacity at constant volume is

$$C_V = C_V^\infty + \frac{C_i}{1 + i\omega\tau}, \quad (1.69)$$

where C_V^∞ is the high-frequency limit of the heat capacity at constant volume. The frequency dependence of the heat capacity is shown in figure 1.8. The heat capacity and ultrasonic velocity are connected by the compressibility. The adiabatic compressibility β_S and the isothermal compressibility β_T are related as follows:

$$\beta_S = \frac{\beta_T}{\gamma(\omega)}. \quad (1.70)$$

Using equations (1.8), (1.15), and (1.70), the ultrasonic velocity can be written as

$$v^2 = \frac{1}{\rho_0 \beta_S} = \frac{\gamma(\omega)}{\rho_0 \beta_T}, \quad (1.71)$$

where $\gamma(\omega)$ is the frequency-dependent specific heat ratio. Here, ρ_0 and β_T are independent of frequency. The ratio of the velocity at the low-frequency limit v_0 and the frequency-dependent complex velocity v^* can now be given by

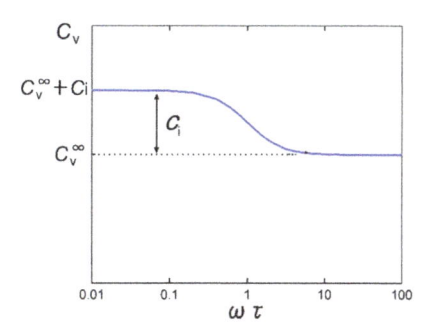

Figure 1.8. Frequency dependence of heat capacity due to relaxation.

$$\frac{v_0^2}{v^{*2}} = \frac{\gamma}{\gamma(\omega)}$$

$$= \frac{C_P}{C_V} \frac{\left(C_V^\infty + \frac{C_i}{1+i\omega\tau}\right)}{\left(C_P^\infty + \frac{C_i}{1+i\omega\tau}\right)} = \left(1 + \frac{C_V^\infty i\omega\tau}{C_V}\right)\left(1 + \frac{C_P^\infty i\omega\tau}{C_P}\right)^{-1}$$

$$= 1 - \frac{C_i(C_P - C_V)}{C_V(C_P - C_i)} \frac{i\omega\tau'}{1+i\omega\tau'} \quad (1.72)$$

$$\left(\tau' = \frac{C_P^\infty}{C_P}\tau\right).$$

Since the complex velocity is given by equation (1.50), a comparison between the real and imaginary parts of equation (1.72) leads to

$$\frac{v_0^2}{v^2} = 1 - \varepsilon \frac{\omega^2 \tau'^2}{1+\omega^2\tau'^2} \quad (1.73)$$

$$\alpha\lambda = \pi\varepsilon \frac{\omega\tau'}{1+\omega^2\tau'^2}, \quad (1.74)$$

where ε is given by the following relation and is called the relaxation strength:

$$\varepsilon = \frac{C_i(C_P - C_V)}{C_V(C_P - C_i)} = \frac{v_\infty^2 - v_0^2}{v_\infty^2}. \quad (1.75)$$

Absorption is usually represented as the absorption per wavelength, $\alpha\lambda$, as in equation (1.74), or as the absorption divided by the square of the frequency, as given below:

$$\frac{\alpha}{f^2} = \frac{2\pi^2\varepsilon}{v_0} \frac{\tau'}{1+\omega^2\tau'^2} = \frac{A}{1+\omega^2\tau'^2}. \quad (1.76)$$

The velocity dispersion and absorption curves are plotted as functions of $\log(\omega\tau')$ in figure 1.9. The arrows in the absorption curves indicate the peak or inflection points at $\omega\tau'=1$. The arrow in the velocity curve denotes the inflection point at $\omega\tau' = v_\infty/v_0$. Measurements of ultrasonic velocity and absorption over a broad frequency range yield the relaxation times and relaxation strengths of various materials.

1.3.4 Examples of the relaxation phenomenon in fluids

Absorption in air is dominated by the relaxation phenomenon at frequencies of less than 10^5 Hz and by shear viscosity and heat conduction (classical absorption) at frequencies of more than 10^5 Hz. The relaxation mechanism in air is vibrational relaxation in nitrogen and oxygen, and the relaxation frequencies are 9 and 24 Hz

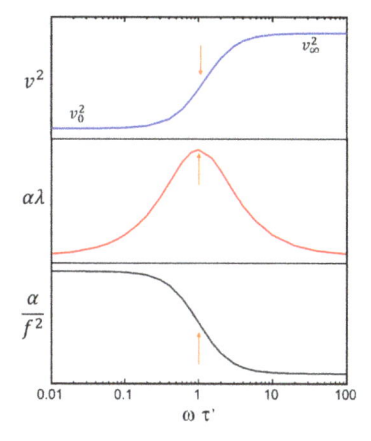

Figure 1.9. Relaxation curves for velocity, absorption per wavelength, and absorption divided by the square of the frequency.

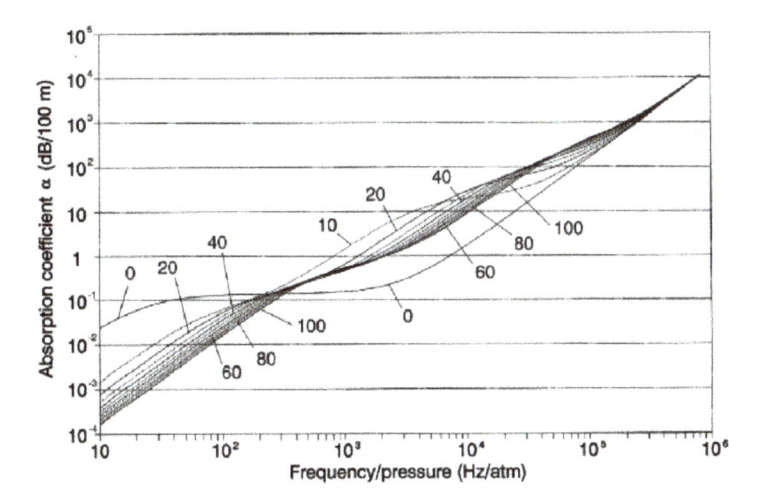

Figure 1.10. Frequency dependence of absorption coefficient α (dB/100 m) in air at various relative humidities (%). Reproduced with permission from [9]. Copyright 1990 American Institute of Physics.

for pure nitrogen and oxygen, respectively. Water vapor influences absorption catalytically. Figure 1.10 shows the absorption coefficient α (dB/100 m) as a function of frequency at 20 °C [9]. The numbers in the figure represent the relative humidity (%). The addition of water vapor shifts the relaxation frequencies to the higher-frequency region, which affects the absorption value significantly and in a complicated manner. For example, absorption at 300 Hz is decreased by approximately one-tenth as the humidity increases from 0% to 20%, while absorption at 3000 Hz increased tenfold as the humidity increases from 0% to 20%. The vibration–translation energy transfer of oxygen is inefficient and is promoted by the efficient energy transfer between the vibrational modes of oxygen and water. For nitrogen, carbon dioxide also participates in the energy transfer. It is very interesting that the propagation of audible sound is directly associated with quantum processes at the molecular level.

Vibrational relaxation in liquids occurs at much higher frequencies in the region over 100 MHz. This is because the collision time between molecules is much smaller than that in gases, which speeds up the vibration–translation energy transfer. Figure 1.11 demonstrates some examples of this phenomenon by showing the velocity dispersions in benzene, pyridine, thiophene, furan, and dichloromethane [10].

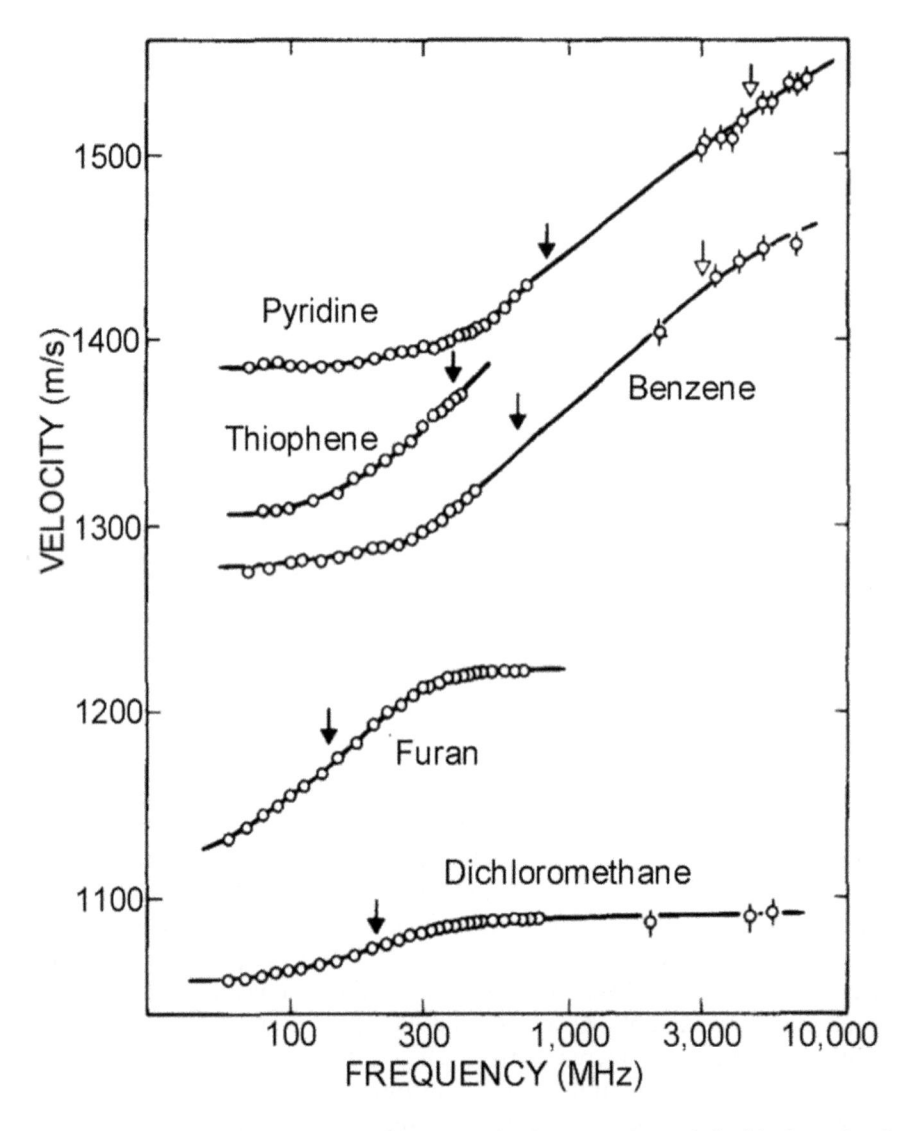

Figure 1.11. Velocity dispersion due to vibrational relaxation in some polyatomic liquids. Reproduced with permission from [10]. Copyright 1980 American Institute of Physics.

The arrows denote the relaxation frequencies. Only one relaxation frequency is observed in many liquids because several vibrational modes are coupled and these modes can be represented by one level, as shown by level B in figure 1.7. In contrast, benzene and pyridine (figure 1.11) exhibit two relaxation frequencies. The lowest vibrational mode of these molecules is decoupled from the other modes, causing a faster vibration–translation energy transfer in the lowest mode.

The temperature and pressure changes associated with ultrasound may perturb the thermodynamic equilibrium between the rotational isomeric forms of molecules, or the equilibrium between monomers and dimers in weakly associating liquids (e.g. acetic acid). Pressure perturbation causes an exchange in the structure or order in highly associated liquids (water and alcohols). These perturbations cause the relaxation phenomenon, resulting in ultrasonic absorption. Rotational isomeric relaxation has been observed in ethane and butane derivatives, esters, aldehydes, and ethers. For instance, the ultrasonic absorption measured in ethyl formate, a typical ester, is shown in figure 1.12 [11]. The temperature dependence of the relaxation frequency, represented by the arrow in the figure, and the relaxation strength, i.e. the maximum value of absorption per wavelength, provide the activation enthalpy, enthalpy difference, and volume difference between *cis* and *trans* isomers.

The absorption spectra of aqueous biomolecular solutions exhibit a different behavior from those of the liquids mentioned above. As shown in figure 1.13, the absorption divided by the square of the frequency (α/f^2) changes by more than four orders of magnitude of frequency in an aqueous solution of bovine serum albumin at a concentration of 0.05 kg L^{-1}. This frequency dependence can be explained by the distribution of the relaxation time. This mechanism was attributed to the perturbation of equilibrium related to multiple degrees of hydration of protein molecules. In the frequency range of 1–10 MHz, the frequency dependence of absorption is expressed as $\alpha = f^n$, with $n = 1.3$–1.4. This value of n is similar to that for bio-tissue, for which the relaxation mechanism has not been exactly specified [13].

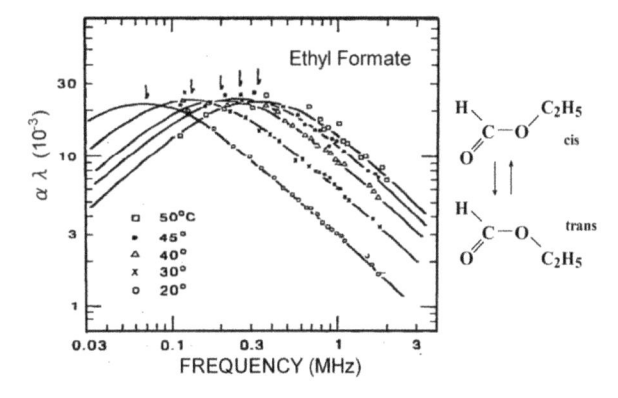

Figure 1.12. Spectra of absorption per wavelength due to rotational isomeric relaxation in ethyl formate. Reproduced with permission from [11]. Copyright 1985 Elsevier.

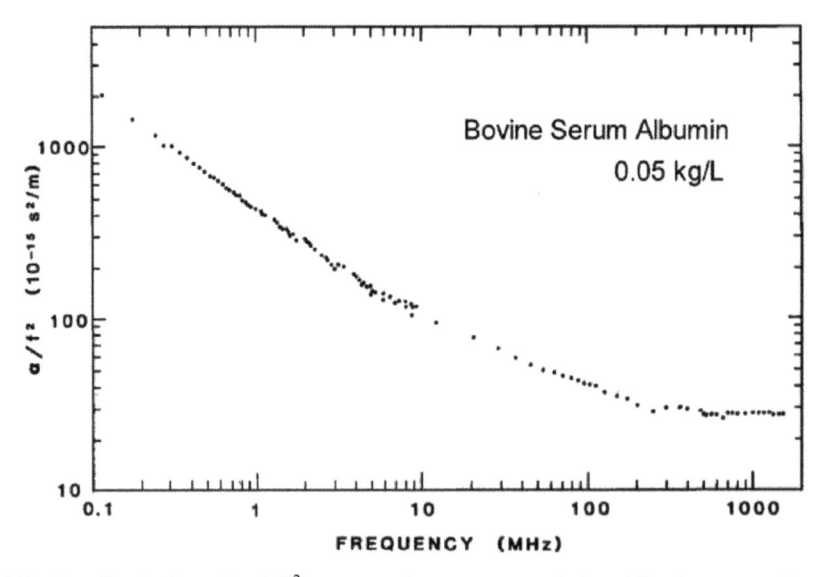

Figure 1.13. Broadband absorption (α/f^2) spectrum in an aqueous solution of bovine serum albumin at a concentration of 0.05 kg L^{-1} with a pH of 7 at 20 °C. Reproduced with permission from [12]. Copyright 1990 American Institute of Physics.

1.4 Sound radiation

The ultrasound field is not homogeneous because of the diffraction effect caused by the finite area of the radiation source. The diffraction effect on ultrasound propagation is more pronounced than on optical propagation because the sound wavelength is much larger than the optical wavelength. In this section, we describe the sound field radiated by a circular rigid plate that performs an alternating motion in the normal direction (a circular piston) and describe the focused sound field radiated by a concave source. Focused sound fields are commonly used in medical applications. The use of high-intensity focused ultrasound is explained in chapter 10.

We first consider the radiation from a point source, i.e. a spherical wave in which the surfaces of the constant phase or wavefronts are concentric spheres. The wave equation (1.14) expressed in spherical polar coordinates is

$$\frac{\partial^2 p}{\partial r^2} + \frac{2}{r}\frac{\partial p}{\partial r} = \frac{1}{v^2}\frac{\partial^2 p}{\partial t^2}, \tag{1.77}$$

where r is the distance between the point source positioned at the origin and the observation point. The solution to this equation can be written as

$$p(r, t) = \frac{\rho_0}{4\pi r}\dot{Q}\left(t - \frac{r}{v}\right), \tag{1.78}$$

where $\dot{Q}$ is the time derivative of the volume velocity $Q(t)$, which is the volume exhausted or taken in per second by the source. For the harmonic oscillation of the source, the volume velocity varies as follows:

$$Q(t) = \hat{Q} e^{i\omega t} \tag{1.79}$$

so that equation (1.78) yields

$$p(r, t) = \frac{i\rho_0 \omega \hat{Q}}{4\pi r} e^{i(\omega t - kr)}. \tag{1.80}$$

Equation (1.80) gives the pressure of a spherical wave.

1.4.1 Sound field produced by a circular piston source

We imagine a circular piston source set flush in an infinite rigid baffle wall, as shown in figure 1.14. The piston, which has a radius of a vibrates harmonically with the normal velocity component:

$$v_n = v_0 e^{i\omega t}. \tag{1.81}$$

Each small-area element of the piston's surface dS originates spherical waves with a volume velocity of $v_n dS$. The sound pressure at the observation point P is obtained by adding the contributions of all spherical waves using equation (1.80)

$$p(r, t) = \frac{i\omega \rho_0 v_0}{2\pi} e^{i\omega t} \iint_S \frac{e^{-ikR}}{R} dS, \tag{1.82}$$

where R is the distance between the element dS and point P, which is determined by its distance r from the center of the piston and its polar angle θ. The difference due to the factor of two in equation (1.82) arises because the radiation is restricted to the half-space for the circular piston. Equation (1.82) must be evaluated numerically, and an example of the solution is presented in the following section. However, a closed-form solution can be obtained for two special cases. One is the case in which the observation point P is located on the central axis z of the piston, that is, $\theta = 0$. The other situation arises when the observation point P is far from the piston. In this case, all the lines connecting the surface elements dS and P are nearly parallel; hence, the relative differences between Rs are negligible.

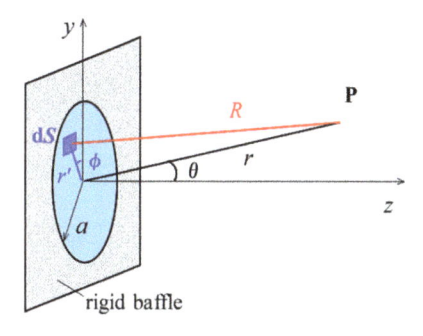

Figure 1.14. Coordinates of the circular piston and the observation point P.

The sound pressure in the first case can be obtained as follows: let the distance between the center of the piston and the surface element dS be r', as illustrated in figure 1.14. The distance R between the surface element dS and the point P on the central axis can then be simplified to

$$R = \sqrt{r'^2 + z^2}. \tag{1.83}$$

The area of the element is given by

$$dS = 2\pi r' dr'. \tag{1.84}$$

Substituting equations (1.83) and (1.84) into equation (1.82) and neglecting the time dependence leads to

$$p(z) = i\omega\rho_0 v_0 \int_0^a \frac{r'}{\sqrt{r'^2 + z^2}} e^{-ik\sqrt{r'^2 + z^2}} dr'$$

$$= \frac{\rho_0 v_0 \omega}{k} \left(e^{-ikz} - e^{-ik\sqrt{a^2+z^2}} \right). \tag{1.85}$$

It is interesting to note that equation (1.85) is composed of two terms of equal amplitude but different phases: the first term represents a wave originated at the center and the second resembles a wave originated at the piston's rim. These waves interfere with each other. Maximum and minimum points exist that depend on their phase differences. However, it should be noted that these interferences are caused by the superposition of spherical waves produced by each element of the piston, i.e. the sound diffraction effect, and not by different waves represented by the two terms. The absolute value of the pressure can be obtained as follows:

$$|p| = \sqrt{pp^*} = \frac{2\rho_0 v_0 \omega}{k} \left| \sin\frac{k}{2}\left(\sqrt{a^2+z^2} - z\right) \right|. \tag{1.86}$$

The sound pressure on the central axis was calculated using equation (1.86), as shown in figure 1.15. The simulation was performed with a sound frequency of 1

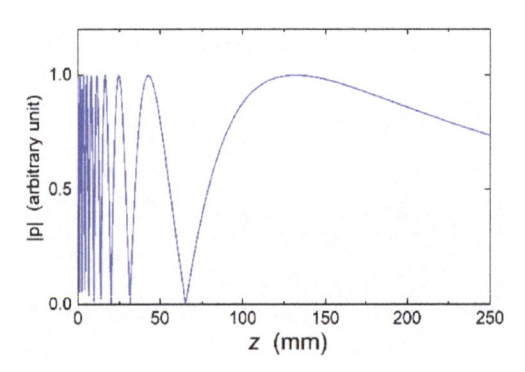

Figure 1.15. Sound pressure on the central axis of the piston source. The ultrasound frequency is 1 MHz and the piston radius is 14 mm.

MHz and a piston radius of $a = 14$ mm. Many maxima and zeros are observed next to the piston source, and the last maximum occurs at $z_0 \approx a^2/\lambda$. The number of maxima increases as ka increases. This range is called the near field of the sound source. Beyond the distance z_0, the sound pressure monotonically decreases because the phase difference between the two terms in equation (1.85) becomes less than the wavelength. In fact, if we assume $z \gg a$, equation (1.86) can be approximated by

$$|p| \approx \frac{\rho_0 v_0 a^2 \omega}{2z} = \frac{\rho_0 Q \omega}{2\pi z}, \qquad (1.87)$$

where $Q = \pi a^2 v_0$ is the volume velocity of the piston source. The dependence of equation (1.87) on z is similar to that of a spherical wave (see equation (1.80)). This region is called the far field.

The second case, in which a closed-form solution of equation (1.82) exists, applies to the far field of the circular piston and characterizes the directional property of ultrasound radiation. The distance R between the surface element dS and the observation point P is approximated under the assumption that $\gg r'$:

$$R = \sqrt{r^2 + r'^2 - 2rr'\cos\phi \sin\theta}$$

$$\approx r - r' \cos\phi \sin\theta. \qquad (1.88)$$

Furthermore, R in the denominator of equation (1.82) is replaced by r. With these approximations, equation (1.82) can be written as

$$p(r, \theta, t) = \frac{i\omega\rho_0 v_0}{2\pi r} e^{i(\omega t - kr)} \int_0^a \int_{-\pi}^{\pi} e^{ikr' \sin\theta \cos\phi} r' d\phi dr'. \qquad (1.89)$$

By employing the integral representation of the nth-order Bessel function

$$J_n(x) = \frac{1}{2\pi} \int_{-\pi}^{\pi} e^{ix(\cos\phi - n\phi)} d\phi, \qquad (1.90)$$

we can obtain

$$p(r, \theta, t) = \frac{i\omega\rho_0 Q}{2\pi r} \frac{2J_1(ka \sin\theta)}{ka \sin\theta} e^{i(\omega t - kr)}. \qquad (1.91)$$

The directional factor of the circular piston is defined as the sound pressure relative to that on the central axis as a function of the polar angle θ:

$$D(\theta) = \frac{p(r, \theta, t)}{p(r, 0, t)} = \frac{2J_1(ka \sin\theta)}{ka \sin\theta}. \qquad (1.92)$$

Figure 1.16 shows the absolute value of the directional factor for the parameters $ka = 20$ (a) and $ka = 59$ (b). The frequency (1 MHz) and piston radius (14 mm) used in the simulation shown in figure 1.15 correspond to $ka = 59$. The quantity $ka = 2\pi a/\lambda$ is equal to the circumference of the piston divided by the wavelength and is used as the parameter expressing the degree of diffraction. For a large value of ka, the radiated

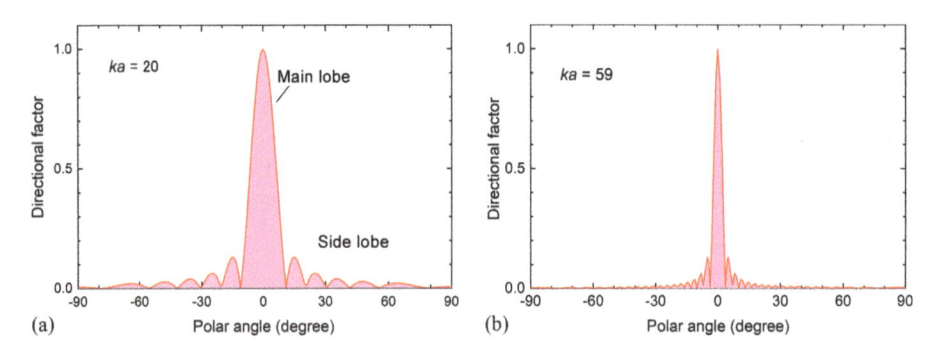

Figure 1.16. Directional factor as a function of the polar angle for (a) $ka = 20$, and (b) $ka = 59$.

sound energy is concentrated in the direction of the central axis. This region of sound concentration is called the *main lobe*. Because the first zero of the first-order Bessel function occurs at $ka\sin\theta = 3.83$,

$$\sin\theta_1 = \frac{3.83}{ka} = 0.61\frac{\lambda}{a} \tag{1.93}$$

gives a measure of the angular half width of the main lobe. Several side lobes are present on either side of the main lobe. The side lobes are undesirable in practical applications such as medical imaging and nondestructive testing. An image or pulse echo originating from the side lobes can interfere with that from the main lobe. The above discussion applies to continuous waves and fixed frequencies. The side lobes become indistinct for pulsed waves that have some frequency bandwidth. Nevertheless, the interference they produce may lead to a false interpretation of the inspection results.

1.4.2 Simulation of a sound field

A detailed sound field can be obtained from a numerical simulation of equation (1.82). We present the simulation results using a parabolic approximation method [14], which is useful for the simulation of an axial symmetric field with a large value of ka. This method provides a sound pressure field from a circular plane source or concave source. We used cylindrical coordinates r and z, and the notation $r' = r$ on the piston at $z = 0$. Equation (1.82) can be transformed into

$$p(r, z) = \frac{i\omega\rho_0 v_0}{z}\exp\left(-\frac{ikr^2}{2z}\right)\int_0^a \exp\left[\frac{ikr'^2}{2}\left(\frac{1}{D} - \frac{1}{z}\right)\right] J_0\left(\frac{krr'}{z}\right) r'\mathrm{d}r'. \tag{1.94}$$

This equation gives the sound field produced by a plane source if we set the curvature radius $D = \infty$, or a focused sound field if we set, for instance, $D = 40$ mm.

Figure 1.17 shows the colored profile of the sound pressure field (a) and its three-dimensional (3D) representation (b) radiated by a plane circular source with a radius of 14 mm at a frequency of 1 MHz. MATLAB® was used for the simulation. The variation in pressure along the line at $r = 0$ corresponds to the curve shown in figure 1.15. Similar plots of a focused sound pressure field are shown in figure 1.18.

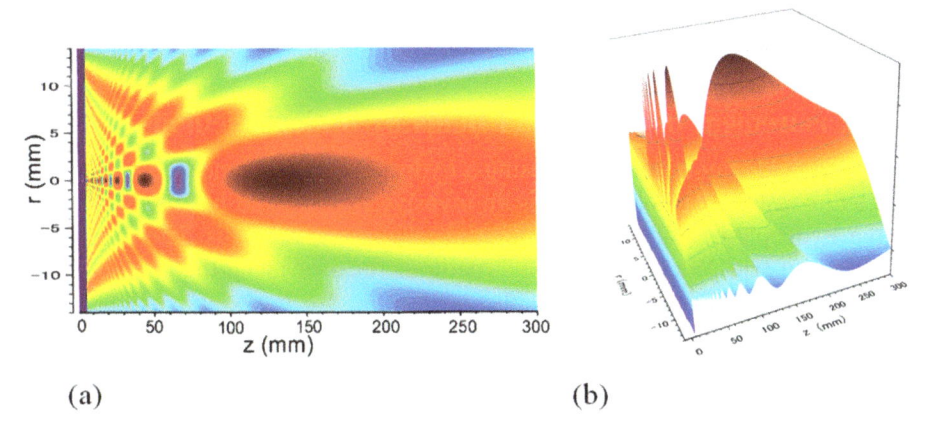

Figure 1.17. (a) Sound pressure field radiated by a plane circular source with a 14 mm radius at 1 MHz ($ka = 59$), and (b) its 3D representation.

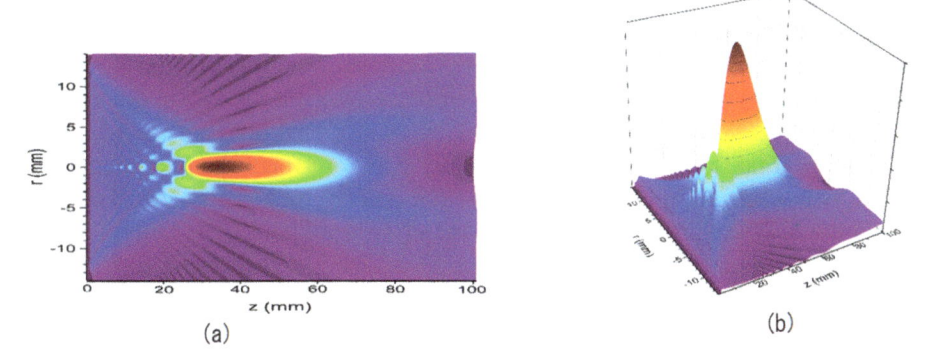

Figure 1.18. (a) Focused sound pressure field radiated by a concave source with a 14 mm radius and a 40 mm curvature radius at 1 MHz [33], and (b) its 3D representation.

The same parameters, except for the curvature radius $D = 40$ mm, were used in the simulation. Some features can be identified compared to the plane-source field. The maximum value of the sound pressure lies at $z = 36.4$ mm on the central axis in the focused field, whereas it lies at $z = 133$ mm for the last maximum in the plane-source field. The focusing gain is defined by a multiple of the maximum pressure relative to the average pressure at the surface of the source, and is given by

$$G = \frac{ka^2}{2D}, \qquad (1.95)$$

which was calculated to be 10.4 in the present case. On the other hand, for the plane-source field, the multiple of the maximum pressure relative to the average pressure at the surface of a source is 2. The sound energy is also concentrated in the lateral direction, and the beam width is subjected to the diffraction limit. The full beam width at 3 dB down at the focal point is

$$W \approx 2\left(\frac{1.62D}{ka}\right) \qquad (1.96)$$

which was calculated to be 2.2 mm in the present case. This value is close to the wavelength (1.5 mm) of ultrasound at 1 MHz in water.

1.5 Measurement of ultrasound fields by optical methods

Ultrasound fields can be measured using a hydrophone that is mechanically scanned in three dimensions. However, this is an invasive method and has the disadvantage that the hydrophone has a limited spatial resolution, which is determined by its active element size. We present optical methods for measuring the ultrasound field, together with some experimental results.

1.5.1 Schlieren method

Density gradients caused by ultrasound give rise to variations in refractive index which, in turn, influence the propagation of light. Figure 1.19 shows the setup of the schlieren method, which is used to visualize ultrasound fields. Light from a laser or an LED is collimated using a lens and a slit, and is perpendicularly incident on ultrasound propagating in a water bath. Ultrasound acts as a phase grating for light when the light beam width is much greater than the wavelength of sound. According to Raman–Nath theory, light is diffracted in oblique directions, which are dependent on the wavelengths of light and sound [15]. Non-diffracted light is focused by a lens positioned beyond the point at which the light passes through the ultrasound, and is blocked by a 'stop,' which is a small black spot painted on a glass plate. The camera detects only diffracted light and visualizes the ultrasound field. A motion picture that captures the propagation of pulsed ultrasound can be obtained using a stroboscopic light and a time-delay generator. The stroboscopic light emission is synchronized with the excitation of the ultrasound pulse, and the trigger time of the light emission is controlled relative to the ultrasound pulse. This procedure creates a slow-motion picture of ultrasound propagation in various environments. Figure 1.20 depicts two frames from a video that demonstrates ultrasonic-pulse transmission through a brass cylinder immersed in water. In figure 1.20(a), an ultrasound pulse at a frequency of 10 MHz with a duration of 1 μs is incident on a brass cylinder. Figure 1.20(b) shows the reflection and transmission of the ultrasound pulse. The ultrasound reflected from the cylinder's surface is indicated in the upper part of the figure. The ultrasound

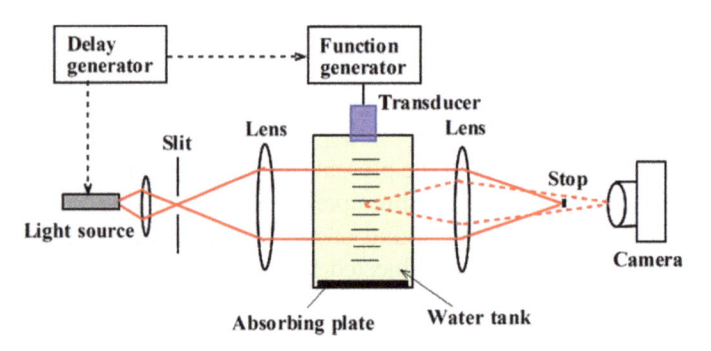

Figure 1.19. Experimental system that visualizes an ultrasound field using the schlieren method.

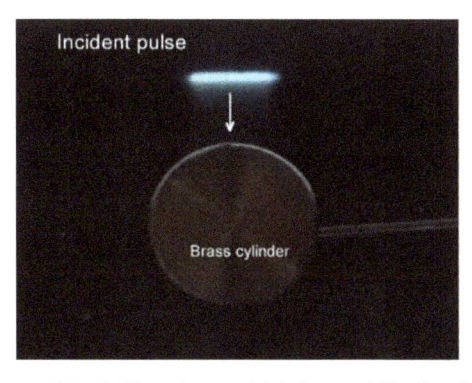

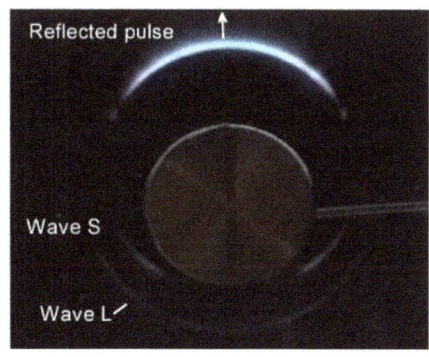

Figure 1.20. Schlieren images (a) before and (b) after the transmission of an ultrasonic pulse through a brass cylinder (courtesy of K Yamamoto, Kansai University) (frames extracted from video available at https://doi.org/10.1088/978-0-7503-4936-9).

refracted into the cylinder is not only a longitudinal wave (L) but also a shear wave (S) which is excited by a tangential force acting at an oblique angle of incidence (mode conversion). Both waves are transmitted through the cylinder and propagate as longitudinal waves in water; they are denoted by Wave L and Wave S, as indicated in figure 1.20(b). Wave S appears after Wave L because the shear-wave velocity is smaller than the longitudinal-wave velocity in the cylinder. In addition to these two waves, circumferential waves can propagate around the cylinder surface [16].

Ultrasound diffraction and ultrasonic-pulse reflection and transmission by a plate were visualized and analyzed by Negishi [17]. Tomographic reconstruction of the sound pressure amplitude and phase at 3 MHz was performed by Reibold and Molkenstruck [18] using the light diffraction method. Neighbors *et al* [19] performed quantitative sound pressure measurements of a line-focused field using schlieren images. Yamamoto *et al* [20] obtained schlieren images of phase conjugate waves that had the time-reversal property and the capability to correct wavefront distortion. Recently, background-oriented schlieren imaging was applied to measure an ultrasound field [21]. In this method, a textured background pattern (random dots or a grid of lines) located in front of a water tank was projected by a light source. The pattern was viewed by a camera located on the other side of the water tank. The pattern image was blurred after passing through the spatial variation of the refractive index caused by the ultrasound. Subtracting images with and without the ultrasound provided a visualization of the sound field.

1.5.2 Photoelasticity imaging method

The variation in refractive index caused by ultrasound in solids is very small compared to that in liquids. The photoelasticity imaging method is useful for visualizing sound fields in transparent solid materials. This method utilizes the stress birefringence of solid media, in which the refractive indices for light polarized along orthogonal axes change with differences in stress between axes [22].

The experimental system used for this method is similar to that of the schlieren method shown in figure 1.19, except for two differences: the first is that two circular polarizers, each consisting of a linear polarizer coupled with a quarter-wave plate, are positioned on each side of the sample. The use of a circular polarizer enables the visualization of both shear and longitudinal waves. The second difference is that the stop used to eliminate the non-diffracted light is removed.

An evanescent wave is generated when ultrasound traveling in water impinges on a solid surface at an angle exceeding the critical angle of the refracted shear wave in the solid. Visualization of an evanescent wave and a Rayleigh wave was performed using the photoelasticity imaging method by Yamamoto *et al* [23], and the results are shown in figure 1.21. An ultrasound pulse at 0.93 MHz traveling in water is incident on a glass substrate (a1). The evanescent wave generated in the glass decays exponentially in the depth direction (a2). In figure 1.21(b1), a Rayleigh wave is generated along the glass surface when the angle of incidence of the ultrasound is smaller than the critical angle. The Rayleigh wave is efficiently excited when the wavelength of the Rayleigh wave is equal to the wavelength in water projected onto the water–glass boundary. The secondary longitudinal wave (leaked wave) is radiated into the water by the Rayleigh wave as it travels along the glass surface (b2).

The Lamb wave mode pattern was analyzed using photoelasticity images in a glass plate [24]. The phase velocities of the symmetric and antisymmetric modes agreed with the theoretical prediction. Recently, high-speed observation of elastic wave propagation in model stones was reported [25] for a study of the fragmentation mechanism of kidney stones in burst wave lithotripsy.

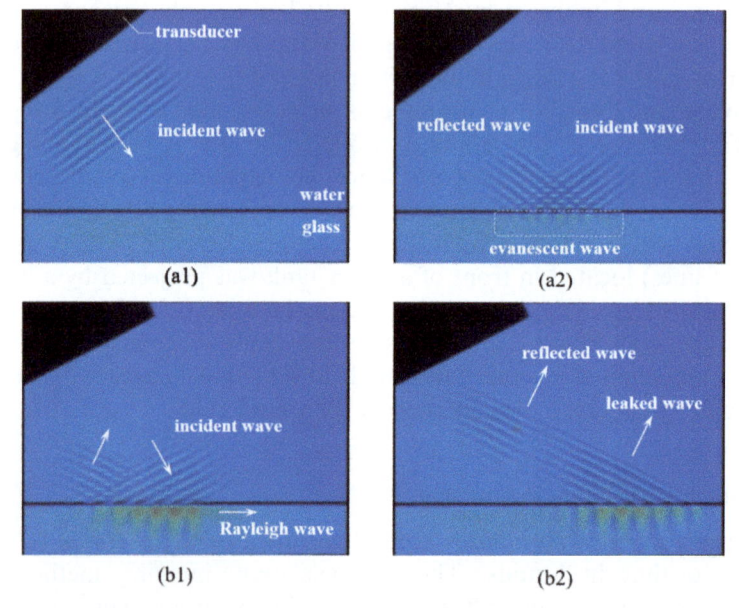

Figure 1.21. Photoelasticity imaging of evanescent (a1 and a2) and Rayleigh waves (b1 and b2) in a glass substrate. They are generated by the oblique incidence of ultrasound traveling in water. Reproduced with permission from [23]. Copyright 2015 Elsevier.

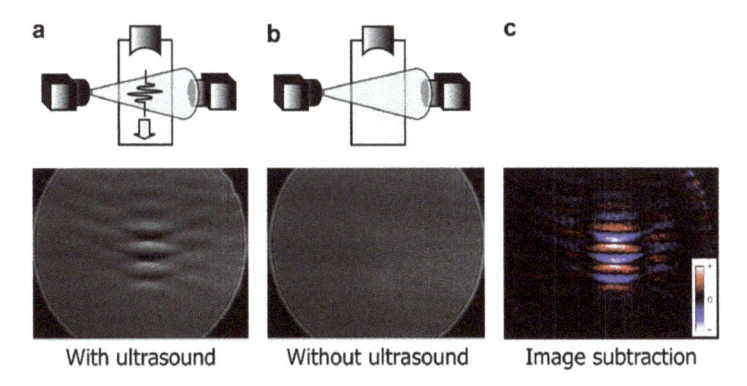

Figure 1.22. Experimental system used for shadowgraphy: (a) an image with ultrasound radiation, and (b) without ultrasound radiation. Subtracted image of an ultrasound pulse that had a three-cycle duration at 1 MHz (c). Reproduced with permission from [27]. Copyright 2015 Elsevier.

1.5.3 Shadowgraphy method

The shadowgraphy method is based on light deflection by the medium, which causes a refractive index gradient [26]. Consider light traveling in a direction perpendicular to the direction of ultrasound. If the variation in the refractive index caused by the ultrasound shows a positive spatial second derivative for the direction of light travel, the variation acts as a defocusing lens. If the variation in the refractive index shows a negative spatial second derivative, the variation acts as a focusing lens. These produce shadowgraph images of the ultrasound on a camera screen. Kudo [27, 28] proposed a simple and highly sensitive shadowgraphy method. Figure 1.22 shows the experimental system and shadowgraph images (a) with ultrasound pulse (three-cycle duration at 1 MHz) radiation and (b) without ultrasound pulse radiation. In figure 1.22(c), ultrasound positive and negative peaks are clearly obtained from the difference between figures 1.22(a) and 1.22(b).

1.5.4 Luminescence due to acoustic cavitation

Irradiation due to intense ultrasound in liquid causes bubble generation, which is called acoustic cavitation. The acoustic bubbles repeat the oscillation of expansion and contraction in phase with the sinusoidal cycle of the acoustic pressure. The violent bubble contraction produces high-temperature and high-pressure conditions of 10 000 K and 1000 atm, respectively, at the time of bubble collapse in the process of adiabatic compression. These conditions induce the formation of hydroxyl (OH) radicals due to the pyrolysis of water molecules and the emission of blue-white light (sonoluminescence, SL) [29–31]. The light-emitting bubbles are trapped at the pressure antinodes of the standing acoustic waves established in a liquid container. Hence, observation of the distribution of the light-emitting bubbles can provide an image of the sound field.

The sound field subjects the acoustic bubble to a force, called the primary Bjerknes force, given by

Side view   Top view

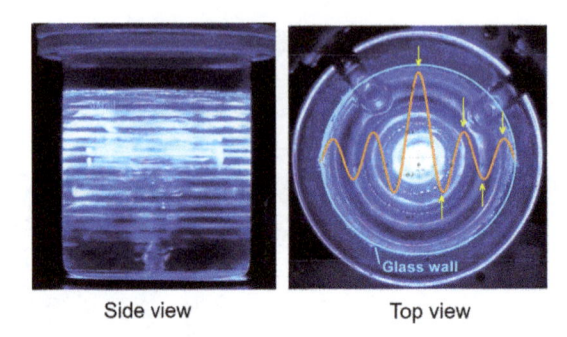

Figure 1.23. Photographs of sonochemiluminescence in a cylindrical container, demonstrating a standing-wave field at 145 kHz. The exposure time was 10 s (frames extracted from video available at https://doi.org/10.1088/978-0-7503-4936-9).

$$F_B = -< V(t)\nabla p >, \quad (1.97)$$

where $V(t)$ is the time-dependent bubble volume, ∇p is the gradient of the acoustic pressure and $< >$ represents the time-averaging operation during an acoustic cycle. In a standing-wave field, if a bubble is smaller than the resonant size, it moves towards an antinode of the acoustic field. Light-emitting bubbles satisfy this condition. To observe the distribution of the acoustic field, it is advantageous to use sonochemiluminescence (SCL), which emits light that is two orders of magnitude brighter than that emitted by SL [32]. The oxidation reaction between OH radicals and luminol is a typical source of SCL. The OH radicals produced in the high-temperature region inside the bubble diffuse out through the bubble–liquid interface and react with luminol molecules in the liquid region adjacent to the bubble. Figure 1.23 shows photographs of SCL produced by a luminol aqueous solution under 145 kHz ultrasound irradiation at an acoustic power of 5 W. The images, which were captured using an exposure time of 10 s, exhibit three-dimensional standing-wave modes in a cylindrical glass container with a volume of 500 ml. The side view shows antinodes of longitudinal modes, and the top view shows antinodes of radial modes, which are expressed by the zeroth-order Bessel function indicated by the orange line in figure 1.23. The arrows denote the peak positions of the Bessel function, which correspond to the antinodes, suggesting good agreement with the light-emitting region. The video in figure 1.23 is a real-time demonstration of SCL. The sample and experimental conditions were similar to those of figure 1.23.

Chapter 8 describes the application of acoustic cavitation to protein aggregation related to Alzheimer's disease.

References

[1] Bhatia A B 1985 *Ultrasonic Absorption* (Dover: New York)
[2] Del Grosso V A and Mader C W 1972 Speed of sound in pure water *J. Acoust. Soc. Am.* **52** 1442–6
[3] Edmonds P D (ed) 1981 *Ultrasonics* (Methods of Experimental Physics vol 19) (Orlando, FL: Academic)

[4] Kuttruff H 1991 *Ultrasonics: Fundamentals and Applications* (New York: Elsevier)
[5] Cheeke J D N 2002 *Fundamentals and Applications of Ultrasonic Waves* (Boca Raton, FL: CRC Press)
[6] Pollard H F 1977 *Sound Waves in Solids* (London: Pion)
[7] Herzfeld K F and Litovitz T A 1959 *Absorption and Dispersion of Ultrasonic Waves* (New York: Academic)
[8] Mason W P (ed) 1965 *Physical Acoustics: Principles and Methods, Vol II, Part A* (New York: Academic)
[9] Bass H E, Sutherland L C and Zuckerwar A J 1990 Atmospheric absorption of sound: update *J. Acoust. Soc. Am.* **88** 2019–21
[10] Takagi K and Negishi K 1980 Measurement of ultrasonic relaxation time and mean free path in liquids *J. Chem. Phys.* **72** 1809–12
[11] Choi P K, Naito Y and Takagi K 1985 Ultrasonic study of rotational isomerism in methyl and ethyl formate *Chem. Phys. Lett.* **121** 169–73
[12] Choi P K, Bae J R and Takagi K 1990 Ultrasonic spectroscopy in bovine serum albumin solutions *J. Acoust. Soc. Am.* **87** 874–81
[13] Dunn F, Edmonds P D and Fry W J 1969 Absorption and dispersion of ultrasound in biological media, *Biological Engineering* ed H P Schwan (New York: McGraw-Hill)
[14] Lucas B G and Muir T G 1982 The field of a focusing source *J. Acoust. Soc. Am.* **72** 1289–96
[15] Breazeale M A 2001 From monochromatic light diffraction to colour schlieren photography *J. Opt. A: Pure Appl. Opt.* **3** S1–7
[16] Neubauer W G 1973 Observation of acoustic radiation from plane and curved surface in *Physical Acoustics: Principles and Methods* vol X ed W P Mason and R N Thurston (New York: Academic)
[17] Negishi K 1982 Visualization of ultrasonic waves by schlieren method *Jpn. J. Appl. Phys.* **21** 3–6
[18] Reibold R and Molkenstruck W 1984 Light diffraction tomography applied to the investigation of ultrasonic fields. Part I: continuous waves *Acustica* **56** 180–92
[19] Neighbors T H, Mayer W G and Ruf H J 1995 Acousto-optic imaging of focused ultrasound pressure fields *J. Acoust. Soc. Am.* **98** 1751–56
[20] Yamamoto K, Ohno M, Kokubo A, Sakai K and Takagi K 1999 Acoustic phase conjugation by nonlinear piezoelectricity II. Visualization and application to imaging systems *J. Acoust. Soc. Am.* **106** 1339–45
[21] Pulkkinen A, Leskinen J J and Tiihonen A 2017 Ultrasound field characterization using synthetic schlieren tomography *J. Acoust. Soc. Am.* **141** 4600–9
[22] Hall G 1977 Ultrasonic wave visualization as a teaching aid in non-destructive testing *Ultrasonics* **15** 57–69
[23] Yamamoto K, Sakiyama T and Izumiya H 2015 Visualization of acoustic evanescent waves by the stroboscopic photoelastic method *Phys. Proc.* **70** 716–20
[24] Li H-U and Negishi K 1994 Visualization of Lamb mode patterns in a glass plate *Ultrasonics* **32** 243–8
[25] Maxwell A D, MacConaghy B, Bailey M R and Sapozhnikov O A 2020 An investigation of elastic waves producing stone fracture in burst wave lithotripsy *J. Acoust. Soc. Am.* **147** 1607–22
[26] Biel J K 2003 Point-source spark shadowgraphy at the historic birthplace *Shock Wave* **13** 167–77

[27] Kudo N 2015 A simple technique for visualizing ultrasound fields without schlieren optics *Ultrasound Med. Biol.* **41** 2071–81
[28] Kudo N 2015 Optical methods for visualization of ultrasound fields *Jpn. J. Appl. Phys.* **54** 07HA01
[29] Brenner M P, Hilgenfeldt S and Lohse D 2002 Single-bubble sonoluminescence *Rev. Mod. Phys.* **74** 425–84
[30] Choi P-K 2017 Sonoluminescence and acoustic cavitation *Jpn. J. Appl. Phys.* **56** 07JA01
[31] Nakajima R, Hayashi Y and Choi P-K 2015 Mechanism of two types of Na emission observed in sonoluminescence *Jpn. J. Appl. Phys.* **54** 07HE02
[32] Grieser F, Choi P-K, Enomoto N, Harada H, Okitsu K and Yasui K (ed) 2015 *Sonochemistry and the Acoustic Bubble* (Amsterdam: Elsevier)
[33] Choi P-K 2022 *Cho-onpa Techno* (Ultrasonic Technology) **34** 19–22 (in Japanese)

IOP Publishing

Ultrasonics
Physics and applications
Mami Matsukawa, Pak-Kon Choi, Kentaro Nakamura, Hirotsugu Ogi and Hideyuki Hasegawa

Chapter 2

Wave propagation in/on liquids and spectroscopy of viscoelasticity and surface tension

Keiji Sakai

In this chapter, we introduce recent progress in ultrasonic spectroscopy and its peripheral technologies, which are used to observe the dynamic behavior of fluids. In the first section, materials are classified into solids, fluids, and viscoelastic fluids from the viewpoint of rheology, and fundamental knowledge about viscosity and its molecular origin is presented using examples. The dynamic properties of the fluid surface are also introduced. Subsequently, we describe recent developments in the experimental approach to thermal phonon observation and its use in investigating the coupling process between translational and rotational viscosities. Furthermore, several recent advances in the methodology of dynamic surface phenomena observation and rheometry are presented.

2.1 Introduction

2.1.1 Viscoelastic properties of, and wave propagation in liquids

2.1.1.1 Solids, fluids, and viscoelastic fluids
As described in the previous chapter, ultrasonic wave propagation is determined by the mechanical properties of the medium. Here, we classify wave propagation media as solids, fluids, or viscoelastic fluids from the viewpoint of rheology [1]. The deformation of a medium due to a longitudinal elastic wave consists of both the volume and shear deformation modes; rheology particularly focuses on the shear aspect. The velocity of an elastic wave is given by the longitudinal elastic modulus M and the density ρ according to $v = (M/\rho)^{1/2}$, where M includes the contributions of the volume and shear moduli, K and G, respectively, as follows:

$$M = K + (4/3)G. \tag{2.1}$$

(a) solid & shear deformation

(b) fluid

(c) visco-elastic fluid

(d) visco-elastic solid

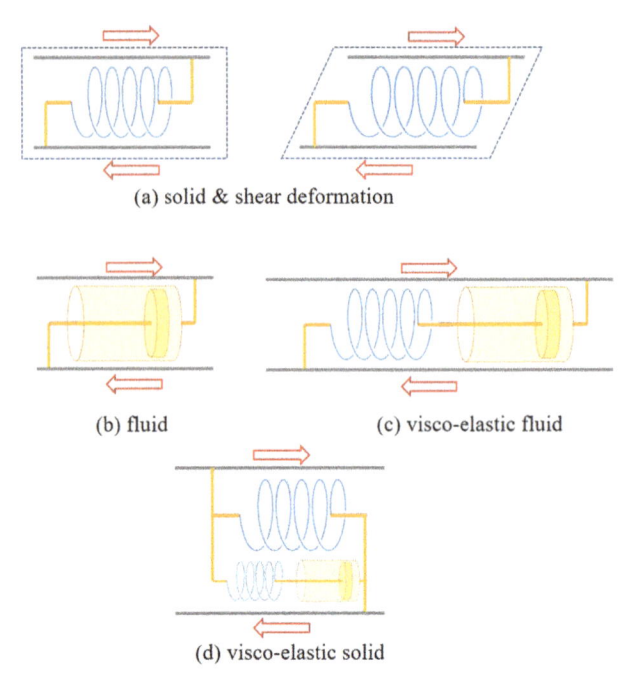

Figure 2.1. Schematic illustration representing the mechanical response to shear deformation of a solid (a), a fluid (b), a viscoelastic fluid (c) and a viscoelastic solid (d).

In this chapter, we focus on the viscous term that represents energy dissipation, which is described by introducing the imaginary part of the moduli. For example, $G = G' + iG''$.

First, we classify media into solids and fluids. Solids are defined as media that possess non-zero G'; this contrasts with fluids, which possess zero G'. While the elastic modulus that determines the propagation of longitudinal ultrasonic waves is given by the summation of the volume and shear components, as described in equation (2.1), we only consider the contribution of the shear mode in this section. Figure 2.1 shows a schematic illustration representing the mechanical responses to shear deformation of a solid (a), a fluid (b), a viscoelastic fluid (c) and a viscoelastic solid (d). A transverse-mode elastic wave can propagate in a solid using the shear elastic modulus as a restoring force, whereas shear deformation localizes in a fluid, since the shear elasticity is zero: the viscosity is the resistant force; it cannot store the energy of deformation, but only dissipates it. In addition to the simple viscous fluids shown in (b), there are many types of viscoelastic fluid, such as polymers, colloids, liquid crystals, and surfactant solutions. The mechanical response of these materials is described by a model composed of a spring and a dashpot (c). Hereafter, we consider the molecular mechanisms of viscosity and viscoelasticity.

2.1.1.2 Viscosity of simple fluids
Here, we consider a viscosity model of a simple liquid at the molecular level. In the previous chapter, we discovered relaxation phenomena that occur with increasing

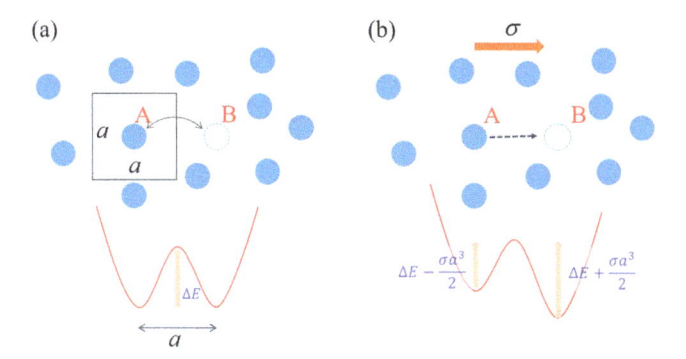

Figure 2.2. Schematic of the translation of molecules under shear stress.

frequency, namely, an increase in the real part and a decrease in the imaginary part of the complex elasticity. The deformation of a medium caused by a longitudinal ultrasonic wave is composed of volume and shear deformation modes. The former leads to a change in the temperature and pressure, which modulates the distribution of the molecular states from equilibrium and then causes energy dissipation through a repeated relaxation process to the equilibrium state. This mechanism of energy dissipation does not work in the higher frequency region, where the period of the ultrasonic wave is much shorter than the time required for relaxation.

The situation is the same for shear viscosity. Here, we consider the molecular mechanism of the shear viscosity of a simple liquid to estimate its relaxation frequency. Figure 2.2 shows a schematic of the translation of molecules under shear stress, which is the elementary process of shear viscosity [2]. Molecules in fluids are randomly located, and a fluid includes vacancies, as shown in figure 2.2(a). A molecule can move to a vacancy via thermal motion. The initial positions of molecule A and vacancy B are separated by an energy barrier of ΔE; the potential energy can be regarded as a double-well type. The molecule at position A attempts to overcome the barrier energy ω_0 times per unit time, where ω_0 is approximately given as the fundamental lattice vibration frequency $\omega_0 \sim k_B T/\hbar$, in which k_B is the Boltzmann constant, T is the temperature, and $\hbar$ is the Planck constant. The probability of a molecule translating from A to B during a unit time is then given by

$$p = \alpha \omega_0 \exp\{-\Delta E/k_B T\},$$

where α is the probability that position B is not occupied by other molecules.

Given the above, we can apply a shear stress σ to a fluid. Let us consider that a molecule occupies a cubic volume with a side length a. For simplicity, the distance between the double well is also a. The force applied to a molecule by the shear stress is then σa^2, and the potential change of σa^3 is added between positions A and B. The double-well potential is then modified to the shape shown in figure 2.2(b); the apparent barrier energies observed from positions A and B are changed to $(\Delta E - \sigma a^3/2)$ and $(\Delta E + \sigma a^3/2)$, respectively. The numbers of molecules per volume of a^3 moving from A to B and B to A are calculated by

$$N^+ = \alpha\omega_0 \exp\{-(\Delta E - \sigma a^3/2)/k_B T\},$$

$$N^- = \alpha\omega_0 \exp\{-(\Delta E + \sigma a^3/2)/k_B T\}.$$

By assuming $\sigma a^3/2 \ll \Delta E$, we obtain the flow speed of the fluid:

$$V = (N^+ - N^-)a = \alpha\omega_0 \exp\{-\Delta E/k_B T\}(\sigma a^4/k_B T), \quad (2.2)$$

where the length of one step a is multiplied by the number of molecules moving rightward.

On the other hand, viscosity is defined as the proportion coefficient between the shear deformation rate and shear stress; therefore, the viscosity η is defined by

$$\sigma = \eta(V/a). \quad (2.3)$$

By substituting equation (2.2) into equation (2.3), we obtain

$$\eta = \frac{\exp(\Delta E/k_B T)}{\alpha\omega_0 a^3/k_B T}.$$

By considering the relation $\hbar\omega_0 \sim k_B T$, η can be given as

$$\eta = \frac{\hbar}{\alpha a^3} \exp\{\Delta E/k_B T\}.$$

This result shows the temperature dependence of fluid viscosity, from which we can estimate the barrier energy ΔE.

Let us consider octane as a sample fluid, in which the molecular interaction can be regarded as the van der Waals type. From the temperature dependence of viscosity at approximately room temperature, ΔE is estimated to be 2.2×10^{-20} J, which results in $\exp\{\Delta E/k_B T\} \sim 10^2$ at around room temperature. Assuming $\alpha = 0.1$ and $a = 10^{-28}$ m^3, we obtain $\eta = 10^{-4}$ Pa·s as the viscosity.

The order of magnitude of the calculated viscosity agrees with the actual value, despite the fact that above calculation is a mere approximation. Discussions were carried out to investigate how high-frequency ultrasonic waves respond to the relaxation of simple shear viscosity. The relaxation time is estimated to be $\tau \sim (1/\omega_0)\exp\{\Delta E/k_B T\}$, which is almost the phonon frequency at the edge of the Brillouin zone. From the viewpoint of ultrasonic spectroscopy, shear viscosity can be considered a constant. However, several simple liquids are known to exhibit a decrease in viscosity in the GHz frequency region [3]. This could be due to the relaxation of the existence of long-range interactions through the hydrogen bond, for example. Younger researchers of ultrasonic spectroscopy may someday reveal the entire relaxation spectrum of viscosity for common but strange liquids, such as water.

2.1.1.3 Viscoelastic fluids
In the previous section, we discussed the dynamic process of energy dissipation in the viscous flow of simple liquids; this process involves an energy transfer from the

high-quality energy of the medium's translational motion to the poor-quality thermal motion of molecules. In materials with various internal degrees of freedom, the magnitude of viscosity is determined by the variety of paths to thermal energy. In other words, materials with higher viscosities possess more degrees of freedom, which can correlate with deformation of the medium.

The energy dissipation process requires a finite time τ_η; therefore, the viscosity changes with respect to the timescale of the deformation, and from an experimental viewpoint, the viscosity should be measured as a function of the periodic shear deformation frequency, in which the viscosity decreases as the frequency exceeds the relaxation frequency of $1/\tau_\eta$.

The frequency spectrum of the viscosity has been studied in rheology and by ultrasonic measurements using various methodologies. In addition, theoretical models of relaxation are required to understand the mechanism of viscosity at the molecular level. Here, we introduce one of the most successful theoretical approaches to the relaxation phenomenon of shear viscosity, namely, the molecular model of the entangled polymer system. Figure 2.3 shows a schematic view of the entangled polymer system, which is a common model for melted long-chain molecules. Each polymer chain is randomly bent and entangled with the other polymer chains. The system is complex, and it is impossible to completely describe all the chain motions. Doi and Edwards [4, 5] proposed a sophisticated model to describe the dynamic mechanical response of a polymer system, which focuses on one chain of polymers (a). The polymer is surrounded by other polymers and therefore cannot move across the crossing chain but can move along the direction of the polymer chain, as represented by a tube (b). When shear deformation is applied, the polymer is deformed, and the force is applied from the neighboring polymer chains, which indicates that the circles maintain the position of the polymer chain and the force applied by the circles counters the shear stress (c). The chain is stretched, as seen in (c), and thereafter, the stress is gradually released by the shrinkage of the polymer chain. In addition, the Brownian motion of the chain along the tube contributes to reducing stress. This simple model successfully explained the frequency spectrum of viscoelastic relaxation, and the theoretical prediction agreed well with the results of the rheological measurements.

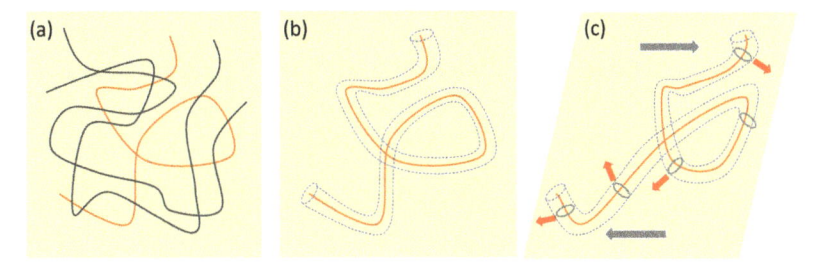

Figure 2.3. Schematic view showing the mechanical response of the entangled polymer system against shear deformation.

The relaxation process of shear stress through molecular motion is known for a wide variety of materials, which are called viscoelastic fluids [6–8]. The characteristic timescale of relaxation depends on the molecular dynamics, and various methodologies are required to reveal the entire relaxation spectra. In section 2.2, we present a method for investigating the behavior of viscoelastic relaxation using the observation of thermal fluctuations.

2.1.2 Dynamics of liquid surface properties

Liquids and gases are widely used materials in various industrial fields. Their advantage as raw materials is that they can flow and be transported via pipelines. With recent developments in high-resolution temporal and spatial fluid processes, such as microfluidics and inkjet technologies, the role of surface properties is increasing. As an example, let us consider the emission of a small liquid droplet in the inkjet process. In an inkjet system commonly used for printing, the typical size of a liquid droplet is approximately 1 pL, and therefore, a droplet with a radius of 10 μm is emitted with an initial velocity of approximately 10 m s^{-1}. The initial velocity is determined by the requirement that the emitted droplets should reach the paper at a distance of at least 1 mm from the emission nozzle. The droplet is affected by the viscous resistant force of the surrounding atmosphere, and the equation for the particle's motion is given as

$$\frac{4}{3}\pi R^3 \rho \frac{\mathrm{d}v}{\mathrm{d}t} = 6\pi \eta_{\mathrm{air}} R v, \qquad (2.4)$$

where R, ρ, and v are the radius, density, and velocity of the flight of the droplet, respectively, and η_{air} is the viscosity of the atmosphere. The flight velocity exponentially decreases with respect to time according to $\sim \exp(-t/\tau)$, and from equation (2.4), we obtain $v\tau \sim 2R^2\rho/9\eta$. Based on the requirement that the penetration length $v\tau$ is greater than 10^{-3} m and the droplet size R is less than 10^{-5} m (required to realize high-quality image printing), together with the assumption that water has $\rho = 10^3$ kg m^{-3} and $\eta = 10^{-3}$ mPa·s, $v > 10$ m s^{-1} is required.

However, the spatial and temporal scales are not determined by the above requirements, but by the occasional agreement in the kinetics of droplet emission. During the inkjet emission process, a pulsed stress is applied to the liquid confined in the emission nozzle. This is similar to the violent blow of a hammer; however, a droplet can be successfully emitted because of the equipartition law of energy. The kinetic energy of the droplet is $(4/3)\pi R^3 \rho v \sim 4 \times 10^{-11}$ J, and the surface energy is $4\pi R^2 \sigma \sim 6 \times 10^{-11}$ J in when the surface tension $\sigma = 50$ mN m^{-1}.

As shown, the energy is almost equally distributed to two degrees of freedom, the surface and inertia in the emission process, and this is the key to the success of inkjet printers. As seen in this example, the surface plays an important role in the micro- and high-speed fluid processes. In this process, typical values of the Reynolds number $R_e \sim R v \rho / \eta$ remain below 100, and the flow field can be accurately regarded as laminar flow. This corroborates the reproducibility of the emission process, even though the typical shear deformation rate of the inkjet emission exceeds 10^6 s^{-1}.

In section 2.4, we introduce a new experimental method that allows observation of the dynamic surface phenomena of liquids through wave phenomena, and in section 2.5, we describe a recent experimental approach to viscous flow that uses a new methodology for noncontact manipulation of picoliter droplets.

2.2 Recent progress in the light-scattering approach to viscoelasticity

2.2.1 Accurate Brillouin scattering experiment based on an optical heterodyne technique

Various types of method have been developed to measure ultrasonic velocity and absorption. Almost all of these methods employ an ultrasonic transducer, which converts the electric signal to/from mechanical vibrations, as a device to excite and/or receive ultrasonic waves. They have direct contact with the sample and apply stress to excite mechanical vibration.

Noncontact measurement of ultrasonic propagation is also effective under extraordinary conditions, such as high/low temperatures and pressures. Brillouin scattering is a noncontact method for the measurement of thermally excited ultrasonic waves, called thermal phonons. In the following discussion, I briefly summarize the principle behind Brillouin scattering measurements [9]. In a medium at a finite temperature, the local pressure and entropy fluctuate owing to the thermal effect. The pressure increase excited by this fluctuation propagates as an elastic wave. Moreover, the local change in entropy relaxes through the diffusion process. These spatial and temporal modulations of pressure and entropy can be detected by optical observation, because these modulations cause local changes in the refractive index. The light incident on the medium in which the local refractive index fluctuates is scattered. We now explain the principle of detection of thermally excited modulation in the refractive index and an experimental method of determining the ultrasonic velocity and absorption as functions of the wave number.

Thermally excited modulation is a random phenomenon, which can be expressed as an ensemble of coherent waves with various wave number vectors K_i and frequencies ω_i, where i denotes the different phonons, and ω_i and K_i can be related to the phase velocity v by $v = \omega_i/|K_i|$. These phonons are not in phase, and the ensemble appears to be a random phenomenon; however, if we experimentally choose only one mode $i = i_0$, we can determine the propagation constant for i_0, which is possible using a light-scattering experiment. Figure 2.4 shows a schematic of the light-scattering detection for the selected wave number of Ki_0 among random ensembles of $\sum K_i$.

Laser light incident on the sample medium propagates with an optical wave number k_{inc} and is effectively diffracted in the k_{sca} direction if the modulation of the refractive index has a periodic structure with wave number vector $K = k_{\text{sca}} - k_{\text{inc}}$. This means that the light scattered in the direction of k_{sca} is converted from the incident light with an optical wave number k_{inc} by the scattering component of K. By determining the directions of the incident and scattered light, we can initially ascertain the propagation direction and wave number of the phonons to be observed. In this process, random fluctuations in space are automatically

$$|\boldsymbol{K}_i| = 2|\boldsymbol{k}|\sin\theta$$

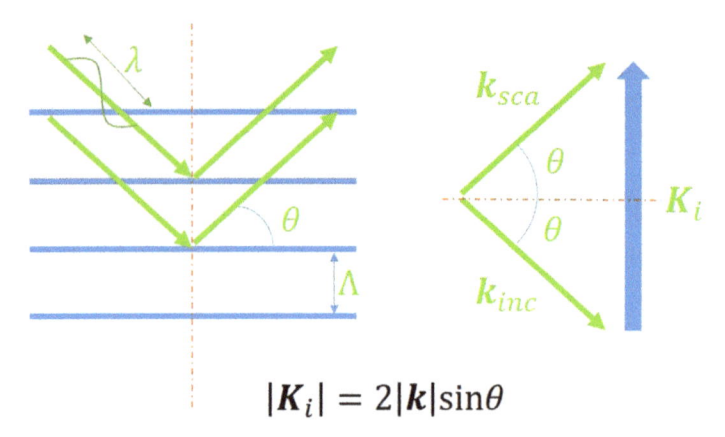

Figure 2.4. Schematic view showing the principle of light-scattering detection of thermal phonons.

decomposed into Fourier components. The thermal fluctuation includes phonons with a wide range of wave numbers; however, the light-scattering configuration detects only one component.

The light is scattered by the propagating phonons; therefore, the frequency of the light is modulated by a Doppler shift; the frequency of the scattered light is shifted by that of the phonons. In addition, the finite correlation time between the light and the phonons, which is restricted by the phonon lifetime, produces an ambiguity in the frequency spectrum of the scattered light. The temporal decay of the phonons can be determined from the peak width of the scattered-light spectrum. It can easily be understood that the spatial area illuminated by the incident laser should be larger than the decay length of the phonons in order to accurately measure phonon absorption.

In the light-scattering experiment, the wave number range is limited by the optical configuration. The upper limit is twice the optical wave number in the sample medium and in common liquids, and the corresponding phonon frequency is less than several GHz. The method used to observe the frequency spectrum of the scattered light is restricted to just an optical resonator, called the Fabri–Pérot interferometer. It is composed of two opposing parallel mirrors, whose separation can be swept by mechanical actuators. The band range, called the 'free spectrum range,' is determined by the distance d between the opposing mirrors in $\Delta f = c/2d$, where c is the velocity of light. The resolution of the interferometer is determined by the reflectivity of the mirrors R to approximately $(1-R)\Delta f$.

The frequency resolution is as high as 100 MHz when a mirror with $R = 0.99$ is employed and the free spectrum range is set to 10 GHz. However, this frequency resolution is not satisfactory for accurately determining phonon decay in the observation of low-frequency phonons. As described, phonons originate from thermal fluctuations, and we can observe various modes of excitation in addition to density modulation, several of which are difficult to artificially excite using mechanical transducers. To observe the slow dynamics of collective molecular

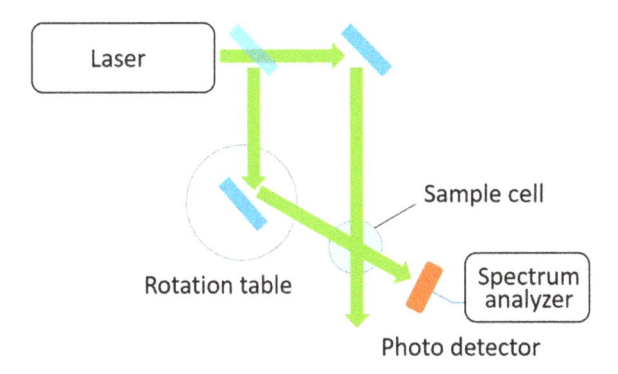

Figure 2.5. Schematic view of the experimental setup used for the optical heterodyne detection of Brillouin scattering.

dynamics, a much greater frequency resolution is required. For this purpose, a new Brillouin scattering measurement method equipped with optical heterodyne detection was developed [10].

Figure 2.5 shows a schematic view of the experimental setup used for optical heterodyne detection of Brillouin scattering. Laser light is divided into two beams, and intense light is used as the incident light. The light scattered by the thermal phonons is superimposed on the local light, and simultaneous detection of these two lights by a photodiode generates a beating signal between the local and scattered lights, which reflects the frequency modulation added through the scattering process. The optical heterodyne detection is carried out automatically because the photodetector generates the output current, which is proportional to the square of the amplitude of the light's electric field. The signal is transmitted to a spectrum analyzer, which displays the power spectrum of the beating signal generated by the superposition of the scattered and local lights. The observation of the phonon spectrum with high frequency resolution achieved using optical heterodyne detection is shown in the following section.

2.2.2 Thermal phonon resonance

As described in the principle behind the optical beating Brillouin scattering measurement, we cannot measure the phonon decay length if it is larger than the width of the detecting laser beam, even though the frequency resolution is remarkably improved by optical heterodyne detection. To understand the contribution of the viscosity over a wide frequency range, especially in the lower region, a technique was invented to determine the long decay length: the observation of thermal phonon resonance [11].

Its principle is similar to that of the conventional ultrasonic resonance method, in which samples are confined in an acoustic cavity. The ultrasonic wave propagates, and the resonance spectrum is observed. In this method, waves that satisfy the resonance condition, namely, that the cavity length is an integer half of the wavelength, are selectively excited.

For the Brillouin scattering measurement, the phonons are equally excited over a wide wave number range, and they propagate between the cavities; the density of the phonons is homogeneous for different wave numbers. However, in the phonon cavity, they repeatedly generate scattered light each time they cross the light beam. The phase of the repeatedly scattered light is not necessarily continuous; for the phonons that satisfy the resonance condition, the phases are continuous, whereas for the phonons of the non-resonant mode, the phase exhibits leaps. Figure 2.6 shows the resonance spectra of the Brillouin scattering observed for liquid toluene; (a) shows the spectrum of the phonons observed without resonator plates, and (b) shows the spectrum obtained using the resonator. As shown, the broad peak in (a) is modified into a series of resonance peaks. By assigning the resonance mode number, we can determine the phonon velocity with an accuracy of 0.1%. Moreover, the width of one resonance peak provides the inverse of the lifetime of the phonons in the resonator, which gives the phonon decay even though the diameter of the laser beam is narrower than the phonon decay length.

To summarize, the frequency resolution obtained from the Brillouin scattering experiment was improved in a step-by-step manner. By employing optical

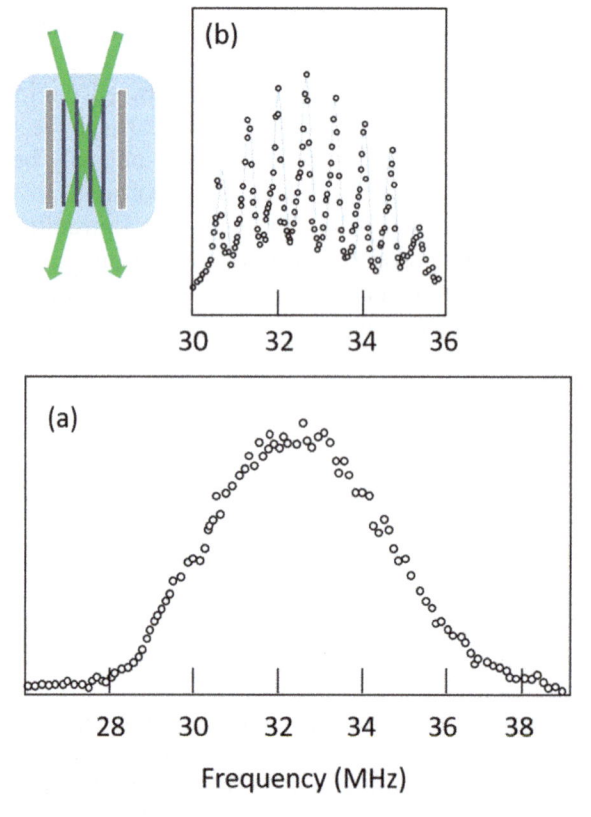

Figure 2.6. Resonance spectra of the Brillouin scattering observed for liquid toluene, obtained for phonons propagating in a free space (a) and in a phonon resonator (b).

heterodyne detection of the scattered-light power spectrum instead of the conventional optical spectrometer, the instrumental ambiguity introduced by the optical resonator was remarkably reduced. The restriction due to the finite beam width of the laser light was solved by employing a thermal phonon resonator. In the next section, we discuss the application of the optical heterodyne Brillouin scattering system to observation of the energy dissipation process through various viscosities.

2.2.3 Determination of shear, orientational, and coupling viscosities in liquids

In the previous sections, we discussed viscosity with respect to the translational motion of fluids. This motion refers to the flow of fluids, and the kinetic energy dissipates through a change in the relative positions of the molecules. In a practical system, actual fluids composed of molecules with shapes other than simple spheres possess other internal degrees of freedom. One of these is the direction of the molecules. Hereafter, we discuss viscosity with respect to rotational motion. Rod-like molecules, whose orientation can be recognized by the direction of the rod's central axis and the rotational motion of molecules, also contribute to energy dissipation.

The observation of rheological phenomena with respect to the orientational mode provides important local information about the molecules. For example, an observation of the local direction of a polymer segment can be related to the anisotropic dielectricity, which is detected by the optical birefringence method. The stress–optical rule (SOR) is one of the most famous guiding principles for investigating local motion in polymers, that is, the proportionality between stress and birefringence.

The optical heterodyne measurement introduced in the previous section can provide information about the dynamics of molecular orientation by combining them with the birefringence technique [12, 13]. In the measurement of longitudinal mode phonons, the light detects the modulation of the isotropic dielectric constant induced by compression and expansion owing to acoustic mode deformation. Conversely, the detection of local fluctuations in the molecular orientation can take advantage of the fact that light experiences anisotropy in the dielectric constant, which is represented by the non-diagonal components of the dielectric tensor. In the experimental system, depolarized light scattering is observed. Linearly polarized light is incident on the media, whose polarization is perpendicular to both the incident and scattering wave number vectors. In a common experimental configuration, the scattering plane is placed horizontally, and the polarization is directed vertically. The incident light is then depolarized by the local fluctuation of the dielectric anisotropy and generates scattered light with polarization in the horizontal direction. This depolarized light scattering from vertical to horizontal is called vertical–horizontal (VH) scattering.

The local orientation of the molecules fluctuates with a typical time constant τ_R, and the frequency spectrum of the scattered light shows an ambiguity of $1/\tau_R$. By observing the peak width of the scattered-light power spectrum in the VH configuration, we can determine the time constant required for molecules to rotate.

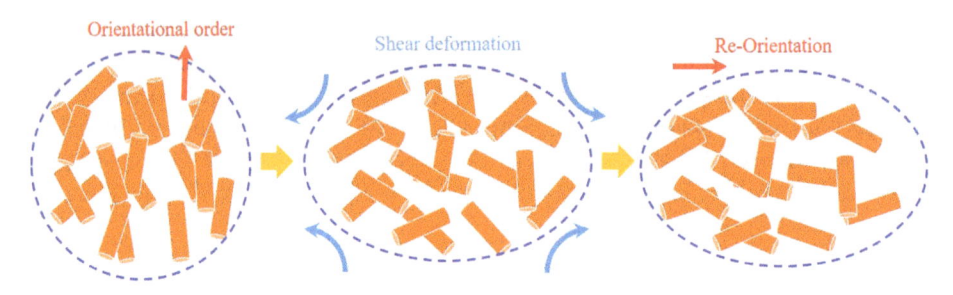

Figure 2.7. Schematic image of the relaxation behavior of orientational order in fluids composed of rod-like molecules.

A high frequency resolution better than 1 kHz achieved by optical heterodyne spectroscopy revealed the behavior of fluids composed of anisotropic molecules, such as rod-like molecules. Let us assume that the alignment of the molecular directions causes shear flow, as shown in figure 2.7, and discuss the consequences of this behavior. Once the collective orientation is excited in the molecule ensemble, it decays with a time constant τ_R. Simultaneously, the decaying motion of the orientation causes shear deformation of the ensemble. It seems reasonable to consider that the shear flow then generates the orientational order of molecules again, which is known as the flow birefringence phenomenon.

The coupling constant describes the degree to which the motion of the orientation causes shear deformation and/or how the shear deformation makes the molecular orientations identical, which is a result of the reciprocity theorem.

Let us estimate the time constant of the motion of molecular orientation and shear deformation in periodical structures that have the wave number K. Generally, the time constant of the molecular orientation is independent of the wave number K and is approximately given by

$$\tau_R = \eta V / k_B T,$$

where η is the viscosity of the surrounding fluid, V is the volume of the molecule, k_B is the Boltzmann constant, and T is the temperature. The time constant of the orientation for a molecule with $V = 10^{-30}$ m^3 and $\eta = 1$ mPa·s is roughly estimated to be 10^{-12} s. It increases with the molecular volume, and several complex fluids that tend to undergo a phase transition to a liquid crystal may exhibit collective motion of the orientation, in which the time constant is known to critically increase toward the phase transition point.

On the other hand, the time constant of shear flow at a wave number K is expressed as

$$\tau_S = \rho / \eta K^2.$$

Substituting $\eta = 10^{-3}$ mPa·s (i.e. considering water), and $K = 10^6$ m^{-1}, we obtain $\tau_S \sim 10^{-6}$ s. These two time constants are quite different in order; therefore, it has been difficult to observe the coupling phenomenon of the orientation and shear flow using

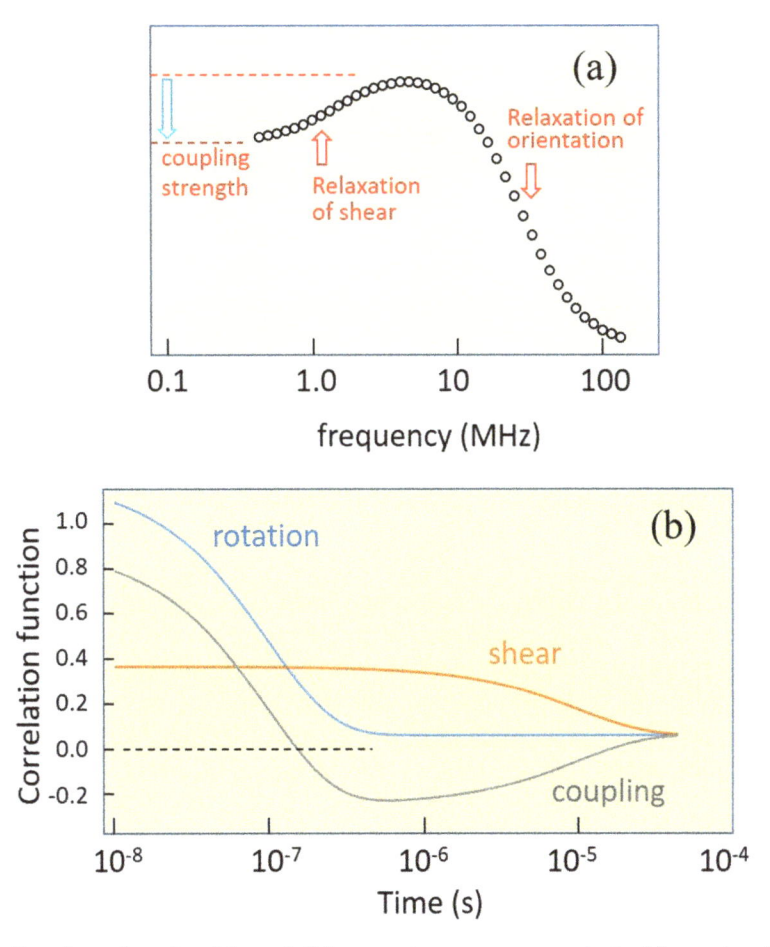

Figure 2.8. Experimental results of dynamic light-scattering measurements obtained for *p-n*-hexyl *p'*-cyanobiphenyl (6CB) with the VH configuration. (a) Power spectrum and (b) correlation function.

only one experimental apparatus. However, the optical heterodyne light-scattering method can simultaneously observe the molecular orientation and coupled shear flow.

Figure 2.8 shows the experimental results obtained for *p-n*-hexyl *p'*-cyanobiphenyl (6CB) with the VH light-scattering configuration. The power spectrum is shown in (a), in which the shape is obtained by the subtraction of the Lorenz function representing shear flow decay from that representing molecular orientation decay. The subtraction can be explained as follows: the excited fluctuation of the molecular orientation decays by $\sim\exp(-t/\tau_R)$, which causes shear flow. The induced shear flow then decays by $\sim\exp(-t/\tau_S)$, causing the orientational order to be perpendicular to the initial direction; this appears as the negative component in the light-scattering spectrum.

$$S(\omega) \sim \frac{1}{1+\omega^2\tau_R^2} - \frac{C}{1+\omega^2\tau_S^2}(C<1). \tag{2.5}$$

This explanation can be directly understood by translating the power spectrum to the correlation function using a Fourier transformation, as shown in figure 2.8(b). The thermally excited orientational order dissipates and overshoots to the negative because the energy transports to the shear flow once, then returns to the orientation in the other direction. Sample 6CB is known to undergo a phase transition to a liquid crystal at the critical temperature $T_C = 29.3$ °C, whereas light-scattering experiments are carried out above T_C, where the sample is regarded as an isotropic liquid. However, because of the collective directional motion of molecules near the phase transition point, the relaxation time increases to approximately 10^{-7} s.

The focus of the experiment was on how the orientational order spontaneously grows toward the phase transition temperature. In this process, it was assumed that the coupling between shear flow and molecular orientation plays an important role. The magnitude of the coupling is given by C in equation (2.5), and the behavior of C was investigated in detail by changing the temperature and the type of liquid. The coupling constant C is related to the third viscosity of μ by

$$C = 2\mu^2/\eta\nu,$$

where η and ν are the shear and rotational viscosities, respectively, and μ is the coupling viscosity, which complementarily determines the shear stress under molecular rotation and the rotational torque under shear flow. By observing the collective motion of the rotation and the translation of molecules using light-scattering experiments, we can determine the third viscosity between the different modes of molecular motion.

2.3 Recent progress in the experimental approach to the dynamic surface phenomena of liquids

2.3.1 Ripplon spectroscopy

2.3.1.1 Light-scattering detection of thermal ripplons

In the previous section, the relationship between the rheological properties of materials and ultrasonic propagation was discussed. In this section, another wave that propagates on the fluid surface is introduced. Surface tension acts as a restoring force that keeps the liquid surface flat. Once the surface is deformed, the displacement propagates as a surface-tension wave, whose phase velocity v_p is given by

$$v_p = \left(\frac{\sigma}{\rho}k\right)^{1/2}, \qquad (2.6)$$

where σ and ρ are the surface tension and the density of the liquid, respectively, and k is the wave number of the wave [14]. The surface-tension wave decays owing to viscosity, which is related to the temporal decay constant as follows:

$$\Gamma = 2(\eta/\rho)k^2, \qquad (2.7)$$

where η is the viscosity of the medium. The surface tension and viscosity of the sample can be obtained by measuring the phase velocity and damping constant of the surface-tension wave. For example, in pure water, the surface-tension wave is expected to propagate at a frequency of up to 100 MHz; therefore, measurements of the surface wave would be an effective tool for understanding the high-speed phenomena of the liquid surface, such as the adsorption process of the surfactant molecules in an aqueous solution.

The temporal resolution of the measurement is determined by the frequency of the surface-tension wave; however, it is difficult to excite the surface-tension wave at very high frequencies. The decay length of the surface-tension wave is of the order of micrometers in the megahertz region, and mechanical contact with the wave transducer causes serious deformation of the surface because of the formation of a meniscus. Therefore, a new experimental system was developed to observe surface-tension waves in the megahertz region: ripplon light-scattering spectroscopy.

A ripplon is a thermally excited surface-tension wave [15–18]. A thermal fluctuation of the surface displacement propagates as surface-tension waves, although the displacement is much less than an angstrom. The measurement principle used in this system is almost the same as that of Brillouin scattering, which is explained in detail in the previous section. The laser light incident on the liquid surface is scattered by periodic surface displacement, and the scattering angle provides the wavelength of the ripplon. The frequency of the laser light is modulated through the Doppler effect upon collision with a propagating ripplon, and the frequency shift results in a ripplon frequency. The lifetime of the ripplon is restricted by the temporal decay. A finite lifetime leads to ambiguity in the ripplon frequency; therefore, the decay constant can be determined by the width of the frequency peak of the scattered component.

However, the frequency range under observation is in the region below 100 MHz, which is much lower than the region associated with thermal phonons; this is because the phase velocity of ripplons is much lower than that of phonons. Therefore, as introduced in the previous section, an optical heterodyne technique is employed to analyze the fine structure of the power spectrum of light scattered by the propagating ripplon. Experimentally, the measurement system is almost the same as that for Brillouin scattering; however, the light is perpendicularly incident in order to detect ripplons propagating along the liquid surface.

Figure 2.9 shows a schematic of the light-scattering configuration and the experimental setup used for the ripplon light-scattering spectroscopy system (a) with a typical spectrum observed for the surface of pure water (b) and that covered with a thin layer of oil (c). The principle is almost the same as that of Brillouin scattering, however, the conservation of momentum holds only with respect to the horizontal direction, because the liquid surface system does not have translational symmetry in the vertical direction.

2.3.1.2 Dynamic adsorption process of surfactants

One of the most important problems in the chemical physics of liquid surfaces in the 1990s was observing the formation process of surfactant molecule surface layers. It is possible to determine the surface tension and viscosity of a liquid using conventional

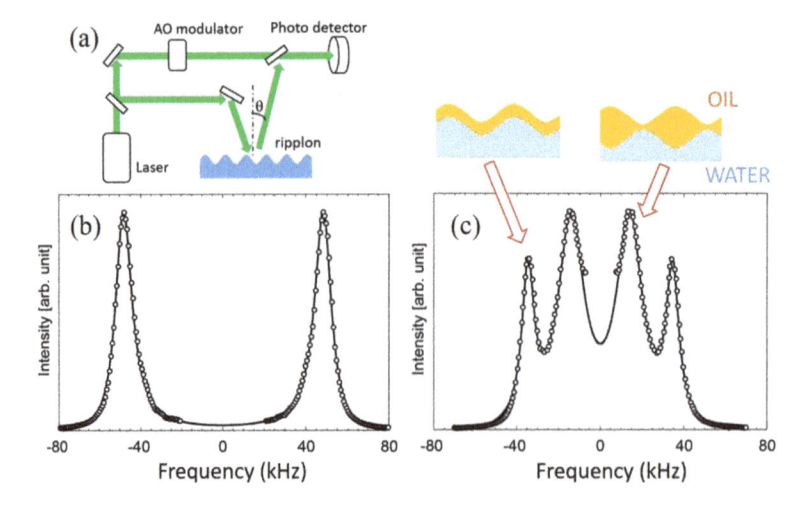

Figure 2.9. Schematic of the light-scattering configuration and the experimental setup used for the ripplon light-scattering spectroscopy system (a) with a typical spectrum observed for the surface of pure water (b) and that covered with a thin layer of oil (c). Reproduced from [18]. © IOP Publishing Ltd. All rights reserved.

methodologies; however, the time resolution of the measurement is not sufficient to capture the dynamic molecular adsorption process. Here, the typical time constant required for the dissolved surfactant molecules to translate to the solvent surface and form a monomolecular layer is considered.

Assuming that the concentration of the surfactant is c and the surface density of the molecular layer in the equilibrium state is Γ, the surfactant molecules within a depth of $l \sim \Gamma/c$ should contribute to the formation of the surface layer. The molecules translate through the thermal diffusion process with the diffusion constant D, which is roughly given by $D \sim k_B T/\eta a$, where k_B is the Boltzmann constant, T is the temperature, η is the viscosity of the liquid, and a is the spatial size of a surfactant molecule. The time required for surfactant molecules to reach the surface through diffusion is approximately given by $\tau \sim l^2/D$. By considering dodecyl sodium sulfate, a very popular surfactant, as a solvent and taking the critical micellar concentration to be c, the time constant of the change in the surface tension can be estimated to be approximately 10^{-5} to 10^{-3} s.

The time resolution of the ripplon light scattering was improved to the order of microseconds by employing a digital oscilloscope to detect the optical heterodyne signal [19]. However, preparation of a fresh liquid surface using a mechanical sweep requires a time that is at least a significant fraction of a second, which is the main problem in directly observing the dynamic change in the surface tension through the adsorption process.

Therefore, we focused on another mechanical property of the liquid surface: surface elasticity. The adsorbed layer of surfactant molecules behaves as a two-dimensional material. A layer of insoluble amphiphile, called a Langmuir film, exhibits a decrease in surface tension when compressed on the surface. The decrease is regarded as a two-dimensional pressure, and the surface elasticity is defined as the differentiation of the surface pressure with respect to the surface area.

As for soluble surfactant molecules, compression of the surface area causes excess molecules to sink into the solution, and the surface elasticity is zero for satisfactorily slow compression. However, surface elasticity emerges as a result of rapid changes in the surface area; the surfactant molecules cannot follow the compression faster than the typical time constant of adsorption or desorption, and the surface exhibits elastic properties.

Ripplon spectroscopy can also detect surface elasticity using the change in the shape of the ripplon spectrum. Therefore, the time constant can be estimated by measuring the surface elasticity as a function of ripplon spectroscopy.

Figure 2.10 shows an intuitive illustration that explains the relationship between surface elasticity, ripplon propagation, and the experimentally observed spectra. The deformation of the surface caused by ripplon propagation accompanies the expansion and compression of the surface area. For pure liquids, the change in the surface area does not cause a change in the surface tension. The surface tension is homogeneous over the entire surface area, as shown in (i) of figure 2.10(a). However, a surface with an adsorbed molecular layer exhibits inhomogeneous surface tension because it is dependent on the local surface density of the surface surfactant molecules, as shown in (ii).

Spatial modulation of the surface tension generates stress directed along the surface, which drives the surface and radiates shear flow into the medium. Note that the dissipation of the ripplon energy is effective for a moderately elastic surface. If the surface layer is very hard and possesses a large surface elasticity, the surface cannot expand or compress via surface deformation. Figure 2.10(b) shows the spectra of ripplons propagating on a pure water surface and an insoluble monomolecular layer of myristic acids. The peak width of the ripplon spectrum on the elastic surface (upper) is broader than that on the inelastic surface (lower). The width of the peaks represents the temporal decay of the ripplon, and the results

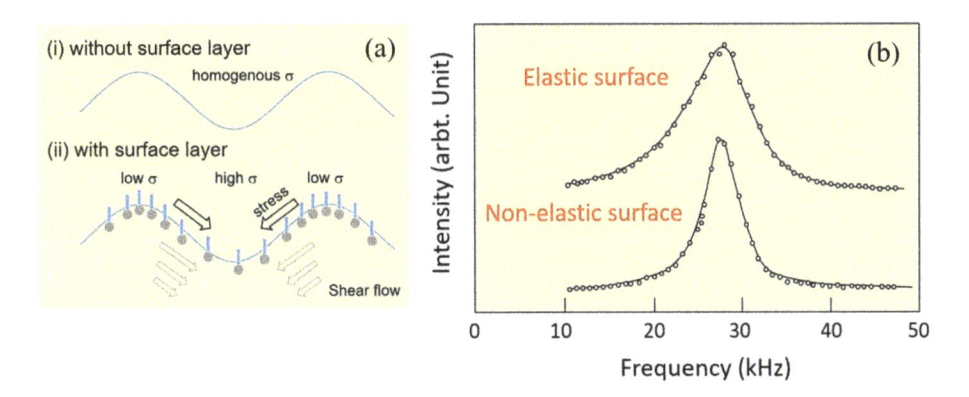

Figure 2.10. Intuitive illustration that explains the relationship between surface elasticity, ripplon propagation, and the experimentally observed spectra. Reproduced from [1]. © 2021 The Japan Society of Applied Physics. All rights reserved.

show that the energy dissipation on the elastic surface increases due to radiation of the wave energy into the bulk medium through shear flow. For an insoluble surface layer, the peak width reaches a maximum value at around the surface elasticity of $\tilde{\varepsilon}\sigma$. This phenomenon can be understood as mechanical impedance matching between the surface layer and the shear flow in the medium beneath the surface. Since a surface without two-dimensional elasticity can only apply the normal stress on the surface as the Laplace pressure due to surface tension, it cannot cause shear laminar flow along the surface. On the other hand, adequate surface elasticity of the adsorbed molecular layer efficiently induces shear stress through the expansion and shrinkage of the surface area, which causes the radiation of the kinetic energy. Harder surfaces with large elasticity cannot be expanded any further and do not cause the shear flow. These are the reasons why the ripplon decay shows a maximum when taken as a function of the surface elasticity. This situation is analogous to impedance matching of surface acoustic waves on solids, bulk waves in contacting liquids, and the phenomenon of leaky surface acoustic waves in the field of ultrasonics.

To summarize, the ripplon can be affected by surface elasticity if it has an adequate amplitude $\varepsilon \sim 10\text{--}30$ mN m^{-1}. Ripplon decay increases with surface elasticity from that predicted by the bulk viscosity, and then decreases. In this process, the phase velocity of the ripplon gradually decreases with surface elasticity. Therefore, we can determine the surface elasticity from the discrepancies of the ripplon frequency and obtain the damping constant from the values calculated by equations (2.6) and (2.7) as well as the surface tension and bulk viscosity.

To observe surface relaxation phenomena through ripplon spectroscopy, a suitable surfactant sample material must be selected. Considering the above conditions, the surface elasticity of an aqueous solution of pentanoic acid was investigated. Figure 2.11 shows the frequency dependence of the surface elasticity of the aqueous solution of pentanoic acid. Pentanoic acid is soluble in water and forms a monomolecular layer on the surface. The concentrations were 3.0×10^{-2} and 1.2×10^{-2} M, which are represented by the closed and open circles, respectively. The measurements in the lower frequency region below 10 kHz were carried out by the capillary wave excitation method. As can clearly be seen, the surface elasticity increases with frequency, and the arrows show the relaxation frequency above which the adsorption and desorption process cannot follow the modulation of the surface area. One can estimate the time required to form the surface molecular layer to be approximately sub millisecond, using the inverse of the relaxation frequency. A method of artificially exciting surface displacement has been developed, which is also an effective tool with which to investigate liquid surface dynamics.

However, it takes multiple months to obtain relaxation spectra by ripplon light-scattering measurement. In addition, the molecular layer must have adequate elasticity to be observed using ripplon propagation. This restriction is a serious difficulty in applying this technique to the observation of the dynamic adsorption process of surfactant materials in industry. These problems have been solved using a new technique introduced in the next section.

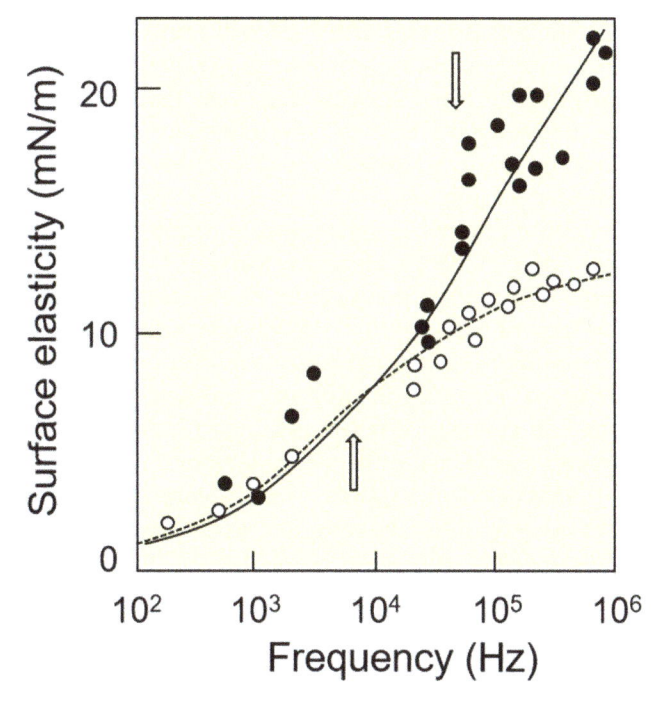

Figure 2.11. Frequency dependence of the surface elasticity of an aqueous solution of pentanoic acid. Concentrations of 3.0×10^{-2} and 1.2×10^{-2} M are represented by closed and open circles, respectively. Reproduced from [1]. © 2021 The Japan Society of Applied Physics. All rights reserved.

2.3.2 Manipulation and observation of micro liquid particles

The principal fluid properties investigated in the field of rheology are elasticity and viscosity, for which new experimental approaches were introduced in other sections of this chapter. However, surface tension also plays an important role in determining the boundary conditions of the surfaces of moving liquids. Section 2.3.1 introduced an approach to dynamic surface tension that involves observing high-frequency surface-tension waves. As the spatial scale of the liquid process becomes smaller, especially in recent industrial fluid applications and processes, such as inkjet technologies and microfluidics, the role of surface properties becomes more important. The contribution of the inertial energy or energy dissipation caused by viscosity is proportional to the third power of the spatial size, while the surface energy increases linearly with the square of the size. For example, in the case of a liquid droplet with a diameter of 10 μm ejected at an initial speed of 10 m s^{-1} by an inkjet nozzle, the inertial energy and surface energy are of the same order. In other words, this law of energy equipartition provides the most suitable conditions for inkjet ejection.

The miniaturization of the liquid droplet size leads to a higher-speed process. In a high-speed observation of the dynamic surface tension introduced in this section, high temporal resolution can be realized by miniaturizing the spatial size of liquids.

Fluid products contain various ingredients; for example, inkjet ink contains color dyes or pigments that provide color, polymers to avoid aggregation of ingredients, and surfactants to promote rapid soaking in paper. As discussed in the previous section, the typical time constant for the adsorption of surfactant molecules onto the surface is calculated to be of the order of $\tau \approx 10^{-5}$–10^{-3} s, which is expected to change with the surface tension.

The typical time required for the emission of a droplet from an inkjet nozzle is approximately 10 μs, which then travels at a velocity of 1–10 m s^{-1} across a distance of 1 mm between the nozzle and the substrate; this substrate could be, for example, paper. The typical time of flight is 10^{-4}–10^{-3} s, which is almost the same as that required for the formation of the surface-adsorbed layer of surfactants that wets the substrate. Therefore, it is doubtful that the surfactant molecules added for satisfactory wetting can contribute to the practical wetting phenomenon in inkjet printing. It is important to measure the actual temporal change in surface tension with a time resolution better than 10^{-4} s. This knowledge is also important for other industrial processes, such as spray painting and emulsification.

Section 2.3.1 introduced experimental results for the surface relaxation phenomenon accompanying the adsorption and desorption processes of surfactants, which complementarily provides the dynamic surface tension in the frequency domain. However, observable targets are limited. Here, a new method for measuring the dynamic surface tension is proposed, which can be applied to almost all surfactant solutions. The time resolution of the measurement was successfully extended to better than 100 μs using inkjet technologies [20, 21].

In this method, the resonant oscillation of a droplet of a surfactant solution generated by the continuous-mode emission of microdroplets is observed. In recent years, various types of generation, manipulation, and observation method have been developed for micro liquid droplets. Several of these methods are introduced to explain the new method of dynamic surface-tension measurement.

The first is a droplet emission system made of glass materials in which a glass capillary is employed as an emission nozzle. Figure 2.12 shows photographs of droplet emissions. The sample liquid is contained in a capillary with an aperture of

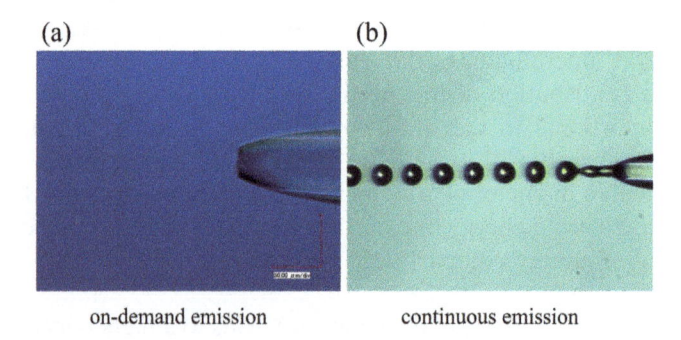

Figure 2.12. Photographs of droplet emission. (a) on-demand and (b) continuous emission. Reproduced from [1]. © 2021 The Japan Society of Applied Physics. All rights reserved (movie available at https://doi.org/10.1088/978-0-7503-4936-9).

10~50 μm. Two piezoelectric actuators sandwich the nozzle to apply impulse compression. A pulsed ultrasonic wave propagates along the capillary and emits a liquid droplet at the aperture using the radiation pressure of the elastic wave. Figure 2.12(a) shows photographs of on-demand and continuous emissions from a glass nozzle taken during the implementation of a stroboscopic method.

A second method of generating a microdroplet is the continuous mode. The emission nozzle, consisting of a glass capillary and piezo actuators, is the same as for the on-demand emission; however, a liquid jet is continuously ejected by a constant pressure applied to the nozzle. Piezo actuators add slight harmonic modulation to the applied pressure, and the ejected liquid jet has a small periodic modulation in its diameter. By adjusting the frequency of the pressure modulation, the fluctuation in diameter spontaneously increases, and the liquid jet is equally divided into a series of flying droplets due to Rayleigh instability. Figure 2.12(b) shows a photograph of the continuous emission of liquid particles with typical diameters of 15–30 μm.

These two emission methods were employed for the purpose of the experiment. For the measurement of dynamic surface tension, the continuous mode was used, whereas the on-demand method was used to observe the dynamic behavior of liquid droplets on substrates.

In continuous-mode emission, the surface of the droplet is created at the time of emission. The surface then ages as the droplets flow. The time-dependent surface tension can be obtained by measuring the surface tension of the flying droplet in a noncontact manner, which is carried out as follows: a gate consisting of two electrodes is set in front of the flying droplets, between which a local electric field is formed. The liquid droplet traveling through the electrodes is stretched by the dielectric force because the permittivity of the sample liquid is larger than that of air. Figure 2.13 shows examples of the behavior of droplets caused by the dielectric force. In figure 2.13(a), the expansion of a flying liquid droplet is shown.

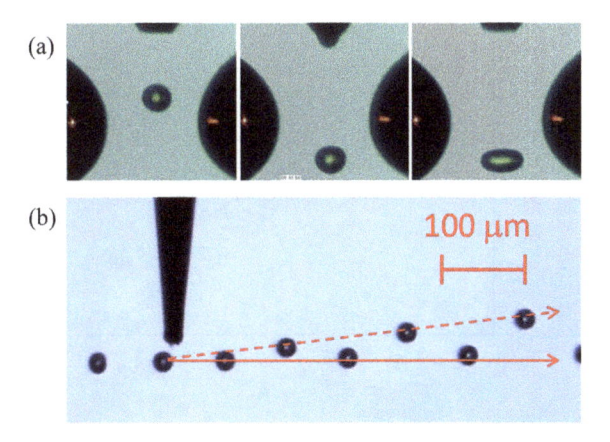

Figure 2.13. Photographs showing the behavior of droplets subjected to the dielectric force. Reproduced from [1]. © 2021 The Japan Society of Applied Physics. All rights reserved.

The dielectric force can also be used to manipulate the flight conditions of the droplet. Figure 2.13(b) shows that the droplets are alternately deflected from the original direction of flight by the application of a harmonic electric field whose frequency is half that of the droplet emission. Acceleration and deceleration are also possible.

After the deformation of the droplet by the dielectric force, it begins to oscillate freely. The resonant frequency of the oscillation is determined by the surface tension as the restoring force, with the droplet radius and density as the inertia. The amplitude of the oscillation decays due to the viscosity of the liquid and the angular frequency, and the decay constant of the oscillation between prolate and oblate spheroids is given by

$$\omega = \sqrt{8\sigma/\rho R^3}$$

$$\Gamma = 5\eta/\rho R^2,$$

where σ is the surface tension, ρ is the density, R is the radius of the droplet, and η is the viscosity.

The dynamic surface tension is measured as follows: a series of continuously generated droplets is emitted by a glass nozzle and introduced into the gap between the electrode pair, where resonant oscillation is excited. A video camera synchronized with the emission of a strobe light takes a video of the droplet oscillation, which is sent to an image analysis system. The eigenfrequency and temporal damping constant are then determined. The age of the emitted droplet surface is determined by the distance between the nozzle and the observation point, and the time-dependent surface tension is obtained by measuring the droplet oscillation over a wide range of distances.

Figure 2.14 shows a typical example of the dynamic surface tension measured for a solution of a well-known surfactant material: sodium dodecyl sulfate (SDS). The

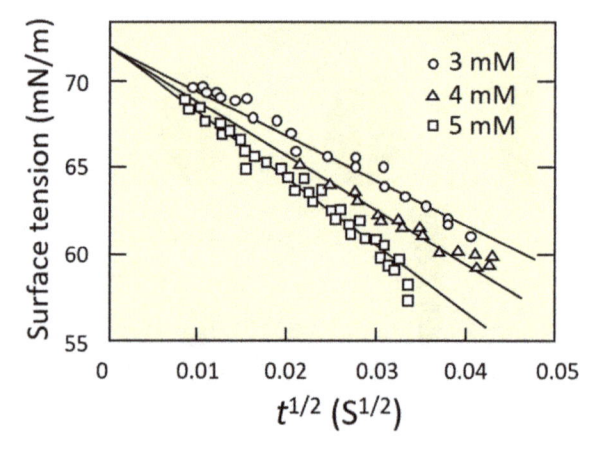

Figure 2.14. Dynamic surface tension obtained for aqueous solutions of sodium dodecyl sulfate. Reproduced from [1]. © 2021 The Japan Society of Applied Physics. All rights reserved.

time required for surfactant molecules to form a surface-adsorbed layer depends on the mobility of the molecules that arises through diffusion, which is faster for smaller molecules. The molecular weight of SDS is one of the smallest among various kinds of surfactant, and the behavior of its surface tension shown in figure 2.14 has almost the fastest change. It is clear that the initial change in surface tension is proportional to the square root of time, indicating that the decrease in surface tension is roughly proportional to the amount of adsorbed surfactant, and the diffusion length is given by $l \sim \sqrt{Dt}$.

As shown, recent technologies in micro-fluid engineering can also be utilized for the measurement of the physical properties with high time resolution: the measurement and facilitation processes are making complementary progresses.

2.4 Introduction to recent progress in rheometry

2.4.1 The electromagnetic spinning (EMS) rheometer system

In the previous sections, new techniques for measuring the mechanical properties of fluids were introduced. However, almost all viscosity measurements in industry are carried out using the conventional and established measurement methods of rheology [22]. Rotational-type viscometers are mainstream and are classified into various types, such as parallel circular plates, cone plates, and double cylinders, although they have several problems in practical use. This is because the driving torque is transmitted mechanically from the main body of the viscosity meter to the probe. One problem is sealability. It is difficult to insert a driving shaft into high-pressure vessels. In the evaluation of viscosity, we measure the torque required to rotate the probe rotor at a constant speed; the frictional torque applied to a commercially available seal would be larger than that induced by the viscosity. In addition, heat conduction through the shaft is harmful when applied to a low-temperature environment.

Knowledge of the rheological properties of bio-systems is also important for the application of ultrasonic investigations in the medical field. One problem is that the measurement of biohazardous material is difficult because the mechanical probe of the viscometer should be in direct contact with the sample. Pollution from/to the sample is inevitable, and the cost of cleaning the measurement apparatus is not negligible. An additional problem is that such measurements can hardly be carried out in extraordinary environments, such as at high/low temperature and pressure.

In this section, a unique method of viscosity measurement is introduced [23, 24]. It belongs to the rotational type; however, the probe and the main body of the viscometer are separated. The probe is driven remotely through electromagnetic interaction. The methodology is called the 'electromagnetic spinning' (EMS) method.

First, the measurement principle of the EMS method is briefly discussed. Figure 2.15 shows a schematic image that explains the principle behind the remote driving of the probe rotor through electromagnetic interactions. The rotor is composed of a conductive material; aluminum is usually chosen for its high conductivity and low density. The weight of the rotor is preferably small because the accuracy of the measurement is restricted by the mechanical friction caused by the probe's rotation.

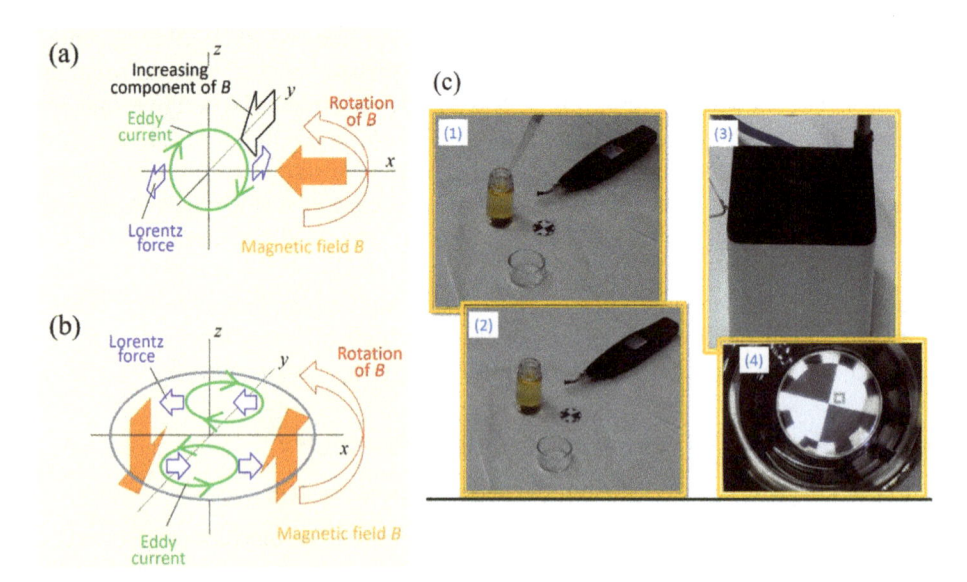

Figure 2.15. Schematic image that explains the principle behind the remote driving of the probe rotor through electromagnetic interactions. Reproduced from [1]. © 2021 The Japan Society of Applied Physics. All rights reserved (movie available at https://doi.org/10.1088/978-0-7503-4936-9).

In the EMS method, friction only occurs at the contact point between the probe support and the bottom of the sample container. In figure 2.15(a), a homogeneous and horizontal magnetic field **B** is shown to rotate. In this configuration, the differentiation vector d**B**/dt is perpendicular to **B**, which generates an eddy current **i**. The Lorentz interaction between **i** and **B** generates the force $\mathbf{F} = \mathbf{i} \times \mathbf{B}$, and the integration of **F** works as a torque, as shown in the figure. In this configuration, the rotor should have a certain depth. In figure 2.15(b), the magnetic field is inhomogeneous, and vectors **B** and d**B**/dt are parallel. Assuming that the distribution of the magnetic field moves, currents are induced, as shown in the figure. The Lorentz force operates such that the probe follows the motion of the distributed magnetic field.

The viscosity is obtained by calculating the ratio between the viscous torque and the shear rate, which is proportional to the rotational speed of the probe rotor. At a constant driving speed, the viscous torque is equal to the driving torque, which is proportional to the difference between the rotational speeds of the magnetic field and the probe rotor. Therefore, by measuring the rotational speed of the probe at a certain rotational speed of the magnetic field, we can determine the viscosity at a related shear rate. The flow curve, which reveals the viscosity dependence on the shear rate, can be obtained by measuring the viscosity while changing the rotational speed of the magnetic field.

From a technical viewpoint, the accuracy of the EMS viscometer depends on the shape of the probe rotor. We employed a metal sphere as the rotor in the initial version of the EMS viscometer. This has the advantage that it is easy to prepare the measurement apparatus; the sample liquid can simply be poured into the sample tube and then a metal sphere can be inserted. The key technical point influencing the accuracy of this viscosity measurement is the spatial size of the sphere.

The resistance torque resulting from the viscosity is proportional to the volume of the sphere, which is the cubic radius, whereas that caused by the friction between the rotor and the bottom of the sample container increases with the fourth power of the radius. This means that the contribution of the sample viscosity increases as the radius decreases. In an industrial EMS viscometer, an aluminum sphere with a diameter of 2 mm is utilized for convenient and easy operator handling, although this restricts the accuracy to approximately 10% for the measurement of pure water with a viscosity of 1 mPa·s.

Additionally, the value of the shear deformation rate cannot be uniquely determined. At present, the mainstream rotor shape is an auto-standing rotor, which can reduce the harmful contribution of mechanical friction and achieve an accuracy of 1% for water. The configuration of the auto-standing rotor is compatible with the conventional and most popular parallel plate, cone plate, and double cylinder types. Frames extracted from a video that show the actual measurement can be seen in figure 2.15(c). The details of the rotor are discussed elsewhere; here, recently developed peripheral technologies are introduced instead.

2.4.2 Measurement of viscoelasticity using the EMS system equipped with quadruple electromagnets

The EMS viscosity measurement system is already commercially available, in which the driving magnetic field is generated by the mechanical rotation of permanent magnets attached to the motor. The configuration of this apparatus is simple and immune to breakdown, and the driving mode of the magnetic field is only limited to simple rotation. By changing the driving torque, we can obtain the shear rate dependence of the viscosity, which is called the 'flow curve'.

To observe the viscoelastic properties of materials, as introduced in section 2.1.1, the elasticity and viscosity can be obtained by measuring the amplitude and phase retardation of the probe rotor under the application of periodic torque [25]. The spectrum of the complex elastic modulus can then obtained by changing the frequency of the oscillatory torque. To measure the viscoelasticity, quadruple electromagnets are employed to apply harmonic torque to the probe rotor. Two pairs of electromagnets are used to generate the perpendicular and horizontal components of the magnetic fields. The magnets alternate the rotational direction of the synthesized magnetic field between clockwise and counterclockwise, and oscillatory rotation of the probe rotor is observed.

Figure 2.16 shows a typical example of the relaxation spectrum of the viscoelasticity observed in the entangled system of the worm-like micellar solution of cetyltrimethyl ammonium bromide (CTAB) salt sodium salicylate (NaSal). In addition, the mechanical behavior of the sample is shown, in which we can see that the sample is vibrating under mechanical stimulation.

The observed spectrum is a good fit for the single relaxation curve, which is represented by the viscoelastic fluid model shown in figure 2.1(c). The EMS system can be improved to measure the viscoelastic properties in addition to the flow curves of materials.

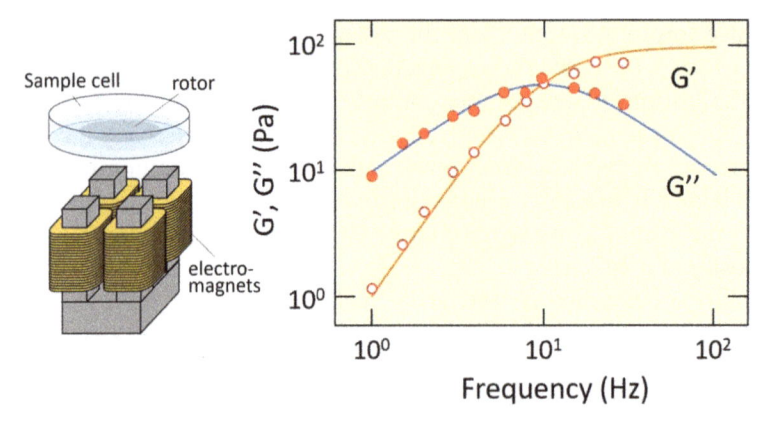

Figure 2.16. Schematic view of an EMS system equipped with quadruple electromagnets and a typical example of the relaxation spectrum of the viscoelasticity observed in the entangled system of the worm-like micellar solution of cetyltrimethyl ammonium bromide (CTAB) salt sodium salicylate (NaSal) (movie available at https://doi.org/10.1088/978-0-7503-4936-9).

2.4.3 Examination of the quantum standard for viscosity

In this section, the possibility of a new standard for viscosity measurement is discussed. At present, the standard method of viscosity measurement is the capillary-type viscometer, in which the quantity of fluid falling due to gravity in a capillary is measured. In addition, the traceability of the viscosity originates from the viscosity of pure water. All physical quantities were redefined in terms of quantum standards in 2019; the kilogram prototype, as the standard of mass, was replaced by the Planck constant. Hence, it is surprising that the rheology standards still depend on such a classic methodology.

The unit of viscosity is [Pa·s], namely [kg m^{-1} s^{-1}] in SI base units, whereas the unit of the kinetic viscosity representing the transportation coefficient of momentum is simple; it is represented as [m^2 s^{-1}] using basic units for space and time. These were defined in the early stage of quantum standardization; therefore, the standard for rheology should follow the trend of physics. The reasons for the standard are accuracy and traceability. Here, a plausible candidate for the new standard of viscosity is examined, that is, the magnetically levitated EMS system [26].

We now consider the viscosity of gases from the viewpoint of the kinetic theory of molecules. To understand the rheology of gases, their viscosities are calculated using an elementary knowledge of physics. If we consider N molecules of gas with mass m contained in a cubic chamber with a spatial size of L and a molecule has an average velocity of c_0 (the velocity component in a specific direction is $\sqrt{3}\, c_0$), the frequency at which a molecule collides with the wall of the cubic chamber is $c_0/2L$. The number of molecules that cross an imaginary area S located in the chamber per unit time can be calculated using $K = (c_0/2L) \cdot N \cdot (S/L^2)$. By defining the molecular density n as $n = N/L^3$, K can be expressed as $K = c_0 n S/2$.

A uniform shear flow is considered, as shown in figure 2.17. The gradient of the flow velocity is $(\partial v/\partial z)$ in the z-axis direction. By assuming that all the molecules

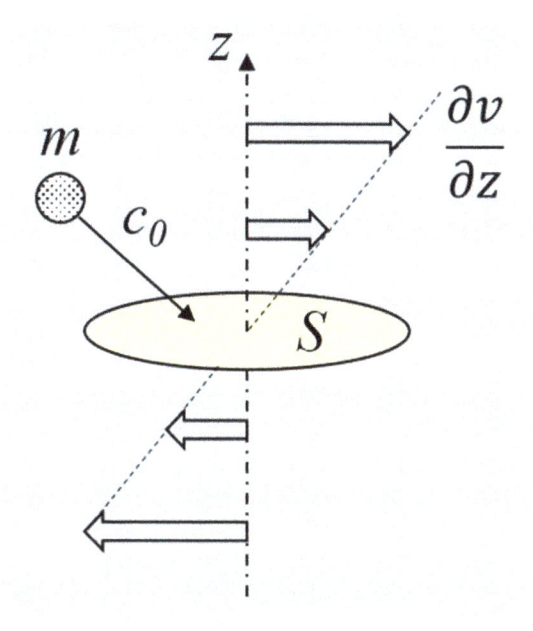

Figure 2.17. Model used to explain gas viscosity. Reproduced from [1]. © 2021 The Japan Society of Applied Physics. All rights reserved.

crossing area S move from a position that is the mean free path l away, molecules moving downward across S have a momentum of $m(\partial v/\partial z) l$, whereas those moving upward across S carry a momentum of $-m(\partial v/\partial z) l$. The entire momentum M crossing S downward per unit time is given by

$$M = K \times 2 \times m(\partial v/\partial z)l = c_0 nS\, m(\partial v/\partial z)l.$$

It is assumed that the shape of a molecule can be regarded as a sphere with a radius b, and that the relationship between the mean free path and the molecular density is given by $l = 1/4\pi n b^2$. The momentum M is expressed as follows:

$$M = c_0\, m(\partial v/\partial z) S/4\pi b^2.$$

The momentum M is the impulse applied to the area S per unit area; therefore, S receives a shear stress of $T = M/S = c_0\, m(\partial v/\partial z)/4\pi b^2$. By comparing this equation to the definition of the viscosity coefficient $T = \eta(\partial v/\partial z)$, the gas viscosity can be expressed as follows:

$$\eta = c_0\, m/4\pi b^2.$$

Important knowledge regarding gas viscosity can be obtained from these equations. Gas viscosity is independent of the density if a gas can be regarded as a fluid, that is, a continuous medium. In other words, gas viscosity is constant if the typical spatial scale is sufficiently larger than the mean free path of the gas molecules. In the above discussion, the transportation of momentum is considered to understand viscosity. Molecules act as the carriers of the gas momentum. In the low-density region, the number of carriers decreases, whereas the mean free path increases. These two factors cancel each other out, and the viscosity remains constant when the characteristic spatial size is larger than the mean free path.

However, the viscosity is proportional to the square of the temperature, because the viscosity is proportional to the molecular velocity c_0, which is related to the temperature through the law of equipartition of energy, $m(\sqrt{3c_0})^2/2 = (3/2)k_BT$. The tendency is the opposite for liquids: the viscosities of liquids generally decrease with temperature.

Although this discussion is based on a very simple model of the kinetic theory of gases, the calculation accuracy can be improved by strictly applying the Boltzmann equation for the momentum transportation phenomenon. In the calculation, a differential cross section with respect to the collision of molecules is required. The molecules of rare gases (group 18 elements) are spherically symmetric and therefore promising candidates for use as standard materials for the measurement of viscosity.

However, it is quite difficult to measure gas viscosity using the conventional rotational method, because its accuracy is unsatisfactory. A major factor preventing accurate measurement is mechanical friction at the rotor support. Even if an air bearing is utilized, the viscosity of the air used to lift the rotor cannot be ignored when the gas viscosity is measured.

The reduction of mechanical friction is also important to improve the accuracy of liquid viscosity measurement. For this purpose, a magnetic levitation EMS system was developed. In this system, a disk composed of diamagnetic material was employed, which floats with the aid of a static magnetic field (i.e. without mechanical support) that is in contact with the rotor.

Figure 2.18 shows a schematic of the magnetic levitation EMS system (a) and a photograph of the probe rotor disk floating above the supporting magnets (b). The rotor is made of graphite and has a radius of 5 mm and a thickness of 1 mm. It floats

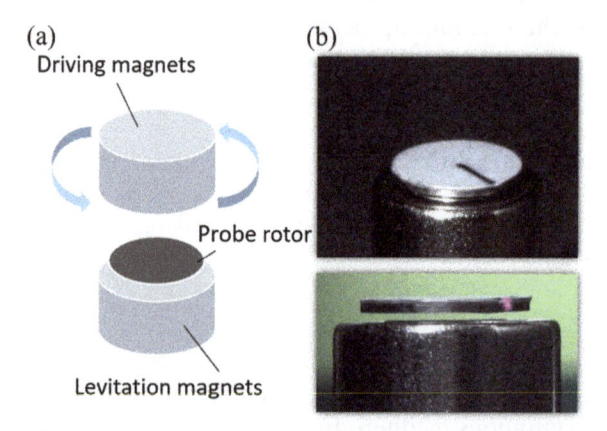

Figure 2.18. Schematic of the magnetic levitation EMS system (a) and a photograph of the probe rotor disk floating above the supporting magnets (b). Reproduced from [1]. © 2021 The Japan Society of Applied Physics. All rights reserved (movie available at https://doi.org/10.1088/978-0-7503-4936-9).

in the static magnetic field and detects the torque from the rotating driving magnets located above it.

The viscosity can be measured without generating any mechanical friction in the system. The viscosities of various types of gas, which were typically one hundredth as viscous as water, were successfully determined. To examine the capability of the system, the gas pressure was reduced to decrease the apparent resistance force resulting from the gas, and the rotation of the probe rotor was measured. The gas viscosity is independent of pressure when the gas is regarded as a fluid, whereas it begins to decrease when the density of gas molecules decreases and the ballistic properties of the molecules appear. In the present case, the pressure began to decrease when the mean free path of the gas molecules approached the typical spatial scale, that is, the gap between the probe rotor and the substrate below.

Figure 2.19 shows the pressure dependence of the viscosity of argon at room temperature. The viscosity is constant at pressures higher than 10^2 Pa, whereas it decreased below this pressure value. Assuming that the radius of an argon molecule is 2×10^{-10} m, the mean free path at atmospheric pressure is approximately 10^{-7} m. It increases inversely with pressure and reaches a gap of 10^{-3} m at approximately 10 Pa, which is clearly shown in figure 2.19.

The lower limit of the viscosity in this experiment was determined by the ultimate pressure of the vacuum pump, which was of the order of 10^{-8} Pa·s. In principle, measurement of lower viscosities is possible by reducing the driving torque supplied to the rotor, which can be easily carried out by, for example, introducing a longer distance between the driving magnet and the rotor.

As described above, at present, the origin of traceability is the viscosity of water at 20 °C, which is 1.002 07 mPa·s; however, it cannot be adopted in the framework of the quantum standard. In the EMS method, the applied torque can be accurately determined by measuring the magnitude of the magnetic flux density and the conductivity of the probe. Furthermore, by simplifying the shape of the rotor and

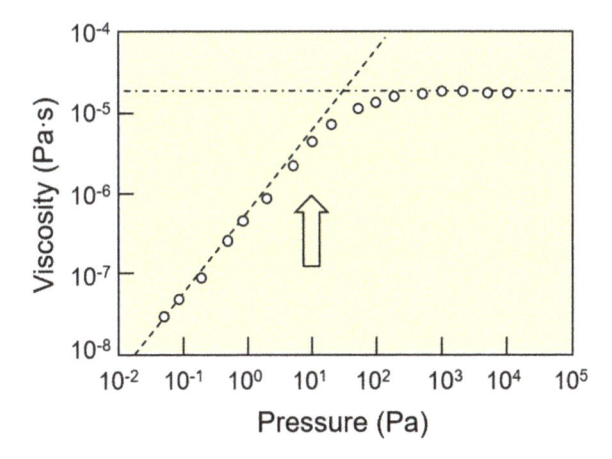

Figure 2.19. Pressure dependence of the viscosity of argon at room temperature. Reproduced from [1]. © 2021 The Japan Society of Applied Physics. All rights reserved..

the boundary condition of the flow field around the rotor, it is possible to accurately calculate the flow field through numerical simulation. An attempt was made to replace the classical standard for viscosity using the EMS method.

In this chapter, we introduced some topics related to viscoelasticity and the related experimental techniques used to observe wave phenomena. Recent progress in this field is remarkable, and we hope that these techniques will be widely employed in the academic and industrial fields.

References

[1] Sakai K 2021 *Jpn. J. Appl. Phys.* **60** 1–11
[2] Laidler K J and Eyring H 1964 *The Theory of Rate Process* (New York: McGraw-Hill) ch 9
[3] Hashitani R, Matsui H, Koda S and Nomura H 1988 *Bull. Chem. Soc. Jpn.* **61** 3087
[4] Doi M and Edwards S F 1978 *J. Chem. Soc. Faraday Trans.* **74** 1818–32
[5] Doi M and Edwards S F 1986 *The Theory of Polymer Dynamics* 1986 (Oxford: Clarendon)
[6] Kato S, Nomura H, Honda H, Zielinski R and Ikeda S 1988 *J. Phys. Chem.* **92** 2306
[7] Ono K, Shintani H, Yano O and Wada Y 1973 *Polymer J.* **5** 164
[8] Mitaku S, Jippo T and Kataoka R 1983 *Biophys. J.* **42** 137
[9] Berne B J and Pecora R 2000 *Dynamic Light Scattering* (New York: Dover)
[10] Matsuoka T, Sakai K and Takagi K 1993 *Rev. Sci. Instrum.* **64** 2136
[11] Sakai K, Hattori K and Takagi K 1995 *Phys. Rev.* B **52** 9402
[12] Matsuoka T, Sakai K and Takagi K 1993 *Phys. Rev. Lett.* **71** 1510
[13] Hirano T and Sakai K 2008 *Phys. Rev.* E **77** 1–5
[14] Levich G L 1962 *Physicochemical Hydrodynamics* (Englewood Criffs, NJ: Prenrice-Hall) p 591
[15] Langevin D 1992 *Light Scattering by Liquid Surfaces and Complementary Techniques* (New York: Dekker)
[16] Earnshaw J C 1996 *Adv. Coll. Interface Sci.* **68** 1
[17] Sakai K, Choi P-K, Tanaka H and Takagi K 1991 *Rev. Sci. Instrum.* **62** 1192
[18] Koga T, Mitani S and Sakai K 2015 *Jpn. J. Appl. Phys.* **54** 041801
[19] Sakai K, Honda H and Hiraoka Y 2005 *Rev. Sci. Instrum.* **76** 063908
[20] Kutsuna H and Sakai K 2008 *Appl. Phys. Express* **1** 1–3
[21] Ishiwata T and Sakai K 2014 *Appl. Phys. Express* **7** 1–4
[22] Viswanath D S, Ggosh T K, Prasad D H L, Dutt N V K and Rani K Y 2007 *Viscosity of Liquid* (Dordrecht: Springer) p 1
[23] Sakai K, Hirano T and Hosoda M 2010 *Appl. Phys. Express* **3** 1–3
[24] Sakai K, Hirano H and Hosoda M 2012 *Appl. Phys. Express* **5** 1–3
[25] Matsuura Y, Hirano T and Sakai K 2017 *Rev. Sci. Instrum.* **88** 1–5
[26] Shimokawa Y, Matsuura Y, Hirano T and Sakai K 2016 *Rev. Sci. Instrum.* **87** 1–4

IOP Publishing

Ultrasonics
Physics and applications
Mami Matsukawa, Pak-Kon Choi, Kentaro Nakamura, Hirotsugu Ogi and Hideyuki Hasegawa

Chapter 3

Optical measurements of ultrasonic fields in air/water and ultrasonic vibration in solids

Kentaro Nakamura

The first half of this chapter introduces several optical methods used for sound-field measurements in air and water. Three types of fiber-optic acoustic sensors are introduced; these sensors can replace conventional diaphragm microphones and piezoelectric needle hydrophones in some applications. A noninvasive method for measuring the ultrasonic field based on acousto-optic interaction is then explained. In the latter half of the chapter, laser-based interferometric methods used to quantitatively measure the ultrasonic vibrations of a solid body are demonstrated. Typical configurations for heterodyne laser Doppler velocimeters are illustrated for both out-of-plane and in-plane vibrations; furthermore, two special configurations for high-power ultrasonic tools operating at several tens of kilohertz and small displacements of very-high-frequency ultrasonic devices are presented.

3.1 Measurement of ultrasonic fields in air/water

3.1.1 Problems arising in ultrasonic field measurement

Condenser microphone devices are commercially available and commonly used for measuring airborne ultrasound. A small-diameter condenser microphone, such as the 1/8 inch type, provides a wide frequency response of up to around 200 kHz and moderate sensitivity. However, even such a small sensor disturbs the ultrasonic field to be measured because the ultrasonic wavelength in air is comparable to the diameter of the microphone. For example, the wavelength of the commonly used 40 kHz airborne ultrasound is 8.5 mm. The diameter of the 1/8 inch microphone is as large as one-third of the wavelength at this frequency. This causes obvious problems, particularly for standing-wave measurements. In contrast, piezoelectric hydrophones are used in the case of ultrasonic fields in water and other liquids. For megahertz ultrasound, needle-type hydrophones with diameters of 1 mm or less are utilized. However, the wavelength of megahertz ultrasound in liquids is in the submillimeter range, which causes the same problem as in air. Other practical difficulties of piezoelectric needle hydrophones include their high electrical impedance and fragility. The length of the electrical cable that transports the signal to the associated electrical system needs to be limited; otherwise, its electromagnetic immunity is insufficient. Very thin piezoelectric hydrophones have diameters of less than 0.5 mm; however, the mechanical stability and toughness become limited with a decrease in the diameter.

We need a considerably smaller sensor or a noninvasive way of overcoming these difficulties in order to measure ultrasonic fields. In this section, several types of fiber-optic thin probes and fully optical methods for measuring ultrasonic fields in air and liquids are introduced.

3.1.2 Probe sensors using optical fibers

Several types of fiber-optic probe sensors have been developed to eliminate the difficulties associated with conventional electrical microphones/hydrophones. The simplest but most useful sensor for high-intensity ultrasonic fields is the reflection-type fiber-optic sensor, which comprises only the end of an optical fiber. This sensor has absolute sensitivity, which can be theoretically predicted using the relationship between the change in the optical refractive index of the media and the sound pressure; this means that there is no need to calibrate the pressure sensitivity. The reflection-type sensor can be applied to high-intensity airborne ultrasound and focused ultrasonic fields in water. However, its sensitivity is too low to evaluate the sound pressure level at less than 100–120 dB. In comparison, the Fabry–Pérot type of sensor has better sensitivity. A tiny Fabry–Pérot resonator was fabricated at the end of a fiber cable; the sound pressure was detected as a shift in the optical resonance peaks that was proportional to the pressure. Different methods can be used to fabricate resonators at the ends of fibers. The third type is a sensor based on a fiber Bragg grating (FBG); this sensor is suitable for arrayed hydrophone systems and for multipoint measurements.

3.1.2.1 Reflection-type sensors
The configuration of the reflection-type fiber-optic ultrasonic sensor is illustrated in figure 3.1. The reflected light intensity is measured in a simple setup that comprises a light source, a circulator, and a photodetector. The cleaved end of the fiber cable acts as a small sensor that detects the ultrasonic field through a change in the optical refractive index of the media (air or water). The original principle was first proposed by Stardenraus and Eisenmenger [1] to measure the shock waves of focused ultrasound in water. The application of this method in air was reported by Takei *et al* [2], who made some modifications to the setup. Figure 3.1 is based on Takei's setup. A wideband light source based on the amplified spontaneous emission (ASE) of a doped fiber is used instead of a laser to avoid unwanted interferometric noise. The 3 dB fiber coupler is replaced by a fiber circulator to utilize the input and reflected light powers effectively. A high-power ASE source (~20 mW) is used to

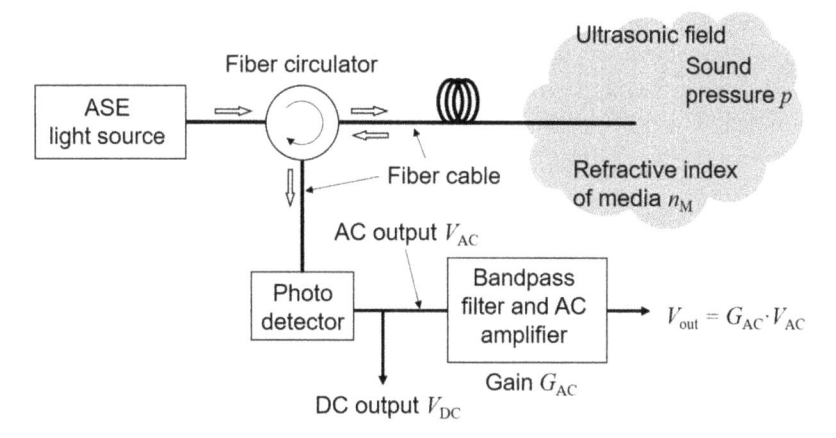

Figure 3.1. Configuration of the reflection-type fiber-optic ultrasonic probe.

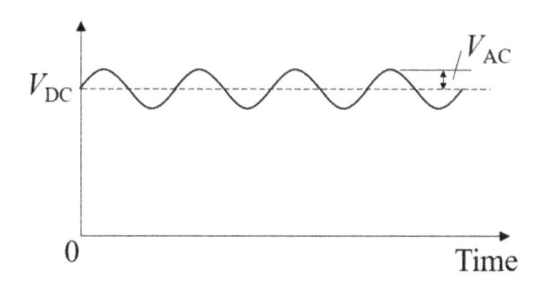

Figure 3.2. Output signal of the photodetector.

obtain a sufficient reflection signal. A telecom wavelength (=1550 nm) is selected as the light source because the fiber-optic components designed for this wavelength are generally common and cost-effective. In addition, this wavelength is believed to be 'eye-safe' because absorption by water or vapor is high. However, most of the light energy is emitted from the fiber end and direct exposure to the emitted light should be avoided.

An InGaAs pin photodiode is used as the photodetector to receive 1550 nm light. The output voltage consists of the DC and AC components illustrated in figure 3.2. The DC component is proportional to the static reflection intensity at the fiber end, whereas the AC component originates from ultrasonic pressure. The absolute value of the sound pressure can be determined by measuring these two components as follows:

First, we consider the relationship between the sound pressure and the resultant deviation in the refractive index of the medium (air or water). Let us assume that the change rate of the volume of air is equal to that of the optical refractive index of the air:

$$\frac{\Delta V}{V} = -\frac{\Delta n}{n_a - 1} \qquad (3.1)$$

Here, n_a and Δn represent the refractive index of air and its variation due to the ultrasonic field, respectively, whereas V and ΔV represent the volume and its change, respectively. A negative sign is necessary because shrinkage causes an increase in the refractive index. The states with and without sound pressure p are related each other as follows:

$$PV^\gamma = (P + p)(V + \Delta V)^\gamma = \text{const} \tag{3.2}$$

because the adiabatic condition is valid for ultrasonic waves. P represents the atmospheric pressure and γ represents the ratio of the specific heat of air (= 1.4). We can derive the relationship that governs the volume change rate by assuming that the sound pressure p and volume change ΔV are infinitesimal compared with P and V, as follows:

$$\frac{\Delta V}{V} = -\frac{p}{\gamma P}. \tag{3.3}$$

The speed of sound in air is expressed using the density ρ as follows:

$$c = \sqrt{\frac{\gamma P}{\rho}}. \tag{3.4}$$

Combining equations (3.1), (3.3), and (3.4), the variation in the refractive index is proportional to the sound pressure in air:

$$\Delta n = \frac{n_a - 1}{c^2 \rho} p = 1.93 \times 10^{-9} p. \tag{3.5}$$

Here, the value used for the refractive index of air $n_a = 1.000\,2736$ at a light wavelength of approximately 1550 nm. A sound speed of 340 m s^{-1} and an air density of 1.226 kg m^{-3} at room temperature and ambient pressure (15 °C and 1013 hPa) were applied.

For the measurement under water, according to Eykman's equation [3], we have

$$\Delta n = \frac{(n_w - 1)(n_w^2 + 1.4 n_w + 0.4)}{(n_w^2 + 0.8 n_w + 1) c^2 \rho} p = 1.60 \times 10^{-10} p, \tag{3.6}$$

where n_w represents the refractive index of water (= 1.333). For the speed of sound c and the density ρ, 1480 m s^{-1} and 1000 kg m^{-3}, respectively, were used.

Next, we calculate the rate of change of reflectivity at the fiber end facing the medium. The static reflectivity R at the boundary between the fiber-end face and the medium is expressed as follows:

$$R = \frac{(n_f - n)^2}{(n_f + n)^2}, \tag{3.7}$$

with the refractive indices n_f and n for the fiber core and the medium, respectively. Then, the rate of change of reflectivity is

$$\frac{\Delta R}{R} = \frac{1}{R}\frac{\partial R}{\partial n}\Delta n = -\frac{4n_f}{(n_f - n)(n_f + n)}\Delta n. \tag{3.8}$$

Applying equations (3.5) or (3.6), equation (3.8) can be rewritten as a function of sound pressure, which gives

$$\frac{\Delta R}{R} = -\frac{4n_f}{(n_f - n)(n_f + n)}\frac{n - 1}{c^2\rho}p \tag{3.9}$$

for air, and

$$\frac{\Delta R}{R} = -\frac{4n_f}{(n_f - n)(n_f + n)}\frac{(n - 1)(n^2 + 1.4n + 0.4)}{(n^2 + 0.8n + 1)c^2\rho}p \tag{3.10}$$

for water. The static reflectivity R and its change ΔR are proportional to the DC and AC components, respectively, and therefore, we get

$$\frac{V_{AC}}{V_{DC}} = \frac{\Delta R}{R}. \tag{3.11}$$

Finally, the sound pressure can be determined by measuring the ratio of the AC to DC components and combining these relationships as follows:

(1) For air

$$p = \frac{V_{AC}}{V_{DC}} \cdot \frac{(n_f - n)(n_f + n)c^2\rho}{-4n_f(n - 1)} = \frac{V_{AC}}{V_{DC}} \times 1.02 \times 10^8 \text{ [Pa]} \tag{3.12}$$

(2) For water

$$p = \frac{V_{AC}}{V_{DC}} \cdot \frac{(n_f - n)(n_f + n)c^2\rho}{-4n_f(n - 1)} \cdot \frac{(n^2 + 0.8n + 1)}{(n^2 + 1.4n + 0.4)}$$
$$= \frac{V_{AC}}{V_{DC}} \times 4.32 \times 10^8 \text{ [Pa]} \tag{3.13}$$

Here, a refractive index of $n_f = 1.47$ was applied to the fiber core. These results indicate that the sensitivity of the reflection-type fiber probe is very low. For example, if the DC component is 1 V, the AC component is 20 µV for a sound pressure level of 160 dB (=2 kPa) in air. This signal level can be detected using a lock-in amplifier or an electrical spectrum analyzer. We observed the waveform of the ultrasonic signal at this level using an oscilloscope after amplification by 40 dB or more combined with bandpass filtering. High-intensity ultrasound in water at pressures of more than 100 kPa can be observed more easily. The noise level of the light source should be carefully examined to achieve a better signal-to-noise ratio. A high-power superluminescent diode (SLD) is another candidate for the light source.

In the above discussions, we focused on airborne ultrasound measurement as well as moderately high-intensity ultrasound measurements in water. For in-water applications, especially for very-high-intensity fields such as shock waves and high-intensity focused ultrasound (HIFU), a more detailed consideration is required. For the in-water applications, the effect of modulating the fiber core's refractive index needs to be considered for accurate measurement because the acoustic impedance of the fiber is not enough different from that of water, although it can be negligible in the case of in-air applications. A good guide to very-high-intensity applications and several 10 MHz applications in water can be found in [4].

The true sensing part of the fiber end is the core, which has a diameter of only 10 μm for standard single-mode fiber. However, the outer diameter of the fiber cladding (=125 μm) is comparable to the ultrasonic wavelength of 10 MHz in water, and the diffraction effect becomes obvious. Thinner fibers should be used for such high-frequency applications. A fiber of 80 μm or thinner, developed for onboard interconnects, can be used. Thinning by chemical etching is another solution for achieving higher frequencies. A tapered fiber tip with a diameter of 7 μm was investigated for an ultrasonic field at up to 100 MHz [5]. Simultaneously, a following circuit with a wider frequency bandwidth is required for the photodetector. The fiber-optic reflection-type sensor exhibits omnidirectivity in the frequency range at which the wavelength of the ultrasound under test is sufficiently larger than the fiber diameter; this is applicable for most in-air applications because the highest frequency practically utilized is hundreds of kilohertz, and the wavelength is in millimeters. However, we need to determine the diffraction effect due to the fiber end if the frequency is higher than 10 MHz in water. Figure 3.3 shows a snapshot of an experimental setup used to measure airborne standing waves excited between a transducer end surface and a reflector. A 1/8 inch condenser microphone was also placed in the photo to compare its diameter with that of the fiber probe.

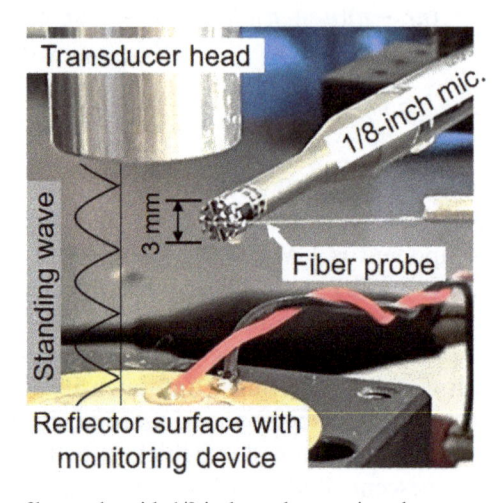

Figure 3.3. Reflection-type fiber probe with 1/8 inch condenser microphone measuring a standing-wave field between a 40 kHz high-power transducer and a reflector.

3.1.2.2 Fabry–Pérot-type sensors

An optical resonance structure causes steep peaks or dips in the wavelength dependence of the reflected light intensity. The simplest one applicable to the end of a fiber is the Fabry–Pérot resonator, which is composed of a pair of tiny parallel reflectors, as shown in figure 3.4. A small cylinder or film of transparent polymer is attached at the end surface of a single-mode fiber, and its acts as an optical resonator and an acoustic sensor. A half mirror of the designed transmittance is inserted between the fiber and the polymer, while the other side of the polymer is sealed with a full mirror to obtain appropriate reflection characteristics.

Figure 3.5 demonstrates one of the methods for fabricating a resonator structure at the end of a fiber [6]. First, a thin gold layer is formulated as a half mirror on the cleaved end of a single-mode fiber by vapor deposition or another method. Second, a dummy fiber is placed in line, and a transparent polymer glue is injected between the two fiber ends. Third, the alignment of the axis, parallelism, and gap is performed using a multi-degree-of-freedom precision manipulator. The transmitted and reflected light is monitored using a superluminescent diode and an optical spectrum analyzer during the adjustment so that clear and strong dips appear in the wavelength dependence. When the spectrum is acceptable, UV light is used to cure the glue. The dummy fiber is then removed. Finally, the end of the polymer cavity is sealed using gold. This method can be too laborious for an acceptable manufacturing yield, and therefore, attaching a thin, small polymer film to the end of the fiber [7] is a better alternative.

An ultrasonic signal can be detected and demodulated into an electrical signal using the setup shown in figure 3.6. The light source in figure 3.1 is replaced by a tunable laser, and the wavelength characteristics of the reflection exhibit periodic dips. The interval between the dips, called the free spectral range (FSR), is determined by the length L and refractive index n of the cavity, whereas the steepness of the dip, called the finesse, is a function of the reflectivity of the half mirror. The wavelength of the light source is set to the middle of the upward or downward slope of the dip. The dip position is slightly modulated by ultrasonic pressure, and the reflected light intensity is altered by the applied ultrasound. Although a higher finesse results in higher sensitivity, the dynamic range is

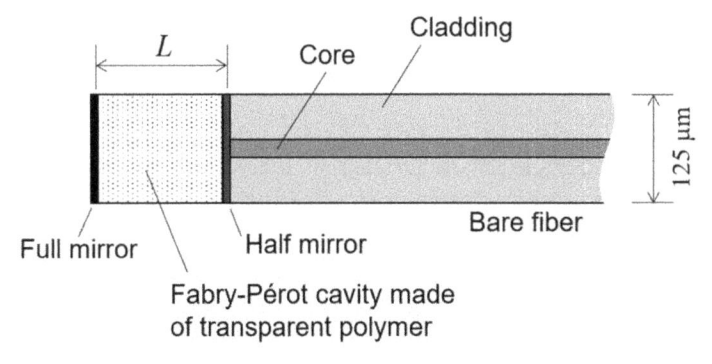

Figure 3.4. Fabry–Pérot resonator fabricated at the end of a fiber.

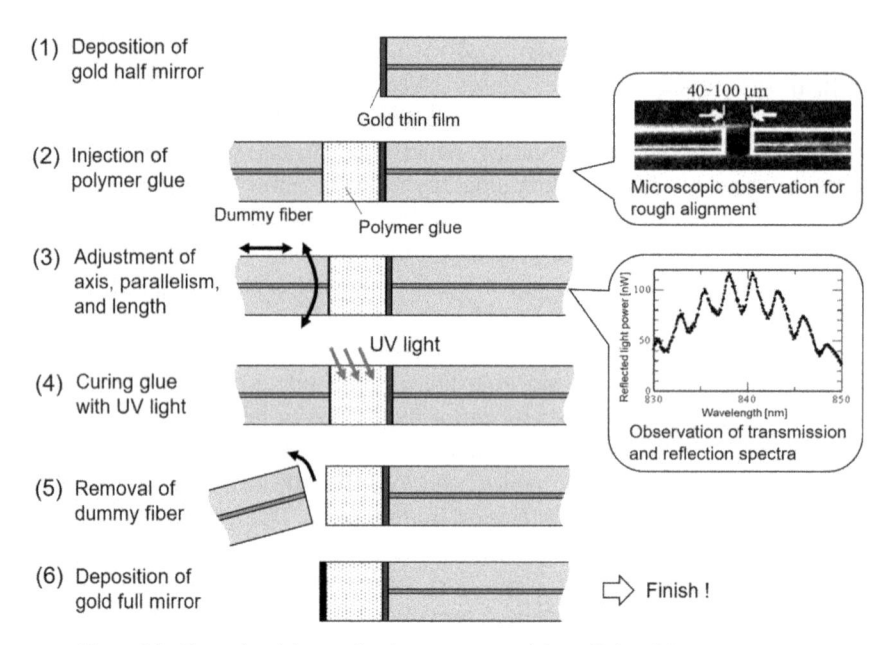

Figure 3.5. Example of the production process used for a Fabry–Pérot-type sensor.

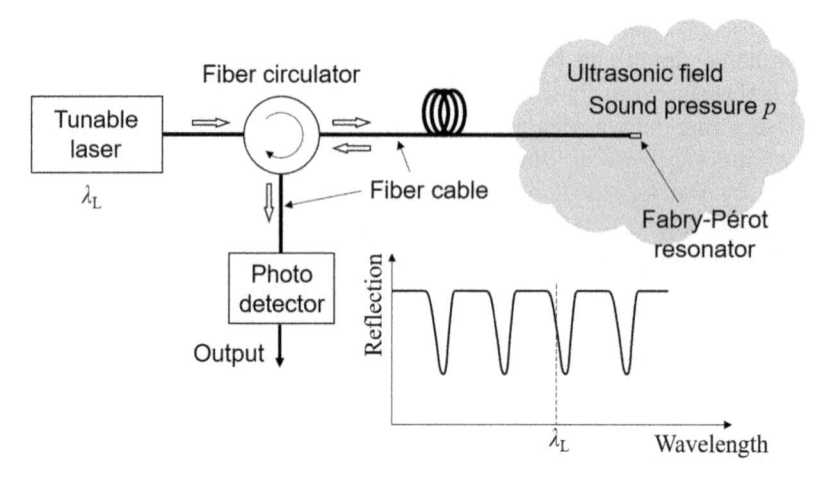

Figure 3.6. Instrument setup for a Fabry–Pérot ultrasonic sensor.

suppressed. The wavelength characteristics of the reflectivity and ultrasonic sensitivity were measured for a prototype sensor, as shown in figure 3.7. The ultrasonic sensitivity is the highest around the middle of the slopes of the reflectivity dip. The phase of the ultrasonic signal is inverted by selecting a slope gradient. The wavelength of the light source, λ_L, needs to be maintained at the optimal operation point to cope with temperature drift. A way of maintaining the operation point is required [8] for practical use. From another point of view, this means the

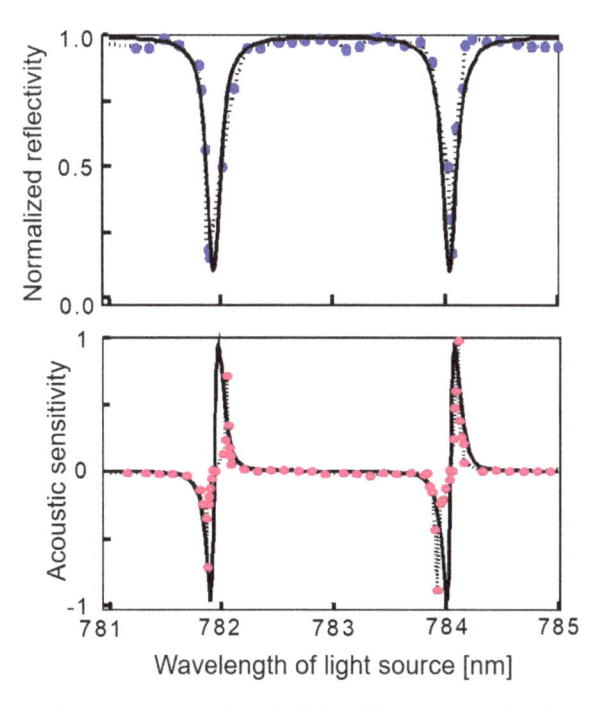

Figure 3.7. Reflectivity and ultrasonic sensitivity of a Fabry–Pérot sensor as functions of optical wavelength.

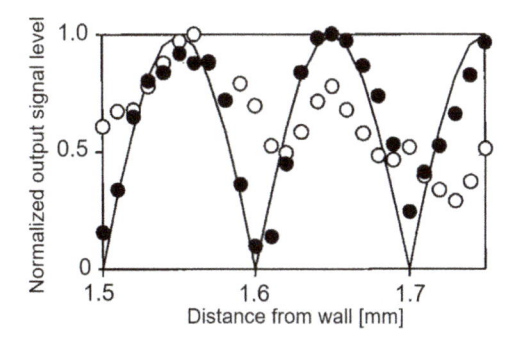

Figure 3.8. Standing wave formed between a 7.5 MHz transducer and a rigid wall. The black solid plots show the results measured using the Fabry–Pérot fiber probe, and the open circles represent the outputs of the piezoelectric needle hydrophone, which was 0.5 mm in diameter. A solid curve is drawn to show the ideal distribution of the standing wave.

temperature can be measured simultaneously with the sound pressure [9]. This could be important for HIFU applications and chemical processing using ultrasonic energy.

A high-frequency standing-wave field (7.5 MHz) was measured using a Fabry–Pérot fiber sensor, as shown in figure 3.8. The results obtained using a piezoelectric needle hydrophone with a diameter of 0.5 mm are also plotted in the figure. The wavelength of the standing wave is calculated to be 0.2 mm, which is considerably

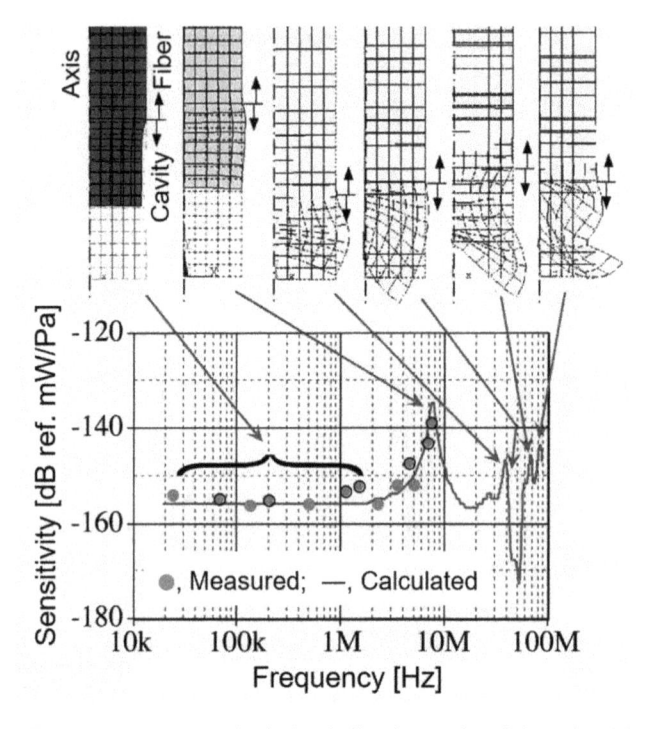

Figure 3.9. Frequency response and calculated vibration modes of the Fabry–Pérot sensor.

smaller than that of the needle hydrophone but almost double that of the fiber. The results indicate that nodal dips are clearly measured using the fiber sensor.

The frequency response is mainly determined by diffraction for reflection-type fiber sensors. However, the mechanical resonance of the polymer cavity plays an important role in the case of the Fabry–Pérot sensor. The forced vibration of the cavity and fiber is simulated through finite-element analysis, as shown in figure 3.9, together with the measured sensitivity. The first resonance appears at approximately 7 MHz, and the highest frequency with constant sensitivity is determined by the resonance. Although the absolute sensitivity has been simulated and theoretically studied [10], calibration of the sensitivity is inevitable, as is the case for conventional piezoelectric probes. A detailed experimental investigation of the sensitivity and directivity was carried out by Beard *et al* and summarized in reference [11].

3.1.2.3 Fiber Bragg grating sensors
FBGs are in-line fiber-optic filters used in telecom applications and, at the same time, they have been actively studied as strain or temperature sensors [12] because of their potential capability for use in arrayed sensor systems. Furthermore, FBGs are sensitive to ultrasonic waves [13] and they are more suitable for use in an array than the Fabry–Pérot type. There have been trials of arrayed ultrasonic probes using the Fabry–Pérot sensor [14, 15]; however, the number of elements was rather limited because of multiple resonance dips.

As illustrated in figure 3.10, the refractive index of the fiber core is periodically modulated along the axis at a pitch of d. This structure works as a Bragg reflector and exhibits a single reflection peak in a typical telecom band at the central wavelength of

$$\lambda_c = 2nd, \qquad (3.14)$$

where n denotes the average refractive index of the core. For example, the modulation depth of the refractive index is approximately 0.3% and the number of gratings is 1000. The gratings are permanently inscribed by illuminating a Ge-doped fiber using UV light [16]. Figure 3.11 shows an example of the reflection

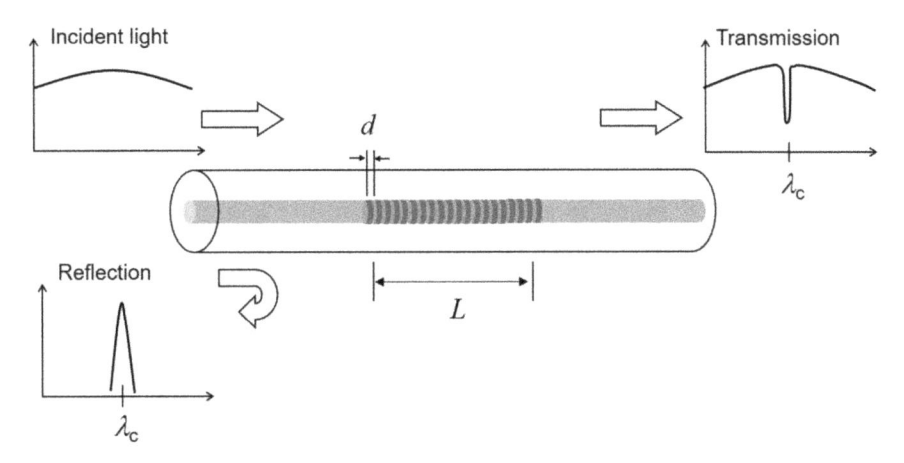

Figure 3.10. Fiber Bragg grating.

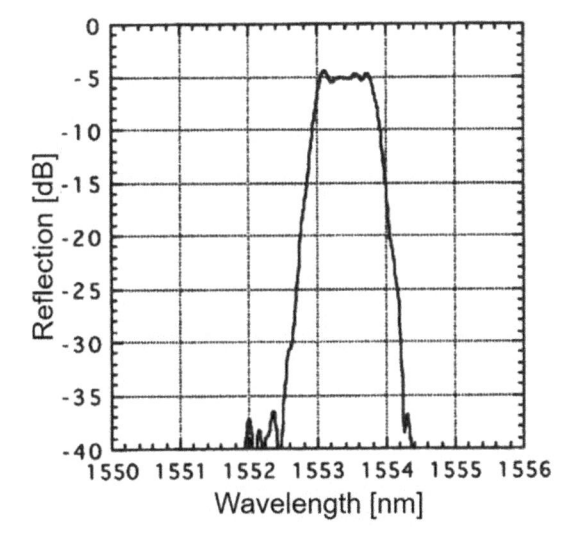

Figure 3.11. Example of the reflection spectrum of a FBG. This is optimized as a flat-top filter with a bandwidth of 0.8 nm in the telecom band.

characteristics for a flat-top telecom filter with a bandwidth of 0.8 nm. The shape and intensity of the reflection spectrum can be controlled by modulating the depth, weight, and number of gratings. Gaussian or other peaky characteristics are used for sensor applications to find the peak shift in a precise manner.

The FBG works as an ultrasonic sensor because the pitch and refractive index are affected by external pressure, and the typical pressure sensitivity is around −6 pm MPa^{-1} at 1550 nm. Using a similar approach to that of the Fabry–Pérot sensor, the ultrasonic signal can be transduced to a voltage using the setup shown in figure 3.6. The wavelength of the tunable laser is set to the middle of one of the slopes in the reflection peak to obtain the ultrasonic modulation signal. The central wavelength of the FBG shows a temperature dependence of 12 pm K^{-1} in the telecom band (1550 nm), and it is necessary to introduce a wavelength-tracking system if a large temperature drift is expected. The FBG is capable of responding to ultrasonic waves at 10 MHz and higher in principle. However, we need to understand that the inscribed FBG length along the fiber is several millimeters and that this finite length of the sensitive section results in directivity in receiving ultrasonic waves.

As shown in figure 3.12, an arrayed senor system can be developed by in-line connecting multiple FBGs with different central wavelengths. Peaks with identical central wavelengths can be observed in the spectrum of the reflected light, in which each peak corresponds to an FBG. The signals of the FBGs are individually monitored by scanning the wavelength of a tunable light source. An external-cavity semiconductor laser is suitable for covering a band of 50–100 nm.

However, this is a quasi-multipoint measurement because it is difficult to observe all points in a truly simultaneous manner. For a real multipoint measurement, a sophisticated demodulation unit (interrogator) is required, which can equip parallel output ports corresponding to all FBGs. Figure 3.13 shows an FBG-based ultrasonic sensor array system that uses an arrayed-waveguide grating (AWG) to analyze the reflected light in real time [17, 18]. The tunable laser in figure 3.6 is replaced by a

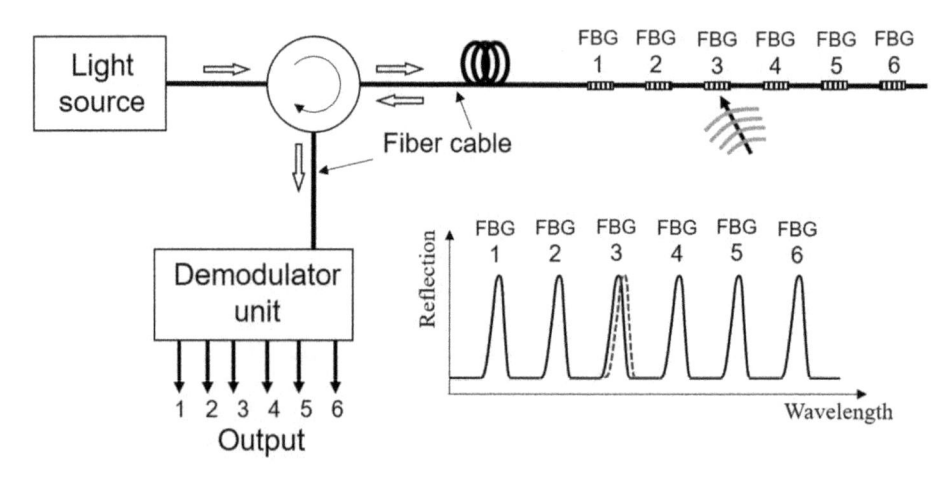

Figure 3.12. Multipoint ultrasound measurement using an FBG array.

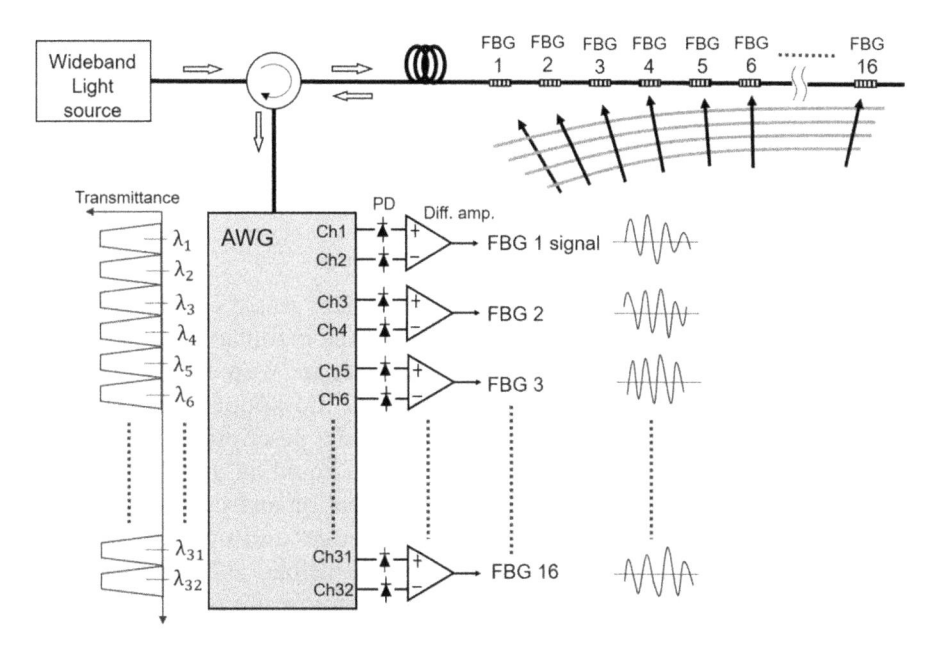

Figure 3.13. FBG hydrophone system using an AWG and differential photodetectors.

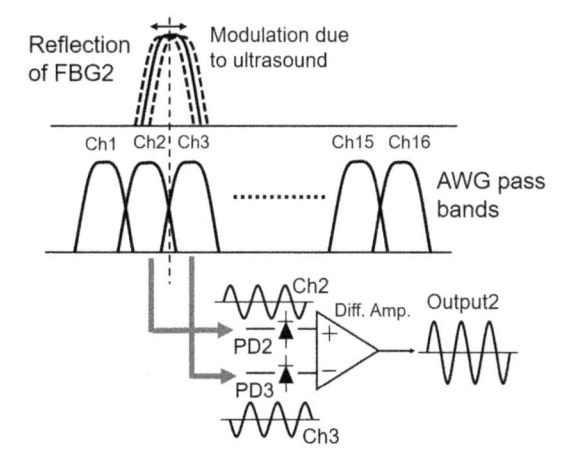

Figure 3.14. Demodulation mechanism used for the ultrasound shown in figure 3.13.

broadband light source, such as ASE or SLD. The FBGs with different central wavelengths act as element sensors in the ultrasonic array and are in-line connected along a fiber cable; the reflected light has a comb-like shape in the wavelength domain because the FBG array is illuminated by broadband light. The AWG functions as a filter bank with many pass-band channels. Each pair of adjacent channels is connected to a differential photodetector to convert the vibratory shift of the FBG reflection wavelength to the corresponding electrical signal, as shown in figure 3.14. The AWG is thermally controlled so that the central wavelength of the target FBG falls in the middle of the spacing between the adjacent passbands of the AWG. AWGs with 32 channels or more are commercially available, and are designed for the standard telecom channels at spacings of 0.4 nm (50 GHz) or 0.8 nm (100 GHz). Considering the usable bandwidth of one light source, the maximum number of multiplexed FBGs in one fiber cable is believed to be 10–20.

3.1.3 Imaging of ultrasonic fields using optical methods

Free-space light with bulk optics is used instead of fiber sensor technology to image the spatial distribution of ultrasonic fields through the modulation in the refractive indices of media. Among the various optical methods used to visualize spatial variation in the refractive indices of media, one of the most popular and useful is the schlieren method [19, 20]. However, we minimize the description of the schlieren method (a tool for visualizing the ultrasonic field in a liquid) in this chapter, as it has already been illustrated in chapter 1. Here, let us mention an example of imaging in air. As a result of the recent progress in imaging devices and signal processing, the visualization of airborne ultrasound has become possible, although the setup of optics such as lenses/concave mirrors and a knife edge is the same as the conventional setup. As an example of the schlieren image in air, a standing wave at 28 kHz is shown in figure 3.15. Standing waves are excited between the vibrating surface of a high-power vibration system driven by a Langevin transducer and a reflector. Styrofoam balls 2–3 mm in diameter are trapped at the nodal planes of the sound pressure because of the acoustic radiation force [21]. The schlieren image is shifted by a quarter wavelength to achieve a spatial distribution of pressure. Pressure nodes, where the gradient of the refractive index is maximal, result in the highest contrast. This is an obvious conclusion because ray deflection is caused by the variation in the refractive index.

Interferometric methods need to be used for higher sensitivity and more quantitative measurement. The ultrasonic field induces variation in the effective

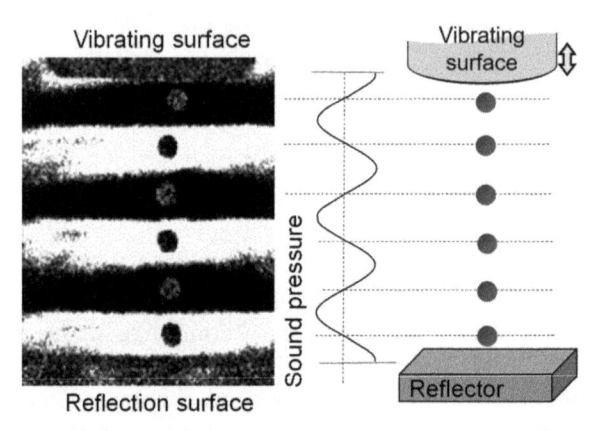

Figure 3.15. Example of a schlieren image: a standing wave excited between a piston-like vibrating surface and a reflector in air at 28 kHz. Small Styrofoam balls are trapped at the nodal planes of the sound pressure because of the acoustic radiation force.

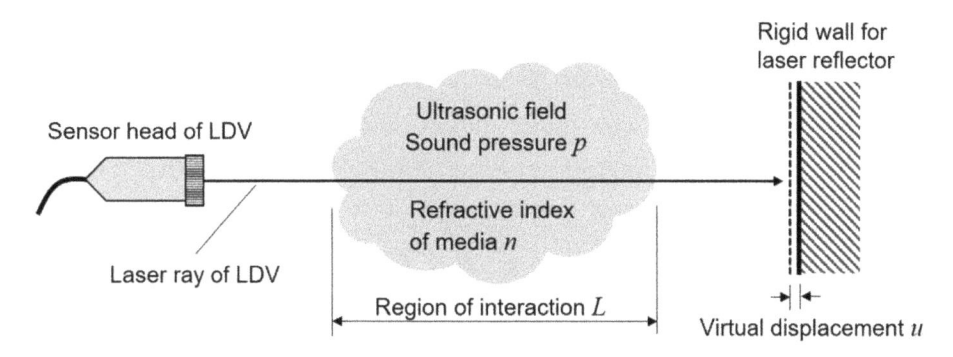

Figure 3.16. Setup used to measure the sound pressure in air/water using an LDV (optical interferometer). © [2002] IEEE. Reprinted, with permission, from [22].

optical path length by modulating the refractive index of the medium. The variation in the path length is small; however, it is easily detected using an optical interferometer, as illustrated in figure 3.16 [22]. In practice, we can utilize a laser Doppler velocimeter (LDV) as a stable interferometer. The configuration and working principle of the LDV are explained in detail in section 3.2.1. The measuring light of the LDV is located such that it runs through the ultrasonic field to be measured and hits a rigid wall; the reflected light is received by the LDV head. This is a common setup for measuring the vibration of the walls. However, in this case, the wall is rigid and has no vibration. Instead, the modulation of the refractive index is detected as if the wall vibrates. Thus, let us assume that the path variation attributed to the refractive-index modulation Δn is equal to that caused by the displacement u.

$$\Delta n \cdot L = n \cdot u. \tag{3.15}$$

The length of the interaction region between the ultrasonic waves and measuring light is denoted by L, and the refractive index of the media is denoted by n. Considering that the output of the LDV is the vibration velocity v, equation (3.15) can be rewritten as

$$\Delta n = \frac{nv}{2\pi f L}, \tag{3.16}$$

where f represents the frequency of the ultrasound. The sound pressure p can be measured by applying equation (3.16) to equation (3.5) for measurements in air. Equation (3.6) is used instead of equation (3.5) in the case of measurements in water.

A two-dimensional image of the ultrasonic field can be obtained by introducing a mechanical scanning system as shown in figure 3.17. A rigid wall is set up as a reflector behind the ultrasonic field under test. A scanning LDV, which is commercially available from various companies, is the most convenient tool for this purpose. An X–Y motorized stage is an alternative practical method for laboratory experiments. The temporal waveforms of the scanned points should be recorded with perfect synchronization in the time domain. As an example of an

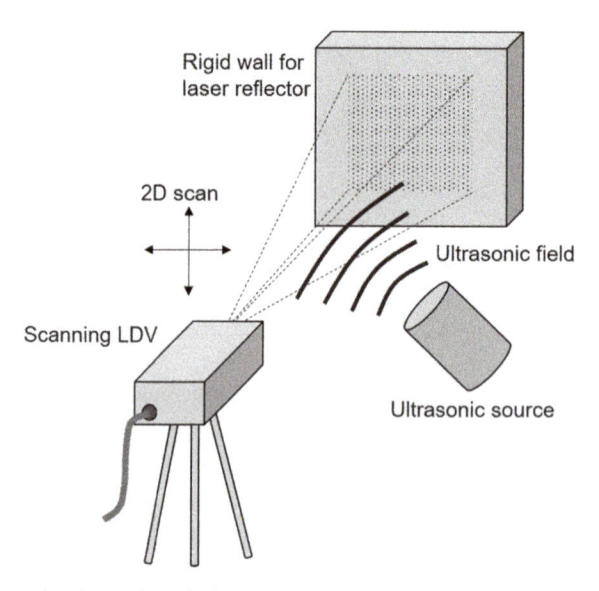

Figure 3.17. Two-dimensional scanning of a laser measurement ray used for the visualization of an ultrasonic field.

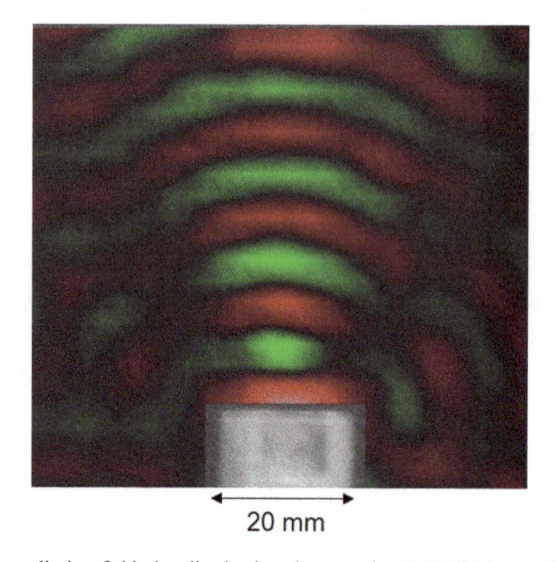

Figure 3.18. Ultrasonic radiation field visualized using the scanning LDV (video available at https://doi.org/10.1088/978-0-7503-4936-9).

ultrasonic field visualized by a scanning LDV, ultrasonic radiation at 28 kHz from a piston-like vibrating surface 20 mm in diameter is shown in figure 3.18; the free field and diffraction around the edge are clearly visualized. A second example is shown in figure 3.19, in which circular standing waves are excited in the inner space of a vibrating aluminum ring at 27 kHz; the ring, which has a diameter of approximately 65 mm, vibrates almost uniformly in all angular directions, and therefore, the

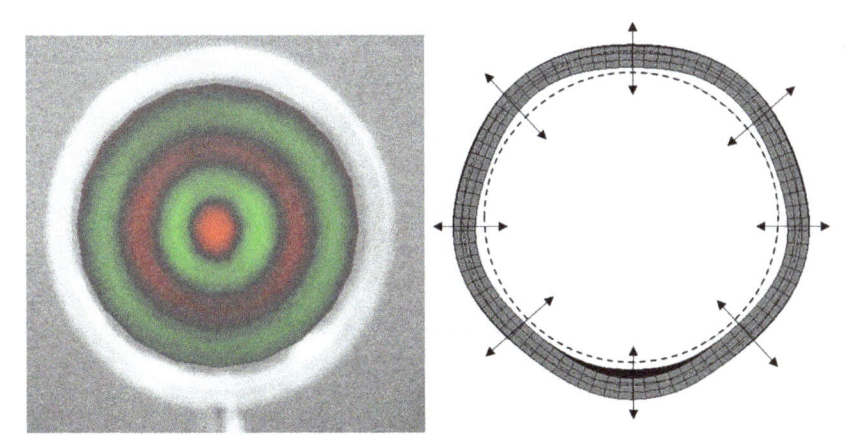

Figure 3.19. Ultrasonic standing wave in a vibrating ring visualized with the scanning LDV (left) (video available at https://doi.org/10.1088/978-0-7503-4936-9), and numerically simulated vibration mode of the ring (right).

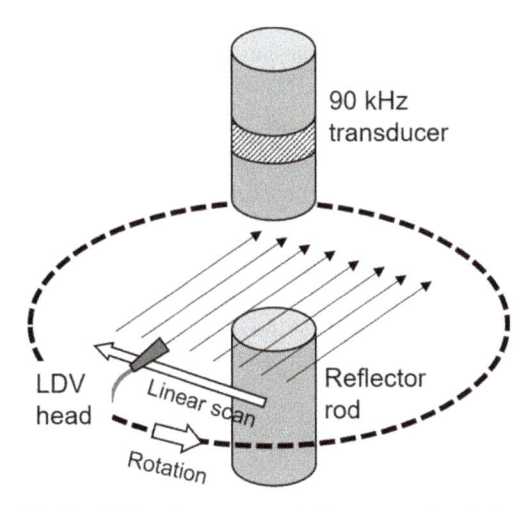

Figure 3.20. Setup used for the CT-based measurement of a cross-sectional view of the ultrasonic field.

resultant ultrasonic field inside the ring becomes axisymmetric. The vibration mode shown in the figure was numerically simulated.

The output signal of the LDV contains all the contributions from region L of the ray. In a special case, for example, the LDV output signal becomes zero when positive and negative pressures at the same level exist together along region L. We need to introduce a computed tomography (CT) algorithm to resolve the spatial distribution in the direction of the measuring ray. Let us illustrate an example of the CT reconstruction of the depth resolution applied for the ultrasonic field measurement. Figure 3.20 depicts a scenario in which a 90 kHz ultrasonic field is measured between a piston-like transducer 6 mm in diameter and a reflection surface of the same shape and size; standing waves are generated between the transducer and the rod. The LDV head is scanned transversely to obtain the cross-sectional distribution

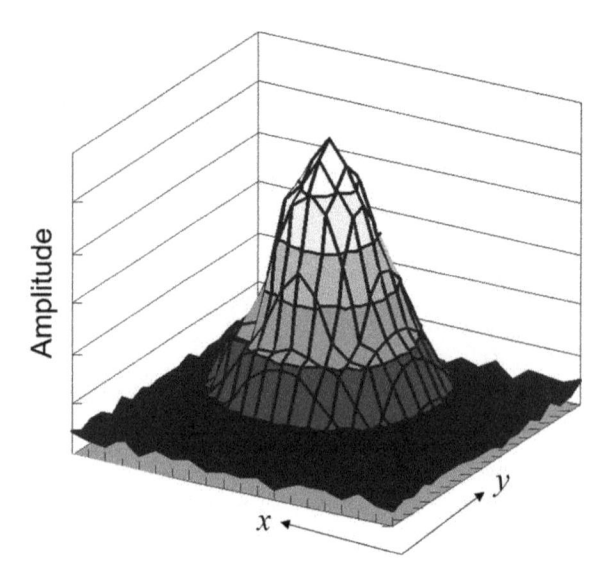

Figure 3.21. Reconstructed sound pressure distribution for the cross section of figure 3.20.

of the ultrasonic field. However, the one-dimensional distribution obtained by the single linear scanning of the LDV does not yield the real field shape, because the LDV output signal is equivalent to the contribution of all sound pressure signals integrated along the ray, as explained above. One-dimensional scanning is repeated many times while changing the angle to obtain the entire data set required for CT-based reconstruction. The resultant two-dimensional distribution for a cross section is shown in figure 3.21. The sound pressure is maximal at the center and decays in the radial direction. A similar visualization in the audible frequency range was demonstrated by Ikeda [23].

The absolute sound pressure level (SPL) can be measured by applying the relationships given by equations (3.5), (3.6), and (3.16), although the length L for the interaction between the ultrasonic field and laser ray should be known. We need to remember that the SPL obtained is one averaged over the length L. Considering the conditions, the minimum detectable SPL is calculated to be 74 dB ($= 0.1$ Pa) for $L = 50$ mm if the resolution in the vibration displacement measurement of the LDV is 10 pm. The LDV method can be applied to ultrasonic fields in water as well as in solids if the media are transparent. The difference in the optical refractive index of the medium should be correctly introduced for the absolute measurement of the sound pressure.

3.1.4 Super directivity in the detection of ultrasonic waves

The measuring laser ray of an LDV system functions as a noninvasive sound pressure sensor with a finite length of L. This means that the sound pressure sensitivity is distributed in space and the output is accumulated over the length L. Therefore, a pencil-beam directivity is obtained for ultrasound detection if the laser ray is extended to a two-dimensional plane, as shown in figure 3.22. The laser ray is

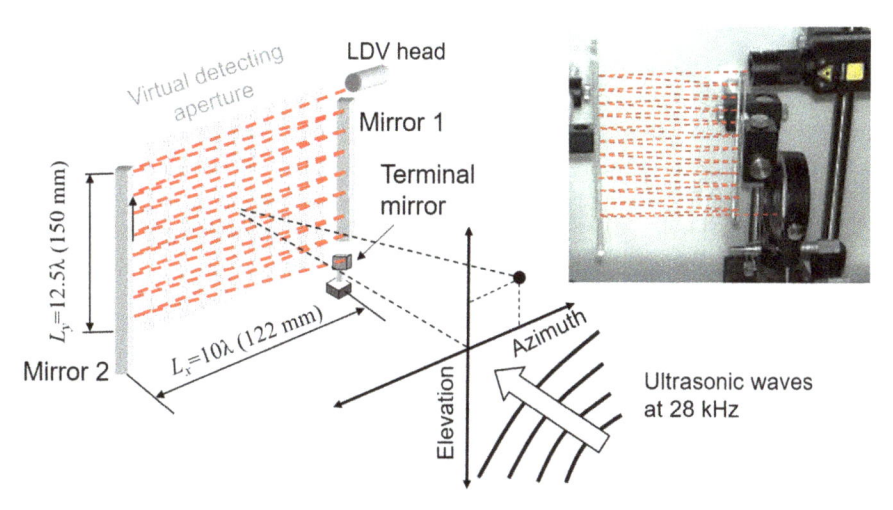

Figure 3.22. Pencil-beam setup used to detect ultrasonic waves.

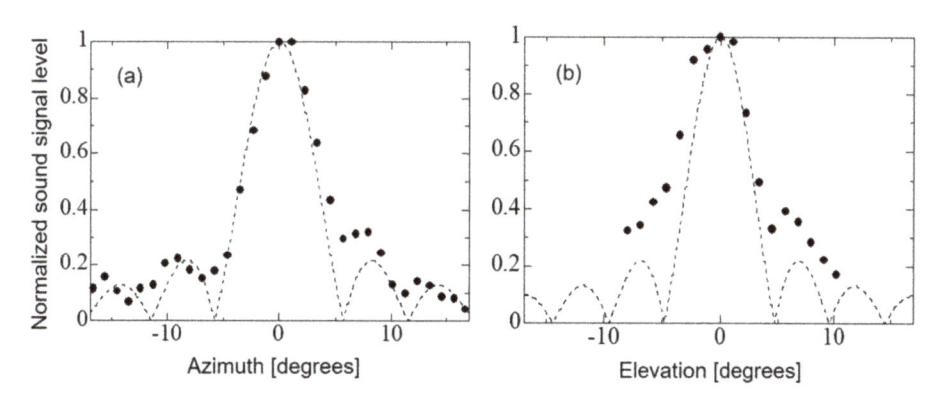

Figure 3.23. Directivity patterns for the (a) azimuthal and (b) elevational directions. The dotted lines represent the theoretical patterns given by equation (3.17).

reflected many times in a zigzag manner between two slender mirrors and returned to the same trace using a third mirror (a retroreflector or corner cube). The spacing between the rays should be shorter than the wavelength of the ultrasound to be measured to suppress the grating lobes in the directivity. The equivalent receiving aperture with a rectangular shape results in a directivity function given by

$$D(\theta, \varphi) = \left| \frac{\sin\left(\frac{\pi L_x}{\lambda}\sin\theta\right)}{\frac{\pi L_x}{\lambda}\sin\theta} \cdot \frac{\sin\left(\frac{\pi L_y}{\lambda}\sin\varphi\right)}{\frac{\pi L_y}{\lambda}\sin\varphi} \right|, \quad (3.17)$$

as functions of the horizontal angle (azimuth) θ and the vertical angle (elevation) φ. The width and height of the aperture are L_x and L_y, respectively. Figures 3.23(a) and (b) show the measured directivity patterns. A 28 kHz ultrasonic source was located at a remote position to fulfil the far-field condition. In the measurement, instead of rotating the setup, the ultrasonic source was linearly moved in both the horizontal and vertical directions using a two-axis motorized precision stage. The width and height of the aperture were 122 and 150 mm, respectively, which are equal to 10 and 12.5 ultrasonic wavelengths, respectively. The full widths at half maximum were 7° and 8° for the azimuth and elevation, respectively, which are in good agreement with the directivity patterns given by theory. The higher side lobes observed in the elevational direction can be attributed to the reflections from the surface of the experimental bench.

3.2 Vibration measurement at ultrasonic frequencies

The non-contact method is ideal for measuring ultrasonic vibration of solid bodies. Electrostatic and electromagnetic methods are possible contactless tools for vibration measurements. However, these methods are rather old-fashioned, and the vibrating body under test is limited to conductive metals. In this section, we focus on optical interferometric methods because of their versatility in practical applications.

3.2.1 Out-of-plane vibration

Figure 3.24 depicts the basic setup used for the Michelson interferometer. The laser light is divided by a half mirror and travels toward a mirror and a target. The former is the reference light and the latter is the object light that hits the target under test. These are combined again by the same half mirror after being reflected by the mirror and the target, and then received by a photodiode. If the target is moving toward the light source at a velocity v, the frequency of the light f_L is changed to f_L' by the Doppler effect.

$$f_L' = \frac{c+v}{c-v} f_L \tag{3.18}$$

The velocity v is sufficiently small in comparison with the speed of light c. Based on this approximation, the Doppler shift Δf_L can be expressed as

$$\Delta f_L \approx \frac{2v}{c} f_L = \frac{2v}{\lambda}, \tag{3.19}$$

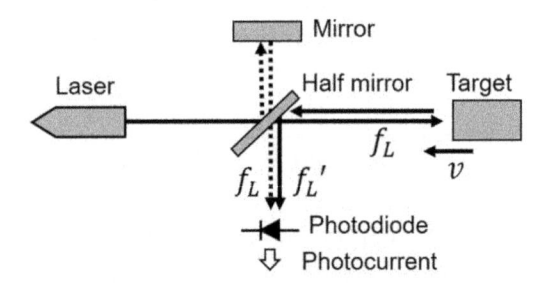

Figure 3.24. Michelson interferometer.

where λ represents the wavelength of light. The Doppler shift is calculated to be 3.16 MHz for a velocity of 1 m s^{-1} when a He–Ne laser with a wavelength of 632.8 nm is used.

Let the electric field of the reference light E_r and that of the measuring light (object light) E_m be

$$E_r = E \cos(\omega t - kx_r), \tag{3.20}$$

and

$$E_m = E \cos(\omega t - kx_m), \tag{3.21}$$

respectively; the superposition of these, E_d, becomes

$$E_d = E_r + E_m = 2E \cos\left[k\frac{x_r - x_m}{2}\right] \cos\left[\omega t - k\frac{x_r + x_m}{2}\right] \tag{3.22}$$

on the photodiode surface. Here, k represents the wave number of light ($= 2\pi/\lambda$), ω represents the angular frequency of light ($= 2\pi f_L$), and x_r and x_m are the optical path lengths for the reference and object lights from the source to the photodiode, respectively. For simplicity, we assume that the two lights have identical amplitude E. The first cosine is the constant amplitude determined by the optical path difference, whereas the second cosine is the alternating electric field at the frequency of light. The output current of photodiode i is proportional to the intensity of the received electric field; however, it never responds to the optical frequency. Thus,

$$i \propto \overline{(E_r + E_m)^2} = \frac{E_1^2 + E_2^2}{2} + E_1 E_2 \cos[k(x_r - x_m)]. \tag{3.23}$$

Here, we denote the amplitudes of the electric fields of the reference and measuring lights by E_1 and E_2, respectively. The current is composed of a constant value related only to the light intensity and a sinusoidal term dependent on the path difference. The photocurrent is shown as a function of the path difference in figure 3.25. The period of change is equivalent to half of the wavelength because of

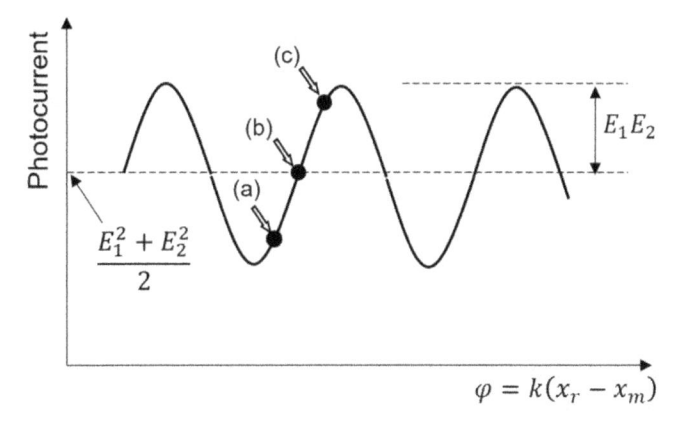

Figure 3.25. Variation of the photocurrent in the setup of figure 3.24.

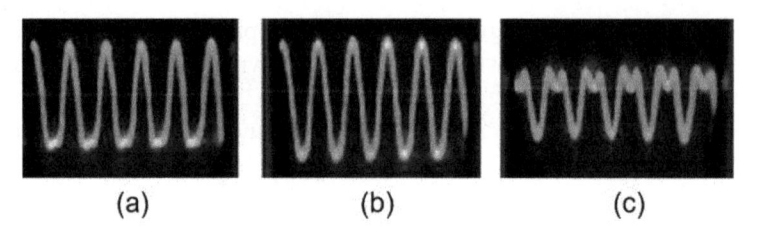

Figure 3.26. Time-domain signals for different operation points: (a), (b), and (c) correspond to the positions indicated in figure 3.25.

the round trip of the measuring light. If the displacement of the object is vibratory with a small amplitude sufficiently smaller than a quarter wavelength, a vibration waveform can be observed in the photocurrent, as shown in figure 3.26. The waveform is distorted if the operation point, which is the neutral position of the object, deviates from the middle of the slope. It is necessary to maintain the position of the vibrating body under test at the center of the slope throughout the measurement; however, this is difficult in practice because the operating point easily drifts due to ambient vibration or temperature variation. Another fatal problem is that the observed amplitude varies depending on the light intensity, and the displacement sensitivity is affected by the optical reflection coefficient of the object under test.

The system explained above is called a homodyne interferometer. A heterodyne system is introduced to overcome the instability of the setup of figure 3.24. The optical frequency of the reference light is shifted by f_B in the heterodyne interferometer. The reference light with the frequency shift is

$$E_r = E_1 \cos\left[2\pi(f_L + f_B)t - kx_r\right], \tag{3.24}$$

and the measurement light with the Doppler shift is

$$E_m = E_2 \cos\left[2\pi(f_L + \Delta f)t - kx_m\right]. \tag{3.25}$$

Thus, the resultant photocurrent becomes

$$i \propto \overline{(E_r + E_m)^2} = \frac{E_1^2 + E_2^2}{2} + E_1 E_2 \cos\left[2\pi(f_B - \Delta f)t + \theta\right]. \tag{3.26}$$

Here, θ represents the phase shift attributed to the path difference. The important point is that the photodiode output is an RF signal at the frequency of f_B, and the Doppler shift is observed as frequency modulation instead of amplitude modulation. If the target object is vibrating at a vibration velocity of V and at a frequency of f_V, the Doppler shift is

$$\Delta f = \frac{2}{\lambda} V \cos(2\pi f_V t). \tag{3.27}$$

The electrical output of the heterodyne system is a frequency modulation (FM) signal with a carrier frequency of f_B modulated by the vibration velocity or a phase

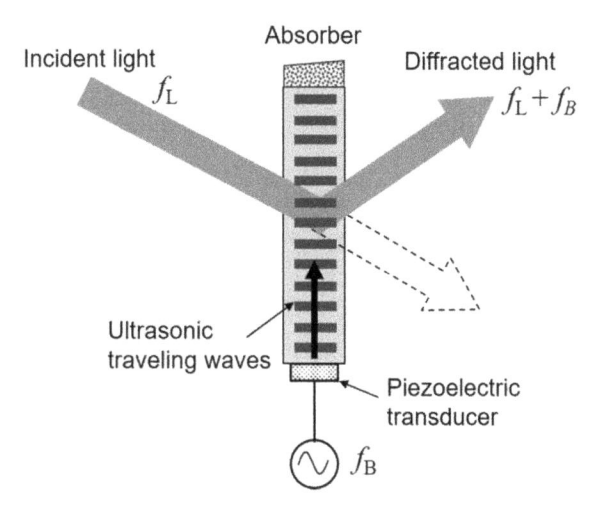

Figure 3.27. Basic structure of an acousto-optic modulator (AOM).

modulation (PM) signal modulated by the vibration displacement. In contrast to the amplitude modulation (AM) output of the homodyne system, the velocity or displacement can be measured precisely, even when the light intensity reflected by the object is weak or fluctuating.

Let us briefly discuss a device that applies a frequency shift to the reference light. As illustrated in figure 3.27, the device comprises a transparent solid bar/plate and a piezoelectric transducer. An ultrasonic traveling wave at a frequency of f_B is excited in the solid and terminated by an absorber. The ultrasonic wave acts as an optical grating because the refractive index is periodically modulated at a pitch identical to the ultrasonic wavelength in the solid. The incident light at a frequency of f_L is deflected by the ultrasonically induced gratings [24], and the frequency of the incident light is simultaneously shifted by f_B because of the traveling motion of the ultrasonic waves. This device is called an acousto-optic modulator (AOM) and is also known as a Bragg cell. Shift frequencies ranging from 40 MHz to several hundreds of megahertz are commonly provided by commercially available AOMs. The target ultrasonic frequency should be sufficiently lower than the AOM shift frequency used to process the heterodyne signal in order to regenerate the ultrasonic vibration waveform during testing. This restricts the applicable range of ultrasonic vibration frequencies under test to several tens of megahertz.

A Mach–Zehnder interferometer is often utilized to insert an AOM into the reference arm, as shown in figure 3.28. Here, a configuration using a polarized interferometer is introduced for practical convenience, and the diagram may appear complicated. A linearly polarized laser is used as the light source, and its polarization direction is adjusted using a half-wave plate (HWP). The light is divided by a polarization beam splitter (PBS) into the measuring and reference lights. The optical frequency of the reference light is shifted by f_B using an AOM, while the measuring light passes through the second PBS without loss and is converted to circular polarization by a quarter-wave plate (QWP). The measuring light then hits the target

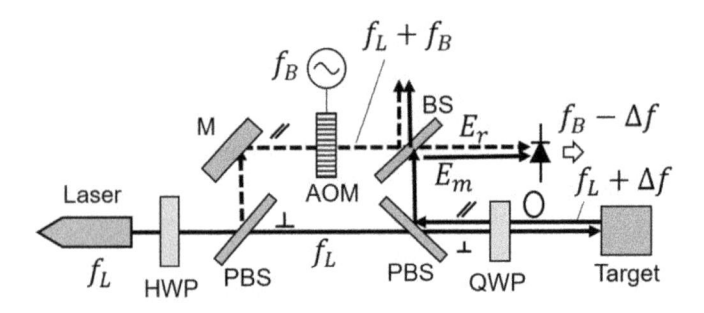

Figure 3.28. Practical configuration of a heterodyne laser Doppler velocimeter based on a polarized Mach–Zehnder interferometer. HWP, half-wave plate; PBS, polarization beam splitter; M, mirror; AOM, acousto-optic modulator; BS, beam splitter; QWP, quarter-wave plate.

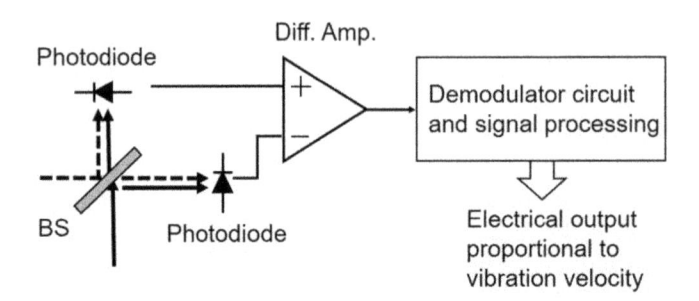

Figure 3.29. Balanced detection of the beat signal.

and experiences a Doppler shift Δf because of the target velocity. The rotation direction of the circular polarization is inverted when the light is reflected by the target, and the reflected light is converted to a linear polarization perpendicular to the incident light by the same QWP. The reflected light is deflected by the PBS and combined with the reference light using a beam splitter (BS). The beat signal of $f_B - \Delta f$ is observed using a photodiode. In practice, a balanced photoreceiver is commonly utilized, as shown in figure 3.29, wherein a pair of photodiodes with identical characteristics and a differential amplifier are installed. The electrical output of the heterodyne interferometer is a radio-wave signal with a carrier frequency of f_B (= 40–200 MHz) modulated by frequency or phase. Various demodulator circuits that are common in radio communications can be applied to retrieve the vibration component from the signal. A phase-locked loop or a quadrature detector is often used in classical analog circuits; direct digital demodulation is applied in some modern LDV systems.

Here, we demonstrate examples of two-dimensional distributions of out-of-plane vibrations. A disk transducer made of piezoelectric ceramics is used as the test sample. One side of the disk is a full electrode, while the other side has a smaller electrode, as shown in figure 3.30. The thickness is adjusted to approximately 1.3 mm to resonate at around 1.68 MHz in the thickness mode; the diameter is

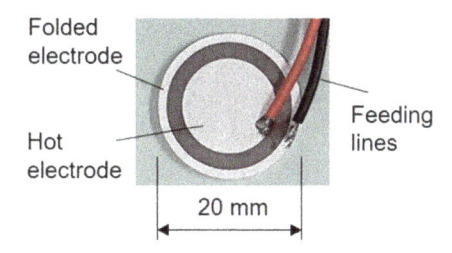

Figure 3.30. Bottom view of a sample transducer: a 1.6 MHz piezoelectric ceramic disk.

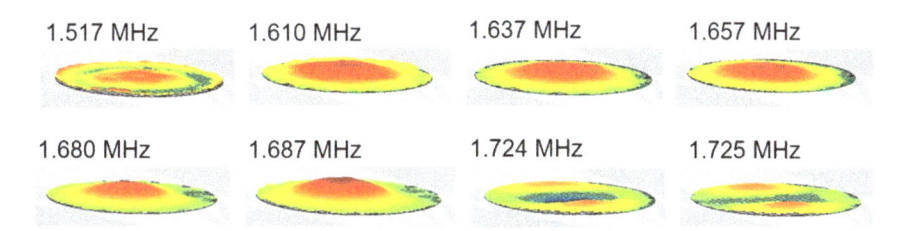

Figure 3.31. Vibration distributions of the disk transducer shown in figure 3.30 measured using scanning LDV (video of the vibration at 1.687 MHz is available at https://doi.org/10.1088/978-0-7503-4936-9).

20 mm. The vibration distribution is obtained using a scanning LDV system. The results for different frequencies are shown in figure 3.31. The vibration amplitude at the peripheral part is suppressed at the frequency around the thickness resonance because of the reduced diameter of the hot electrode on the back surface. Vibration in the radial direction is relatively suppressed when compared to a disk transducer with a full electrode on both sides. However, higher radial modes are excited if the frequency deviates by 3%–9% from the major resonance. A small region on the right edge exhibits little vibration, even at the main resonant frequency. This is believed to be the result of the loading effect of the solder on the back. Synchronization between all the measurement points should be carefully guaranteed by triggering the recording of the temporal waveform using the driving voltage or current of the transducer under test in order to obtain the vibration distribution in this manner.

3.2.2 In-plane vibration

The basic LDV system is sensitive to the velocity component parallel to the measuring light, and it is used to measure out-of-plane vibration. However, we encounter scenarios wherein observation is possible only from the side or when the vibration is originally transverse. Therefore, we must use the in-plane configuration of the LDV system. Two light beams with and without a frequency shift produced by an AOM illuminate the sample surface at an identical angle θ, as illustrated in figure 3.32. The backscattered light is observed through a lens using a photodiode. The electrical output of the photodiode contains the beat signal composed of the shift frequency of the AOM and the Doppler shift, which is similar to that for the out-of-plane case. Considering the directions of the illuminating light beams A and

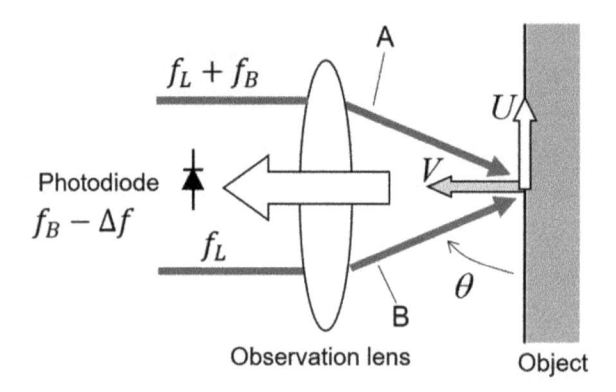

Figure 3.32. Optical setup for in-plane LDV.

B in the figure and the vibration velocity components U and V, the Doppler shift in A is proportional to

$$V \sin \theta + U \cos \theta, \qquad (3.28)$$

and that in B is proportional to

$$V \sin \theta - U \cos \theta. \qquad (3.29)$$

Here, the vibration velocities U and V are components parallel and perpendicular to the object surface, respectively. Only the in-plane (horizontal) component survives, because the output of the photodiode becomes an electrical signal representing the frequency difference between two light beams owing to optical interference; the out-of-plane (vertical) component vanishes. This can be understood if we recall the derivation of the Doppler signal in out-of-plane LDV.

The setup shown in figure 3.32 is intrinsically insensitive to out-of-plane vibration and provides a true in-plane measurement. However, a combination of two or three out-of-plane LDVs targeting the object from different angles can provide both vertical and parallel components via a vector decomposition calculation performed in post-processing. This technique is utilized in a three-dimensional scanning LDV system.

3.2.3 Fringe-counting method for high-amplitude vibration

In industrial applications of power ultrasonic vibrations at less than 100 kHz, such as welding, cutting, bending, homogenizing, and chemical reactions, vibration displacement amplitudes of several tens of micrometers are required. A heterodyne LDV is still an effective and precise tool for measuring such high-amplitude ultrasonic vibrations; however, the use of an AOM and a complicated optical system makes it difficult to reduce the cost. A fringe-counting method that uses a simple interferometer is a cost-effective alternative for measuring high-amplitude vibrations [25, 26].

Let us recall the interferogram of a homodyne interferometer (figure 3.25) and modify it for a wider range of displacements, as shown in figure 3.33. One cycle of the fringe is half of the optical wavelength, and it is equal to 0.316 μm in the case of the He–Ne red laser for the Michelson interferometer shown in figure 3.24. A train of fringes is read out for one cycle of the vibration when the object vibrates with an amplitude much greater than 0.316 μm. The vibration scans the interferogram twice (upward and downward) for one cycle of vibration because the vibration is a round-trip displacement. The output signal of the photodiode is [26]

$$i \propto \cos 2\pi \left(\frac{2u}{\lambda} \cos 2\pi f_V t + \varphi \right). \qquad (3.30)$$

Here, the peak-to-peak displacement of the vibration is $2u$, and the phase determined by the path difference is φ. Figure 3.34 demonstrates a simulated fringe pattern read out for a sinusoidal vibration of 2.50 μm in peak-to-peak displacement. The peak-to-peak displacement is estimated by counting the fringes for one

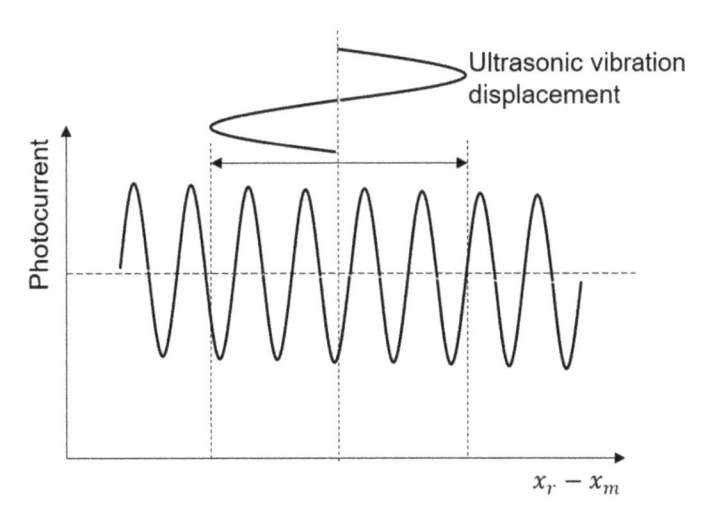

Figure 3.33. The operation of fringe counting, which is used to measure high-amplitude vibration.

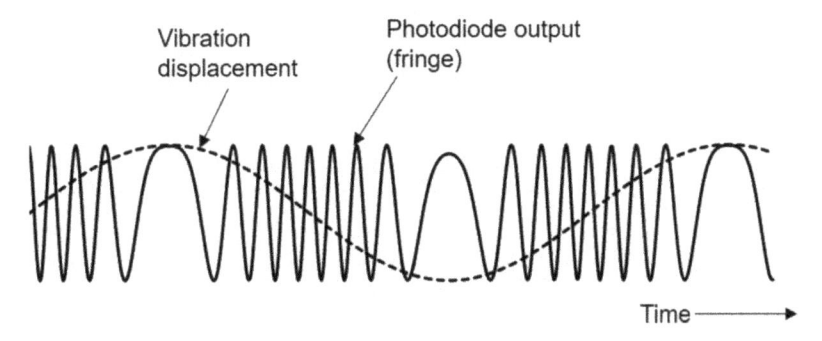

Figure 3.34. Simulated fringe train and vibration displacement.

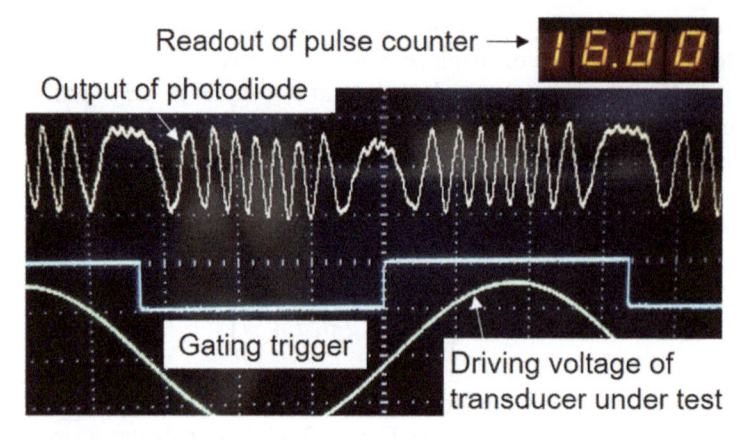

Figure 3.35. Examples of an interferometric signal, the driving voltage of the transducer under test, and the gating trigger signal used for the pulse counter.

cycle of vibration, which gives a value of 2.53 µm. Therefore, it is possible to quantitatively measure the vibration displacement amplitude of industrial ultrasonic transducers using a simple interferometer and a pulse counter gated by a signal synchronized to the ultrasonic vibration under test. A high-stability light source is unnecessary because the counting of fringes is performed for every cycle of the ultrasonic vibration; this means that a slow drift in the phase φ has little influence on the result. The resolution of the peak-to-peak displacement measurement is a quarter of the light wavelength, and it can easily be improved by a factor of two or more by counting the fringes for several cycles of ultrasonic vibration and taking the average. Figure 3.35 shows an example of the observed waveforms and the resultant fringe count. A photodiode with a sufficient response speed is required because the frequency of the fringe pulse reaches 10 MHz, even when the frequency of the vibration under test is less than 100 kHz. For example, a vibration displacement amplitude of 30 µm at 40 kHz results in a fringe train frequency of 7.8 MHz.

3.2.4 Sagnac interferometer for very-high-frequency vibration

Piezoelectric ultrasonic devices for communication and sensors [27–29] such as crystal resonators, film-bulk-acoustic resonators, and surface-acoustic-wave filters are operated at very high frequencies up to the GHz range. However, the maximum applicable frequency of the heterodyne LDV is limited to less than several tens of megahertz because of the beat frequency obtained using the AOM. The vibration amplitude of these devices is on the order of nanometers or picometers; therefore, the fringe-counting technique is not applicable. The homodyne interferometer can be potentially applied to very high frequencies and small displacements, provided the frequency response of the photodiode is guaranteed. However, the stabilization

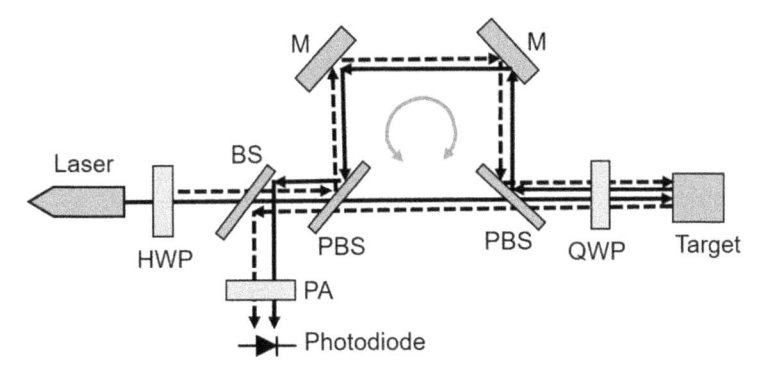

Figure 3.36. Basic configuration of a Sagnac interferometer used to measure very-high-frequency vibration. The solid line represents a counterclockwise path, and the dotted line indicates a clockwise one. HWP, half-wave plate; BS, beam splitter; PBS, polarization beam splitter; M, mirror; QWP, quarter-wave plate; PA, polarization analyzer. © [2011] IEEE. Reprinted, with permission, from [30].

of the operation point against low-frequency disturbance requires further development. The Sagnac interferometer, which is expected to be intrinsically insensitive to low-frequency fluctuations, is a candidate for solving this problem. An optical setup used to explain this principle is illustrated in figure 3.36. The Sagnac method for very-high-frequency ultrasonic devices was studied by Hashimoto *et al* [30] and further improved by his group [31]. The light is divided into a counterclockwise path and a clockwise path using two PBSs and a QWP. Both lights reach the target; however, the former hits the target earlier than the latter by a short time difference. Finally, the lights are combined by a BS and a polarization analyzer (PA) so that the photodiode can observe the interference. The sensitivity is maximized at the vibration frequency corresponding to the time difference generated by the Sagnac loop. The path difference in the Sagnac interferometer is theoretically zero; thus, the sensitivity to unwanted low-frequency vibrations and external turbulence can be suppressed. A low-coherence light source with a moderate power is applicable to this system.

3.3 Conclusions and outlook

Fiber-optic thin probes are useful for measuring ultrasonic fields in air and in water; they are especially effective for the measurement of standing waves with short wavelengths. Air-gap Fabry–Pérot sensors for airborne ultrasound have also been widely investigated for in-air measurements, which we could not include in this chapter. Many of these studies utilized a membrane as the end reflector [32] to enhance the sensitivity. It is necessary to select the right principle among these in order to obtain the required ranges of frequency and sensitivity. The sensitivity of the membrane-based structures is generally high, but they have the drawback of limited frequency responses due to the mechanical resonance of the membrane. The modulation of the refractivity of the air resonator can be employed as a sensing part by using a rigid end reflector instead of a membrane.

Two-dimensional ultrasonic fields can be visualized using a scanning laser Doppler velocimeter through the modulation of the refractive indices of media. However, the visualization process takes a considerable time due to the mechanical scanning of the laser ray. Simultaneous visualization of a two-dimensional sound field distributed over a finite area was demonstrated utilizing a bulk interferometer and computation [33–35]; this can be applied to ultrasonic fields.

LDV is a versatile tool for measuring ultrasonic vibrations and is widely used in many practical applications. Cost-effective and compact LDV configurations are required for high-speed multipoint measurement. Some commercial LDVs utilize semiconductor lasers to replace bulky gas lasers, although precise control of the driving current and temperature of the semiconductor laser is essential. Elimination of the AOM in heterodyne systems is also key to reducing the cost and volume of LDVs.

References

[1] Stardenraus J and Eisenmenger W 1993 Fibre-optic probe hydrophone for ultrasonic and shock-wave measurements in water *Ultrasonics* **31** 267–73

[2] Takei H, Hasegawa T, Nakamura K and Ueha S 2007 Measurement of intense ultrasound field in air using fiber optic probe *Jpn. J. Appl. Phys.* **46** 4555–8

[3] Adler L and Hiedemann E A 1962 Determination of the nonlinearity parameter B/A for water and m-xylene *J. Acoust. Soc. Am.* **34** 410–5

[4] Hurrell A and Beard P 2012 *Ultrasonic Transducers* ed K Nakamura (Oxford: Woodhead) 641–76

[5] Lewin P A, Mu C, Umchid S, Daryoush A and El-Sherif M 2005 Acousto-optic point receiver hydrophone probe for operation up to 100 MHz *Ultrasonics* **43** 815–21

[6] Uno Y and Nakamura K 1998 Fabrication and performance of a fiber optic micro-probe for megahertz ultrasonic field measurements *Trans. IEE Jpn. (E)* **118-E** 487–92

[7] Beard P C and Mill T N 1997 Miniature optical fibre ultrasonic hydrophone using a Fabry–Pérot polymer film interferometer *Electron. Lett.* **33** 801–3

[8] Dorighi J F, Krishnswamy S and Achenbach J D 1995 Stabilization of an embedded fiber optic Fabry–Pérot sensor for ultrasound detection *IEEE Trans. Ultrason., Ferroelect., Freq. Contr.* **42** 820–4

[9] Nakamura K and Nimura K 2000 Measurements of ultrasonic field and temperature by a fiber optic micro-probe *J. Acoust. Soc. Jpn. (E)* **21** 267–9

[10] Uno Y and Nakamura K 1999 Pressure sensitivity of a fiber-optic microprobe for high frequency ultrasonic field *Jpn. J. Appl. Phys.* **38** 3120–3

[11] Beard P C, Hurrell A M and Mills T N 2000 Characterization of a polymer film optical fiber hydrophone for use in the range 1 to 20 MHz: a comparison with PVDF needle and membrane hydrophones *IEEE Trans. Ultrason., Ferroelect., Freq. Contr.* **47** 256–64

[12] Rao Y-J 1997 In-fibre Bragg grating sensors *Meas. Sci. Technol.* **8** 355–75

[13] Takahashi N, Hirose A and Takahashi S 1997 Underwater acoustic sensor with fiber Bragg grating *Opt. Rev.* **4** 691–4

[14] Uno Y and Nakamura K 1998 A fiber optic micro-probe array with wavelength-division-multiplexing technique for ultrasonic field measurements *1998 IEEE Ultrasonics Symp.* vol 2 1273–6 (Cat. No. 98CH36102)

[15] Hijikata Y and Nakamura K 2000 Wavelength-division-multiplexing in fiber-optic micro-probe array for high frequency ultrasonic field measurements *IEICE Trans. Electron.* **E83-C** 293–7

[16] Kashyap R 1999 *Fiber Bragg Gratings* (San Diego, CA: Academic)

[17] Sano Y and Yoshino T Fast optical wavelength interrogator employing arrayed waveguide grating for distributed fiber Bragg grating sensors *J. Lightwave Technol.* **21** 132–9

[18] Fujisue T, Nakamura K and Ueha S 2006 Demodulation of acoustic signals in fiber Bragg grating ultrasonic sensors using arrayed waveguide gratings *Jpn. J. Appl. Phys.* **45** 4577

[19] Kudo N 2015 Optical methods for visualization of ultrasound fields *Jpn. J. Appl. Phys.* **54** 07HA01

[20] Yamamoto K 2012 *Ultrasonic Transducers* ed K Nakamura ed (Oxford: Woodhead))

[21] Hasegawa T and Yoshioka K 1969 Acoustic-radiation force on a solid elastic sphere *J. Acoust. Soc. Am.* **46** 1139–45

[22] Nakamura K, Hirayama M and Ueha S 2002 Measurements of air-borne ultrasound by detecting the modulation in optical refractive index of air *2002 IEEE Ultrasonics Symp., 2002* vol 1 609–12

[23] Ikeda Y, Okamoto N, Konishi T, Oikawa Y, Tokita Y and Yamasaki Y 2016 Observation of traveling wave with laser tomography *Acoust. Sci. Technol.* **37** 231–8

[24] Uchida N and Niizeki N 1973 Acoustooptic deflection materials and techniques *Proc. IEEE* **61** 1073–92

[25] Ueha S, Nakamura T and Mori E 1983 Vibration amplitude measurement using a fringe-counting technique *Ultrasonics* **21** 41–2

[26] Nakamura K 2018 Optical interferometric measurement of vibration amplitude in high power ultrasonic tool through vibration-synchronized fringe counting *Symp. Ultrasonic Electronics* 39 1P4-9

[27] Kakio S 2021 High-performance surface acoustic wave devices using composite substrate structures *Jpn. J. Appl. Phys.* **60** SD0802

[28] Yanagitani T and Takayanagi S 2021 Polarization control of ScAlN, ZnO and PbTiO$_3$ piezoelectric films: application to polarization-inverted multilayer bulk acoustic wave and surface acoustic wave devices *Jpn. J. Appl. Phys.* **60** SD0803

[29] Kondoh J 2018 Nonlinear acoustic phenomena caused by surface acoustic wave and its application to digital microfluidic system *Jpn. J. Appl. Phys.* **57** 07LA01

[30] Hashimoto *et al* 2011 A laser probe based on a Sagnac interferometer with fast mechanical scan for RF surface and bulk acoustic wave devices *IEEE Trans., Ultrason. Ferroelec. Freq. Contr.* **58** 187–94

[31] Takahashi H, Omori T and Hashimoto K 2021 Development of high-speed and phase-sensitive laser probe system for RF SAW/BAW devices with absolute vibration amplitude measurement function *Jpn. J. Appl. Phys.* **60** SDDC10

[32] Zhang W, Lu P, Ni W, Xiong W, Liu D and Zhang J 2020 Gold-diaphragm based Fabry–Perot ultrasonic sensor for partial discharge detection and localization *IEEE Photon. J.* **12** 6801612

[33] Ishikawa K, Yatabe K and Oikawa Y 2020 Seeing the sound of castanets: acoustic resonances between shells captured by high-speed optical visualization with 1-mm resolution *J. Acoust. Soc. Am.* **148** 3171–80
[34] Tanigawa R, Yatabe K and Oikawa Y 2020 Experimental visualization of aerodynamic sound sources using parallel phase-shifting interferometry *Exp. Fluids* **61** 206
[35] Ishikawa K, Yatabe K and Oikawa Y 2021 Physical-model-based reconstruction of axisymmetric three-dimensional sound field from optical interferometric measurement *Meas. Sci. Technol.* **32** 045202

IOP Publishing

Ultrasonics
Physics and applications
Mami Matsukawa, Pak-Kon Choi, Kentaro Nakamura, Hirotsugu Ogi and Hideyuki Hasegawa

Chapter 4

Picosecond laser ultrasonics

Osamu Matsuda and Oliver B Wright

The absorption of picosecond light pulses by a medium can generate gigahertz to terahertz acoustic waves, whose propagation can be monitored by appropriately timed light pulses. This technique, known as picosecond laser ultrasonics, can be used to study the physical properties of nanoscale structures. In this chapter, we discuss the basics of this technique and recent applications involving nanoscale gratings.

4.1 Introduction

To observe and evaluate microscale and nanoscale samples using acoustic waves, one should use a wavelength comparable to or shorter than the length scale of the sample structure. For materials with a sound velocity in the kilometers per second region this corresponds to acoustic waves with frequencies of gigahertz to terahertz order. One method for the generation and detection of such high-frequency acoustic waves is by the use of ultrashort light pulses.

The propagation of laser-generated acoustic waves can be monitored in the time domain by means of delayed light pulses using transient optical reflectivity changes caused by the spatiotemporally varying acoustic field. This measurement technique is an example of the optical pump–probe method: pump-light pulses generate acoustic waves and probe-light pulses are used for transient optical reflectivity measurements. This allows one to evaluate not only the structure and sound velocity of the target sample on a nanometer scale, but also its physical properties such as elasticity, sound absorption, and optical properties as well as transient phenomena such as the ultrafast dynamics of excited electrons. This technique is termed picosecond laser ultrasonics [1, 2].

Using generated longitudinal waves, this technique has been used to study the properties of metals [2–28], semiconductors [1, 2, 29–40], and dielectrics [1, 3, 41–53] in the bulk or in monolayer/multilayer films. It has also been applied to micro/nano structures [54–63] and interfaces [21, 64–66], including quantum wells and superlattices [67–83], biological cells [84–88], quasi-crystals [89], magnetic materials [90–95], multiferroics [96, 97], and materials in which transient spins can be generated [98]. Such measurements have been extended to the high-pressure regime [89, 99–101]. In addition, it has been shown that shear waves can be effectively generated and detected using picosecond laser ultrasonics [10, 14, 16, 20, 23, 25, 27, 28, 37, 77, 102, 103]. Applications also exist in the field of depth profiling [104–106]. This technique has moreover been shown to work for liquids [107–111]. Another important application is in bio-sensing [112–114].

In this chapter, we first discuss the basics of picosecond laser ultrasonics and then some recent applications to metal gratings on transparent substrates, including the generation and detection of shear waves.

4.2 Basics of picosecond laser ultrasonics

4.2.1 Overview

Figure 4.1 schematically shows the stages of a typical picosecond laser ultrasonics measurement. As an example, we choose a thin opaque metal film of submicron thickness deposited on a flat substrate. The film is irradiated by a focused pump-light pulse (figure 4.1(a)). The photon energy is absorbed by the electrons of the film material, and thereafter (within a few picoseconds) this energy is converted to heat. This brings about a quasi-instantaneous temperature rise and sets up a localized thermal stress in the vicinity of the sample surface (figure 4.1(b)). The spatiotemporal variation of the stress launches a strain pulse that propagates in the depth direction (figure 4.1(c)). A static strain distribution is left behind, together with a surface displacement. Part of the propagating strain pulse is reflected at the film/substrate interface and then returns to the surface. The strain field in the sample in

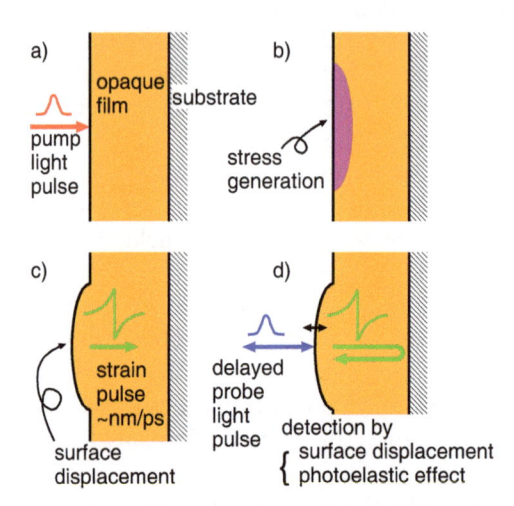

Figure 4.1. Steps in a picosecond laser ultrasonics measurement. (a) Absorption of a pump-light pulse by an opaque thin film. (b) Stress generation by the absorbed light energy. (c) Launching an acoustic strain pulse in the depth direction. (d) Detection of the returning acoustic strain pulse by a delayed probe-light pulse through transient optical reflectivity measurements.

general will modulate the (optical) permittivity through the photoelastic effect: this occurs when the returning acoustic pulse reaches the vicinity of the sample surface, i.e., within the penetration depth of the probe light. This transient modulation can be detected by delayed probe-light pulses as a function of the delay time between the pump- and probe-light pulse arrivals at the sample surface (figure 4.1(d)). Visible, infrared or ultraviolet light can be used for the pump- and probe-light pulses, which typically have at a repetition rate of around 80 MHz. The pump beam is modulated at a low megahertz frequency to allow lock-in detection of the probe intensity, as described in further detail below.

The pump and probe light are usually tightly focused on the sample surface with a spot diameter of ~1–50 μm. The depth of the initial induced mechanical stress is related to the optical penetration depth of the pump light, and is often in the range of 10–100 nm. The propagation depth of the generated acoustic pulses is normally in the submicron range, and is usually smaller than the acoustic Rayleigh length W^2/Λ for acoustic diffraction, where W is the pump-spot diameter and Λ the (usually micron to submicron) acoustic wavelength. A similar argument applies to the probe light, whose optical Rayleigh length is similar to that of the acoustic waves. These conditions imply that little acoustic and optical diffraction occur over the course of the measurements, and thus allow us to simplify the problem to a quasi one-dimensional one in which all the relevant physical quantities, such as temperature increase, stress, strain, light field, etc. depend only on the depth.

Figure 4.2 shows a typical experimental result. The sample is a Cr film with a thickness of 190 nm deposited on a Si (100) substrate [13]. Acoustic pulses are excited in the Cr film's near-surface region by pump-light pulses with a wavelength of 415 nm and a duration of <1 ps at zero pump–probe delay time. The transient optical reflectivity change is monitored by probe-light pulses with a wavelength of 830 nm and a duration of <1 ps by varying the delay time from zero to >150 ps.

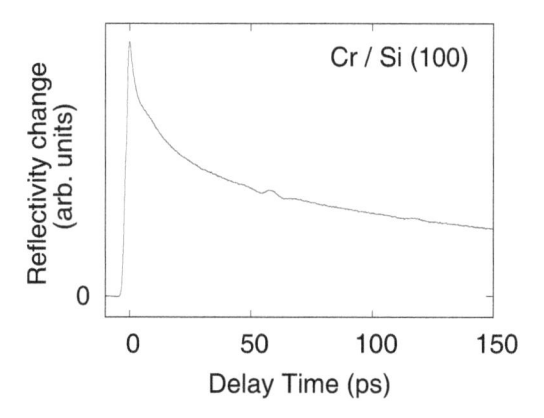

Figure 4.2. Typical experimental transient reflectivity change versus delay time in a picosecond laser ultrasonics measurement of an opaque thin film. The sample is a Cr film that has a thickness of 190 nm deposited on a Si (100) substrate. Adapted with permission from [13], Copyright (2022) by the American Physical Society.

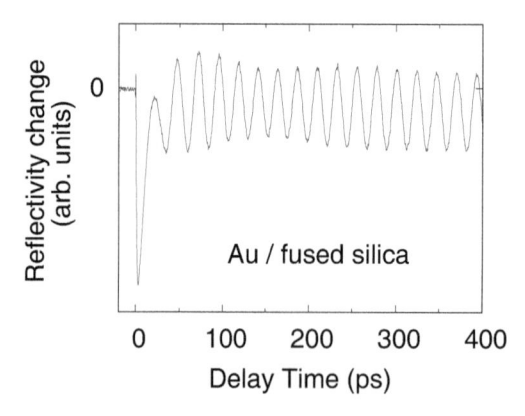

Figure 4.3. Typical experimental transient reflectivity change versus delay time in a picosecond laser ultrasonics measurement involving Brillouin oscillations. The sample is an Au film that has a thickness of 50 nm deposited on a fused silica substrate. The measurement performed from the rear side of the sample.

Propagating acoustic pulses are partially reflected at the Cr–Si interface and return to the surface. The first return to the surface is observed at ~60 ps as a small echo. The acoustic pulse is further reflected at the surface, and gives rise to a second return which is visible as a smaller echo at ~120 ps. From such measurements, one may evaluate the film thickness if the sound velocity is known, or vice versa.

If the sample is transparent or semi-transparent to the probe light, the measured transient reflectivity change becomes very different from that of an opaque substrate. Figure 4.3 shows an example corresponding to an Au film that has a thickness of 50 nm deposited on a fused silica substrate. The measurement is performed from the rear side of the sample (the side without the Au film) using pump- and probe-light wavelengths of 395 and 790 nm, respectively. Acoustic pulses are generated in the Au film, and are transmitted to the substrate. The relatively long-lasting single-frequency signal is known as a Brillouin oscillation. This arises because of the interference between the probe light reflected by the Au/substrate interface and the light reflected (i.e. scattered) by the propagating acoustic pulse in the fused silica substrate. Since the acoustic pulse moves at the speed of sound, constructive and destructive interference conditions periodically arise, leading to oscillations that have a period equal to half the optical wavelength in fused silica divided by the speed of sound. From this measurement one can evaluate the sound velocity if the refractive index of the medium is known, or vice versa. Simultaneous determination of the sound velocity and the refractive index is also possible using a method explained later in this chapter.

4.2.2 Basic experimental setup

Figure 4.4 shows a basic experimental setup. The light source is a mode-locked Ti–sapphire laser which generates light pulses with a central wavelength of 830 nm, a duration of <200 fs, a repetition rate of 80 MHz, and a beam power of >500 mW. An optical second-harmonic generation crystal is used to obtain frequency-doubled light pulses that have a wavelength of 415 (=830/2) nm. The 415 and 830 nm beams

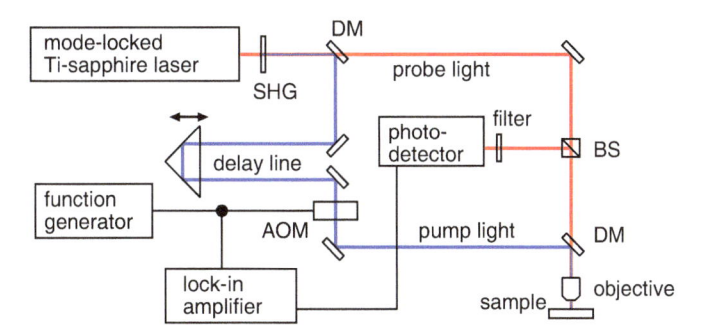

Figure 4.4. Schematic diagram of a basic experimental setup for picosecond laser ultrasonic measurements. SHG: second-harmonic-generation crystal, DM: dichroic mirror, BS: beam splitter, AOM: acousto-optic modulator.

are used as the pump and probe beams, respectively. Dichroic mirrors (DMs) which reflect 415 nm light and transmit 830 nm light are used to split or merge the pump- and probe-light beams. The pump light passes through a delay line, which is a motorized stage equipped with an optical reflector, to control the delay time between the pump and probe arrivals at the sample. Using a microscope objective, the pump- and probe-light beams are focused at the same point on the sample's surface. The probe light reflected from the sample, after a second pass through the microscope objective, is fed to a photodetector by means of a beam splitter (BS).

Since the photoelastic modulation in the optical reflectivity is usually very small (typically corresponding to a fraction 10^{-4}–10^{-6} of the overall reflected probe-light intensity), a modulation technique is commonly used, as noted above: the pump-light pulse train is chopped by an acousto-optic modulator (AOM) at a frequency ~1 MHz, and the modulated reflected probe light is detected by a lock-in amplifier. To avoid contamination of the photodetector output by the modulated pump light, one can use different wavelengths for the pump and probe light, and thereby eliminate any pump-light contamination using a probe-pass/pump-cut optical filter placed in front of the photodetector (a technique known as the two-color method).

It is also possible instead to use, for example, 830 nm light for the pump and 415 nm light for the probe by replacing the optical components appropriately. The optimal choice depends on the target sample, and should be based on a knowledge of the wavelength dependence of the acoustic generation and optical detection efficiencies.

4.2.3 Interferometric setup

Apart from the photoelastic effect, another detection mechanism for picosecond acoustic pulses is to monitor the surface or interface displacements. Surface displacements alter the optical path length of the reflected probe light, and thus its optical phase. To perform such phase detection, one can use an optical interferometer, which converts a phase difference to an optical intensity variation. Several different types of interferometer have been proposed: Mach-Zender [6], Sagnac [7, 9] and Michelson [8, 17, 115], for example. Alternatively, use can be made

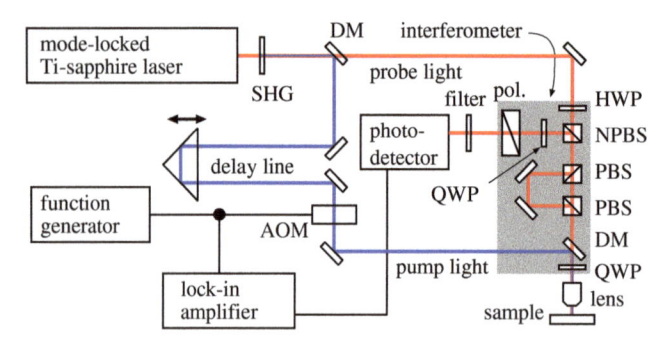

Figure 4.5. Schematic diagram of an interferometric setup used for picosecond laser ultrasonic measurements. The gray shaded zone represents the interferometer. SHG: second-harmonic-generation crystal, DM: dichroic mirror, PBS: polarizing beam splitter, NPBS: non-polarizing beam splitter, AOM: acousto-optic modulator, HWP: half-wave plate, QWP: quarter-wave plate.

of birefringent crystals [116], conoscopic interferometry [117] or probe-beam deflection [118].

Figure 4.5 shows a typical setup using a Sagnac-type interferometer, denoted by the shaded region of figure [7]. A probe pulse entering the interferometer is split into two pulses, temporally separated by 100 ps–1 ns, using straight and detour paths between two polarizing beam splitters (PBSs). The pulse that traverses the former path reaches the sample before the pump-light pulse arrival, whereas the pulse that traverses the latter path reaches the sample after that time. The reflected pulses traverse the straight and detour paths oppositely, and are thus merged into a single pulse. In this way these before-pump and after-pump probe-light pulses interfere, thereby converting the optical phase difference between the two pulses into an intensity variation. To maximize the detection sensitivity, a static phase change of $\pi/2$ is given to one of the two probe pulses. Further details of the interferometer can be found elsewhere [7].

The presence of a positive transient strain of $\sim 10^{-4}$ at the surface of the sample causes the surface to protrude by a tiny distance ζ, typically ~ 10 pm. For optical incidence from the air (or vacuum), the optical path length of the probe light is thus shortened by 2ζ, which introduces a phase advance of $2k\zeta$, where k is the wave number of the probe light in air. Assuming that an extra $\pi/2$ phase difference is introduced between the two probe pulses as described above, the intensity of the probe light is proportional to

$$\overline{|\cos(\omega t + \pi/2) + \cos(\omega t - 2k\zeta)|^2} = 1 - \sin(2k\zeta) \simeq 1 - 2k\zeta, \qquad (4.1)$$

where ω is the optical angular frequency and the overbar denotes a temporal average. The first term in the temporal average arises from the 'reference' probe beam reflected at the surface before the pump-light arrival, and is retarded by $\pi/2$. The second term arises from the 'signal' probe light reflected at the surface after the pump-light arrival, which experiences the surface displacement induced by the pump pulse. The use of the pump modulation technique allows a typical detection sensitivity of $k\zeta \sim 10^{-6}$ or $\zeta \lesssim 1$ pm (0.01 Å).

Here, we define the complex amplitude reflectance of the probe light $r = |r|\exp(i \arg r)$ to be the ratio of the complex electric field amplitudes for the incident and reflected light. Suppose that the reflectance is changed to $r' = r + \Delta r = (1 + \rho)|r|\exp[i(\arg r + \delta\phi)]$ by the transient strain. The amplitude ρ is related to the change in the magnitude of r, whereas the phase change $\delta\phi$ is related to the change in the phase of r. For $|\rho| \ll 1$ and $|\delta\phi| \ll 1$, r' can be written in the following approximate form:

$$r' = r(1 + \rho + i\delta\phi), \tag{4.2}$$

or

$$\frac{\Delta r}{r} = \rho + i\delta\phi. \tag{4.3}$$

The intensity reflectivity R and its modulated value $R' = R + \Delta R$ are related to r and ρ by

$$R = |r|^2,$$
$$\frac{\Delta R}{R} = 2\mathrm{Re}\left(\frac{\Delta r}{r}\right) = 2\rho. \tag{4.4}$$

As expected, ΔR does not depend on $\delta\phi$. Figure 4.6 shows the result of an interferometric measurement for the Cr film of figure 4.2. The temporal variation of the echo in ρ is as shown in figure 4.2. The temporal variation of $\delta\phi$ is larger than that of ρ in this case. The phase change $\delta\phi$ is related to both the surface displacement and the photoelastic effect (see reference [13] for a detailed discussion). By a detailed analysis of the echo shapes, one may obtain information about the ultrafast relaxation of photoexcited electrons in the Cr film and the ultrasonic absorption in the GHz frequency range [13].

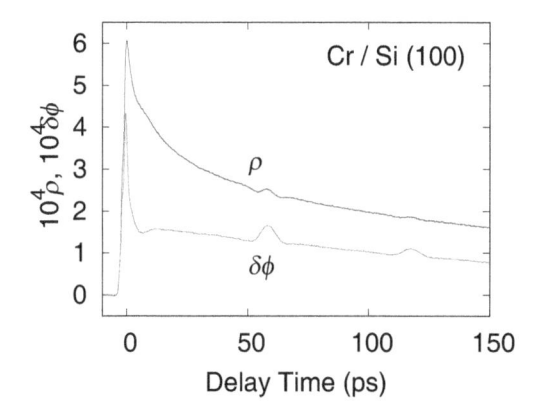

Figure 4.6. Typical experimental transient complex reflectance changes versus delay time in a picosecond laser ultrasonics measurement. The sample is a Cr film that has a thickness of 190 nm deposited on Si (100) substrate. Adapted with permission from [13], Copyright (2022) by the American Physical Society.

4.2.4 One-dimensional model

We now discuss the basic analysis of picosecond laser ultrasonics measurements. It is pertinent to model the excitation, propagation, and optical detection of acoustic waves using a theory based on a knowledge of material and geometrical parameters. Fitting to experimental results always requires one to derive unknown parameters.

Consider the example of a nanoscale multilayer sample [46]. Each layer, including the substrate, is assumed to be isotropic. Both the pump and the probe light are normally incident on the sample via air (or vacuum). As in section 4.2.1, we make use of a one-dimensional approach in the depth (z) direction.

Because of the isotropic nature of the sample and the symmetry of the excitation by the focused pump light, one expects only longitudinal acoustic waves to propagate in the z direction. We take the source of the acoustic wave generation to be thermal stress, although various other mechanisms for stress generation exist [119, 120]. The corresponding acoustic wave equation is given by

$$\rho_0 \frac{\partial^2 u_z}{\partial t^2} = \frac{\partial \sigma_{zz}}{\partial z},$$
$$\sigma_{zz} = c_{11}\eta_{zz} - (c_{11} + 2c_{12})\beta\Delta T$$
$$= 3\frac{1-\nu}{1+\nu}B\eta_{zz} - 3B\beta\Delta T, \qquad (4.5)$$
$$\eta_{zz} = \frac{\partial u_z}{\partial z},$$

where ρ_0 is the mass density, u_z the displacement in z, σ_{zz} the appropriate stress component, η_{zz} the corresponding strain component, c_{11} and c_{12} the elastic tensor components, β the linear thermal expansion coefficient, ΔT the temperature rise, ν Poisson's ratio, and B the bulk modulus. The quantities $u_z, \sigma_{zz}, \eta_{zz}$ as well as ΔT are functions of z and t. The material parameters $\rho_0, c_{11}, c_{12}, \beta, \nu, B$ are spatially characterized by step functions in z, being constant within each layer. Assuming a functional form for ΔT, e.g., that arising from the absorbed energy of the pump-light pulse and the corresponding temperature rise in each layer, the spatiotemporal evolutions of u_z and η_{zz} can be calculated from the above acoustic wave equation.

The optical detection of the acoustic waves relies on the photoelastic effect, i.e., the modulation of the permittivity by the strain, and on the surface or interface displacements. The latter can also be regarded as a modulation of the permittivity distribution caused by the motion of the thin-film boundaries. To find the modulation in the reflected probe light, the electromagnetic wave equation needs to be solved for the given permittivity modulation in space and time. The temporal modulation of the permittivity is, in general, much slower than the optical oscillation, and thus the former can be regarded as quasi-static.

For normally incident linearly polarized monochromatic light (polarized along the x-axis), the non-perturbed electromagnetic wave equation can be simplified to a Helmholtz equation:

$$\left[\frac{\partial^2}{\partial z^2} + k^2\varepsilon\right]E_{0x}(z) = 0, \tag{4.6}$$

where k is the wave number of the probe light in vacuum ($c = \omega/k$ is the speed of light in vacuum). The common time dependence $\exp(-i\omega t)$ is omitted. The relative permittivity ε is a step-like function of z, being constant within each layer. Because each layer is isotropic, the light is x-polarized throughout the whole system. E_{0x}, a function of z, is the x component of the electric field, and involves the incident, reflected and transmitted light. Because of the translational symmetry in the x and y directions, the x and y wave vector components, which are zero in this case, are conserved, i.e., the light always propagates along the z-axis. E_{0x} can be expressed as a linear combination of plane waves using a transfer matrix method.

On modulation of the permittivity, the modulated electric field can be obtained by solving the perturbed equation

$$\left[\frac{\partial^2}{\partial z^2} + k^2(\varepsilon + \Delta\varepsilon(z))\right]E_x(z) = 0, \tag{4.7}$$

where $\Delta\varepsilon(z)$ is the permittivity modulation. This is expressed as

$$\Delta\varepsilon(z) = \Delta\varepsilon_{\text{pe}} + \Delta\varepsilon_{\text{if}}, \tag{4.8}$$

where $\Delta\varepsilon_{\text{pe}}$ is the photoelastic contribution and $\Delta\varepsilon_{\text{if}}$ is the surface or interface displacement contribution. The former is given by

$$\Delta\varepsilon_{\text{pe}} = P_{12}\eta_{zz}, \tag{4.9}$$

where P_{12} is a component of the layer-dependent photoelastic tensor. The latter term in equation (4.8) ($\Delta\varepsilon_{\text{if}}$) may take a nonzero value in the immediate vicinity of the surface or an interface, representing the replacement of the neighboring medium within the region of protrusion or contraction.

The solution for equation (4.7) can be written as an integral in the form

$$E_x(z) = E_{0x}(z) + \int_{-\infty}^{\infty} k^2 G(z, z')\Delta\varepsilon(z')E_x(z')dz', \tag{4.10}$$

using a Green's function $G(z, z')$, which satisfies

$$\left[\frac{\partial^2}{\partial z^2} + k^2\varepsilon\right]G(z, z') = -\delta(z - z'). \tag{4.11}$$

The iterative substitution of the expression for E_x from equation (4.10) for E_x in the integral on the right-hand side of this equation leads to an expansion of $E_x(z)$ in the form

$$\begin{aligned}E_x(z) \simeq{} &E_{0x}(z) + \int_{-\infty}^{\infty} k^2 G(z, z')\Delta\varepsilon(z')E_{0x}(z')dz' \\&+ \iint_{-\infty}^{\infty} k^4 G(z, z')\Delta\varepsilon(z')G(z', z'')\Delta\varepsilon(z'')E_{0x}(z'')dz'dz'' + \cdots.\end{aligned} \tag{4.12}$$

Since $\Delta\varepsilon_{pe}$ is much smaller than ε, or, alternatively, since the region of integration for $\Delta\varepsilon_{if}$ occupies a very short distance, an expansion up to the first order (i.e., up to the second term on the right-hand side of equation (4.12)) is normally sufficient. The reflected light component involved in $E_x(z)$ can be used to calculate the reflectivity for the intensity and the complex reflectance components.

Figure 4.7 shows experimental results for interferometric measurements at normal incidence from air on a thin multilayer sample (the curves labeled as expt.). The sample consists of an amorphous silica (a-SiO$_2$) layer (that has a thickness of ~1 μm) on a polycrystalline Cr layer (that has a thickness of ~100 nm), both deposited on a fused silica substrate. Long-lasting Brillouin oscillations are observed on a step-like background: the step at around 200 ps corresponds to the acoustic pulse generated in the Cr film reaching the sample surface, and the step at around 400 ps corresponds to the return of the acoustic pulse to the (buried) surface of the Cr film.

The results of theoretical simulations based on the model described above are also shown in figure 4.7 (the curves labeled as calc.). Good agreement between the experimental and simulated results is obtained after parameter fitting for the a-SiO$_2$ and Cr film thicknesses and photoelastic constants and for the a-SiO$_2$ longitudinal sound velocity.

The above light-scattering theory has been extended to handle probe light with arbitrary polarization and incident angles for the case of anisotropic multilayers [27]. It has been further extended to handle two- and three-dimensional inhomogeneities [121].

The theoretical simulation could be improved by considering a more realistic model of the optically induced acoustic wave generation. In general, the absorbed photon energy is first transferred to electrons, and their excess energy is then transferred to the lattice within ~1 ps. For some metals, such as Au, the electrons diffuse over relatively long distances, ~100 nm, before the energy is fully distributed to the whole system of electrons and lattice [4]. This process can be treated with a two-temperature model (TTM) in which the electrons and lattice are considered as

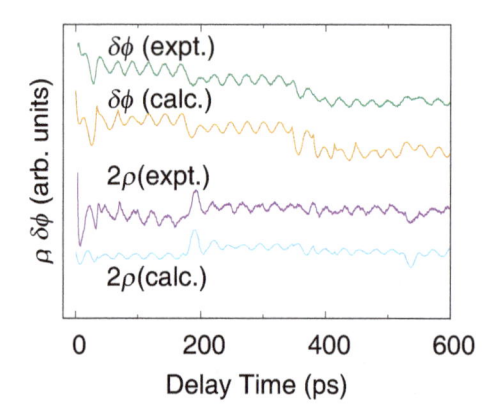

Figure 4.7. Experimental (expt.) and theoretical simulation (calc.) results for the complex transient reflectance changes versus delay time for an a-SiO$_2$/Cr/glass sample. Adapted with permission from [46], Copyright (2002) by The Optical Society.

systems with separate well-defined temperatures, having their own separate thermal diffusion processes and interacting with one another [122].

More details of the art of picosecond laser ultrasonics can be found in references [123, 124] and references therein.

4.3 Extensions of picosecond laser ultrasonics

In this section, we describe some recent developments in laser picosecond ultrasonics involving Brillouin oscillation measurements in transparent media coated with metallic gratings.

4.3.1 Time-resolved Brillouin-scattering measurements assisted by metallic gratings

As described in section 4.2.1, measurements on transparent media may show a single-frequency long-lasting Brillouin oscillation. For probe light normally incident on the sample surface, the interference between the light reflected at the surface and that reflected by the moving acoustic pulse becomes repeatedly constructive and destructive with a period of T:

$$2vT = \lambda/n, \tag{4.13}$$

or

$$f = \frac{1}{T} = \frac{2nv}{\lambda}, \tag{4.14}$$

where v is the sound velocity of the medium, λ the probe-light wavelength in vacuum, n the refractive index of the medium, and f the Brillouin oscillation frequency (see figure 4.8(a)), typically on the order of a few tens of gigahertz.

This can be interpreted in a more general way using the following steps: (1) the incident probe light is scattered by the phonons, so that the total momentum of the photons and phonons is conserved; (2) the scattered photon energy is increased or decreased (anti-Stokes and Stokes scattering, respectively) by the absorbed or created phonon energy; and (3) the beating of the scattered light and the non-scattered

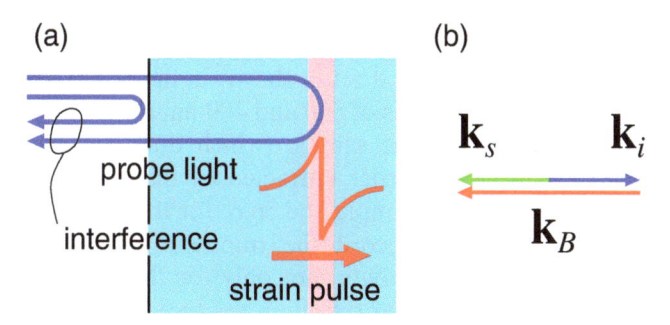

Figure 4.8. (a) An explanation of how Brillouin oscillations occur. (b) Schematic of the conservation of photon and phonon momenta in Brillouin scattering.

reflected light results in Brillouin oscillation. For normally incident and scattered light (wave vector parallel to z), momentum conservation is expressed as

$$k_{sz} = k_{iz} \pm k_{Bz}, \qquad (4.15)$$

where $k_{iz} = nk$ is the z component of the incident photon wave vector in the medium, k_{sz} the z component of the scattered photon wave vector in the medium, and k_{Bz} the z component of the absorbed (+ for ± on the right-hand side) or created (− for ± on the right-hand side) phonon wave vector (see figure 4.8(b)). Because the phonon energy is small compared to the photon energy, one can approximate the scattered photon wave number to be the same as the incident photon wave number, i.e., $k_{sz} \simeq -nk$:

$$2nk = |k_{Bz}|. \qquad (4.16)$$

Since the phonon angular frequency is given by $v|k_{Bz}|$, equation (4.16) is equivalent to equation (4.14).

A single measurement of a Brillouin oscillation with normally incident probe light leads to a temporal variation at the Brillouin oscillation frequency f. As shown in equation (4.14), this frequency is not sufficient to determine n and v simultaneously. To achieve this, one should perform additional measurements, for example, by using different probe-light incident angles. Although such measurements are possible, high focusing accuracy is required [104, 105].

However, such multiangle data can be obtained in a single measurement using a metallic grating structure fabricated on a transparent medium [62]. A proper analysis of the data allows one to determine the sound velocity and refractive index simultaneously. Several other picosecond laser ultrasonic studies for grating-like structures have been reported, but their main aims were different, e.g. measurement of the vibration of the structure itself [125] or the observation of buried structures [126, 127].

The sample used in reference [62] is a fused silica substrate that has a thickness of 1 mm coated with two Au grating structures fabricated by electron-beam lithography and lift-off techniques. The grating pitches are $p = 587$ and 479 nm, the grating thickness is 50 nm, and the nominal grating widths are 294 and 240 nm, respectively. A Cr film that has a thickness of 2 nm is used between the Au grating bars and the fused silica substrate to improve adhesion. Measurements are performed using a standard picosecond laser ultrasonics setup similar to that shown in figure 4.4 with the modified optical setup shown in figure 4.9. Pump and probe light that have respective wavelengths of 800 and 400 nm are focused on the grating structures from the rear side of the sample (which does not contain a grating structure). The probe light is first-order diffracted by the grating structure (to an angle of 42.8° for the $p = 587$ nm sample and 56.6° for the 479 nm sample), and is then fed to a photodetector to record the transient reflectivity changes. For convenience we use the term 'reflectivity' not only for the reflected light but also for the diffracted light. In fact, specular reflection produced by a grating corresponds to the zeroth diffraction order.

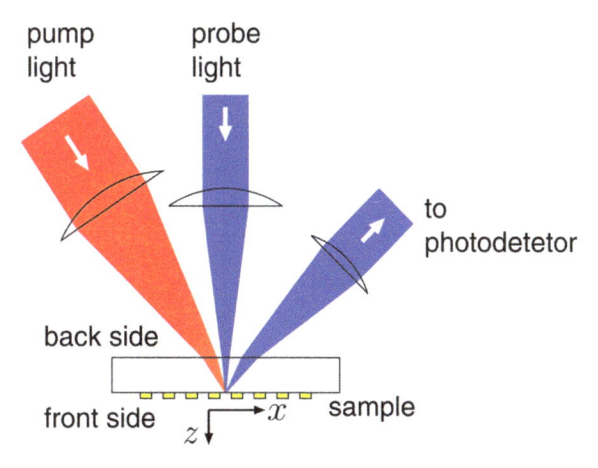

Figure 4.9. Setup used for transient reflectivity measurements for a sample consisting of an Au grating on fused silica. The probe light is normally incident on the sample from the rear side, and the first-order diffracted beam intensity is monitored. The incident probe light is linearly polarized along the grating bars (y direction). Adapted with permission from [62], Copyright (2018) by the American Physical Society.

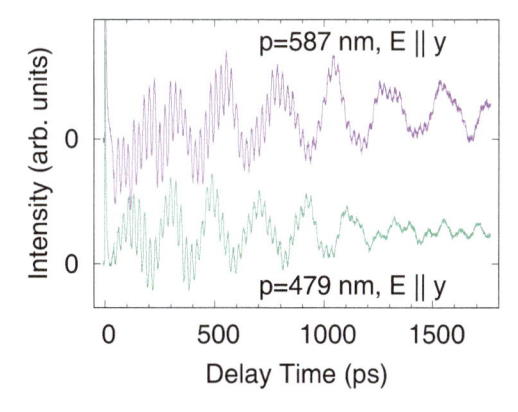

Figure 4.10. Transient reflectivity changes versus delay time for Au gratings on fused silica using rear-side normal-incidence probing with y polarization (along the bars) and detection of the first-order diffracted beam. Adapted with permission from [62], Copyright (2018) by the American Physical Society.

Figure 4.10 shows the raw transient reflectivity data for probe polarization along the grating bars (y direction). Unlike the simple single-frequency Brillouin oscillation of figure 4.3, data for both grating pitches show complicated long-lasting oscillations involving relatively low-frequency components at ~5 GHz and high-frequency components at ~50 GHz.

The modulus of the Fourier amplitude of the transient reflectivity is shown in figure 4.11. The frequency resolution is determined by the measured range of the delay times; in this case, the range is about 1500 ps, and thus the resolution is $1/1500 \text{ps}^{-1} \simeq 0.67$ GHz, which corresponds to the frequency step of figure 4.11. The maximum apparent Q factor is given by the product of the frequency of the peak in question and the range of the delay time, i.e. $Q \simeq 60$ for the peak at 40 GHz. The

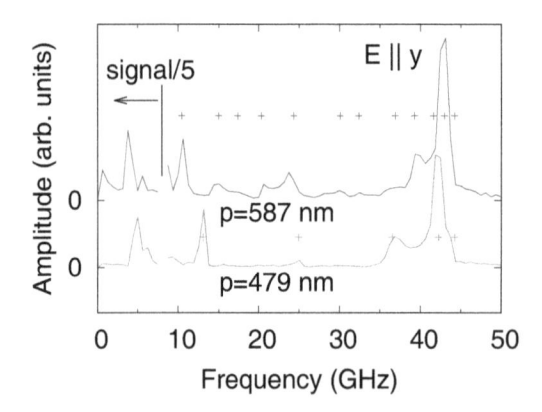

Figure 4.11. Modulus of the Fourier amplitude of the transient reflectivity versus frequency for Au gratings on fused silica. The + symbols indicate the expected peak positions based on the calculations described in the text. The vertical scale to the left of the vertical black line has been changed to reduce the signal in the region <10 GHz by a factor of five. Adapted with permission from [62], Copyright (2018) by the American Physical Society.

accuracy of the peak frequency is not necessarily equal to the frequency resolution. For a single frequency peak, a frequency accuracy of <0.1 GHz is possible by the use of a zero-padding technique or by curve fitting.

The spectra in figure 4.11 are much richer than those for a simple single-frequency Brillouin oscillation. Comparing the data for $p = 587$ and 479 nm, the former pitch exhibits an even richer spectrum.

When the pump-light pulse is absorbed by the metallic grating, the absorbed photon energy is converted to a temperature increase and thus to thermal stress. Each metallic bar launches acoustic waves into the glass substrate. The angular distribution of the acoustic wave propagation is determined by the diffraction of acoustic waves by the periodic grating structure. In the following, we consider both acoustic waves and probe light within the respective diffraction Rayleigh lengths, and regard both these wave types as plane waves. Here, the objective is to derive the observed Brillouin oscillation frequencies rather than to develop a full theory of the acoustic frequency spectrum.

In contrast to the approach adopted in section 4.2.4, we also consider variations in the lateral (x) direction. Taking the x-axis perpendicular to the grating bars and the z-axis in the depth direction (directed from the back surface to the front surface of the sample), the x component of the wave vector $\mathbf{k}_B$ of the generated acoustic waves is given by

$$k_{Bx} = Nq, \qquad (4.17)$$

where $q = 2\pi/p$ is the wave number of the grating and N is an integer. These acoustic waves can be regarded as forming a moving grating-like strain field by a simple consideration of the acoustic wave vectors involved, i.e., through a superposition of waves with different Ns. One should keep in mind, however, that this is an approximate picture. In fact, the grating-like strain field formed just after the generation of the acoustic waves does not retain its shape perfectly during propagation since the z component of the sound velocity is dispersive for $k_{Bx} \neq 0$.

The multiple Brillouin oscillation frequencies observed in experiments result from the scattering of the probe light by the acoustic waves propagating in various directions. To explain these frequencies, we consider the light diffracted by the grating structure as well as the light scattered by the propagating acoustic waves. Since the diffraction efficiency at the grating (>0.1) is much higher than that associated with the scattering by the acoustic waves ($\lesssim 10^{-4}$), multiple diffraction processes (e.g. double diffraction) in addition to single diffraction processes may be involved in the overall probing process. On the other hand, scattering that occurs more than once as a result of the acoustic waves can be ignored, since its effect is extremely weak in comparison.

The possible sequences of diffraction by the grating and scattering by the acoustic waves are depicted in figure 4.12. The simplest sequence involves the incident probe beam being scattered by the acoustic waves in the direction of the first-order

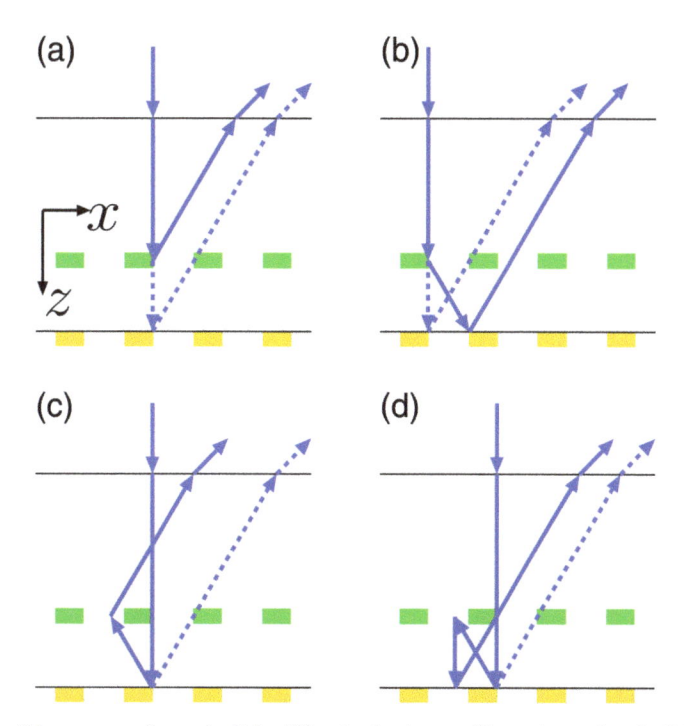

Figure 4.12. Possible sequences for probe-light diffraction by the metallic grating and probe-light scattering by the acoustic waves. The yellow rectangles indicate the cross section of the metallic bars. The green rectangles indicate the (assumed, see text) grating-like strain distribution produced by the generated acoustic waves. The dotted blue arrows show the light diffracted by the metallic grating without any interaction with the acoustic waves. The solid blue arrows indicate the diffraction (if any) and scattering of light by the acoustic waves. (a) Simple backward scattering by the acoustic waves only. (b) Forward scattering followed by diffraction. (c) Diffraction followed by forward scattering. (d) Diffraction followed by backward scattering and subsequent diffraction. Adapted with permission from [62], Copyright (2018) by the American Physical Society.

diffraction of the probe light by the metallic grating (figure 4.12(a)). The sequences involving single diffraction by the grating and scattering by the acoustic waves are shown in figure 4.12(b) and (c). They differ in the order of their events: (b) first scattering then diffraction, and (c) first diffraction then scattering. The sequence involving two diffractions by the grating and scattering by the acoustic waves is shown in figure 4.12(d). These occur in the following order: diffraction, scattering, diffraction.

Among these four sequences, (a) and (d) involve backward scattering, in which the signs of the z components of the wave vectors of the light before and after scattering are opposite. On the other hand, (b) and (c) involve forward scattering, in which the sign of the z components of the wave vectors of the light before and after scattering are the same. Forward scattering measurement is possible only when the probe light comes from the rear side of the sample. In all four sequences, first-order diffracted light that does not interact with the acoustic wave is mixed with scattered light. The latter is frequency shifted by the frequency of the acoustic wave involved. This mixing results in temporal beating, and thus the diffracted light intensity oscillates at the frequency of the acoustic wave involved in the scattering.

For each diffraction at the metallic grating, the x component of the light wave vector is altered by an integer multiple of q. The light frequency is not altered, so the wave number is conserved during the diffraction.

Equation (4.15) for momentum conservation on scattering can be generalized to

$$\mathbf{k}_s = \mathbf{k}_i \pm \mathbf{k}_B, \tag{4.18}$$

where $\mathbf{k}_i$ is the wave vector of the light before scattering, $\mathbf{k}_s$ is that after scattering, and $\mathbf{k}_B$ that of the acoustic wave scattering the light. The plus sign on the right-hand side indicates phonon absorption on scattering, whereas the minus sign indicates phonon creation. The angular frequencies are related through energy conservation:

$$\omega_s = \omega_i \pm \omega_B, \tag{4.19}$$

where the suffixes i, s and B denote the frequencies of the light before and after scattering and that of the acoustic wave, respectively. Since $\omega_B \ll \omega_i$, we approximate $|\mathbf{k}_s| \simeq |\mathbf{k}_i|$ when considering momentum conservation (equation (4.18)).

The probe-light wave vectors before and after scattering as well as the related acoustic wave vectors based on the predictions of equations (4.17) and (4.18) are depicted in figure 4.13. To distinguish the wave vectors, we introduce the notation (m, d), where m specifies the x component of the light wave vector, $k_x = mq$, and d takes the values ± 1 according to the sign of the z component of the light wave vector. The suffixes i and s specify the quantity before and after scattering, respectively, and are used for both m and d. The sequences in figure 4.12 correspond to (a) $d_i = 1$, $d_s = -1$, (b) $d_i = 1$, $d_s = 1$, (c) $d_i = -1$, $d_s = -1$, and (d) $d_i = -1$, $d_s = 1$. They are depicted in the top-left, top-right, bottom-left, and bottom-right regions separated by the thick horizontal and vertical lines in figure 4.13, respectively.

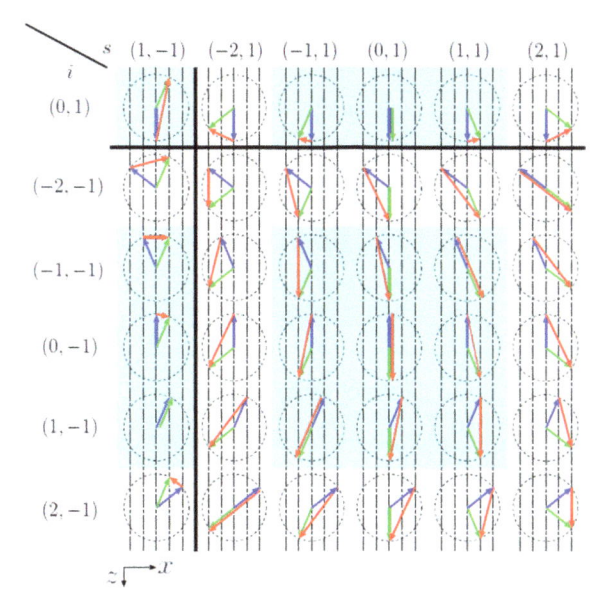

Figure 4.13. Probe-light wave vectors before and after scattering ($\mathbf{k}_i$ in blue, and $\mathbf{k}_s$ in green, respectively) and absorbed-phonon wave vectors ($\mathbf{k}_B$ in red). The labels on the left-hand side show (m_i, d_i) (before scattering), whereas the labels at the top show (m_s, d_s) (after scattering). The dash-dotted vertical lines indicate the possible k_x values for the probe light that can result from diffraction. The blue shaded region shows possible scattering processes that include only first-order optical diffraction. Adapted with permission from [62], Copyright (2018) by the American Physical Society.

The probe-light wave vectors are given by

$$\mathbf{k}_j = \left(m_j q,\, 0,\, d_j \sqrt{k_j^2 - (m_j q)^2}\right), \quad (4.20)$$

where $j = i,\, s$. The wave number k_i of the probe light before scattering is equal to nk, where n is the refractive index of the substrate (k being the probe-light wave number in vacuum). As previously mentioned, the wave number k_s of the probe light after scattering is slightly different from k_i because of the frequency shift given by equation (4.19), but we approximate $k_s = k_i$ as before. In order for the square root in equation (4.20) to have a real value, m_j should fulfill $-nk \leqslant m_j q \leqslant nk$. In the case of the sample under study, for the $p = 587$ nm grating $|m_j| \leqslant 2$, whereas for the $p = 479$ nm grating $|m_j| \leqslant 1$. In figure 4.13, the blue shaded regions show possible scattering processes that include only first-order optical diffraction, corresponding to the $p = 479$ nm grating. The $p = 587$ nm grating allows all the scattering processes shown in figure 4.13, and should result in a larger number of different Brillouin oscillation frequencies compared to the $p = 479$ nm grating. This prediction agrees with the experimental observations in figure 4.11.

The Brillouin oscillation frequency f_B is given by

$$f_B = \frac{v|\mathbf{k}_B|}{2\pi} = \frac{v}{2\pi}\left\{[(m_s - m_i)q]^2 + \left[d_s\sqrt{k_i^2 - (m_s q)^2} - d_i\sqrt{k_i^2 - (m_i q)^2}\right]^2\right\}^{1/2}, \quad (4.21)$$

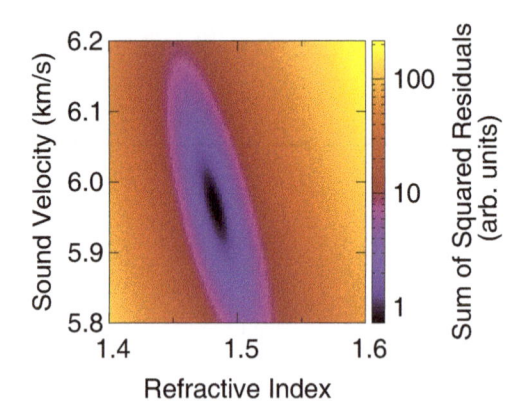

Figure 4.14. The sum of the squared residuals versus n and v for the predicted Brillouin oscillation frequencies compared with the experimental ones in figure 4.11.

where v here denotes the longitudinal sound velocity of fused silica. As explained later, we are not able to observe shear acoustic modes in this specific configuration.

The Brillouin oscillation frequencies obtained from equation (4.21) for a given n and v are compared with the experimentally obtained peak frequencies shown in figure 4.11. The most probable n and v are obtained by locating the minimum of the sum of the squared residuals for the estimated and experimental frequencies. Figure 4.14 shows a map of the sum of the squared residuals versus n and v. The optimal values $n = 1.482$ and $v = 5.968 \times 10^3$ m s^{-1} are in good agreement with the values found in the literature, $n = 1.471$ (at 400 nm) and $v = 5.968 \times 10^3$ m s^{-1} for fused silica at room temperature [128]. These values are used to plot the + symbols in figure 4.11, and good agreement with the experimental peaks is obtained. The results indicate that it is possible to estimate n and v from a single measurement without changing the probe incident angle.

It is also possible to use obliquely incident probe light for such a grating sample. Suppose the incident plane of the probe beam is perpendicular to the grating bars: the wave vector of the probe light incident on the sample is then $\mathbf{k} = (k_x, 0, \sqrt{k^2 - k_x^2})$. The form of the possible probe-light wave vectors in the sample is then slightly modified from that in equation (4.20), as follows:

$$\mathbf{k}_j = \left(k_x + m_j q, 0, d_j \sqrt{k_j^2 - (k_x + m_j q)^2}\right). \quad (4.22)$$

The Brillouin oscillation frequency is now given by

$$f_B = \frac{v}{2\pi}\left\{[(m_s - m_i)q]^2 + \left[d_s\sqrt{k_i^2 - (k_x + m_s q)^2} - d_i\sqrt{k_i^2 - (k_x + m_i q)^2}\right]^2\right\}^{1/2}. \quad (4.23)$$

A convenient configuration is to choose the probe-light incident angle that satisfies $k_x = q/2$: in this case, the negatively directed first-order diffracted light from the sample returns in exactly the reverse direction to that of the light entering the sample. (The experimental setup appropriate to this case is similar to that shown in figure 4.4.)

Deposited gratings can be used to study both the optical and acoustic properties of samples in cases in which optical access is limited, such as in high-pressure environments related to diamond anvil cells. The general method could potentially also be extended to the study of anisotropic and inhomogeneous samples in cases in which the physical properties vary with depth.

4.3.2 Generation and detection of shear acoustic waves assisted by metallic gratings

Picosecond laser ultrasonic measurements are often focused on the detection of longitudinal waves because of the use of isotropic or high-symmetry samples or high-symmetry optical excitation and detection configurations. The generation and detection of shear acoustic waves is, however, preferable for a more complete probing of elastic properties. In addition, shear waves are slower than longitudinal waves, and thus possess shorter wavelengths more suitable for nanoscale probing at a given acoustic frequency.

To generate shear acoustic waves, one may use anisotropic media [10, 14, 20, 27, 77, 102, 111, 129–133] or acoustic waves propagating in oblique directions [16, 23]. It also has been theoretically suggested that grating-like optical excitation using the interference between non-parallel pump-light beams may generate shear acoustic waves [134, 135]. This implies that pump-light irradiation of metallic gratings can generate shear acoustic waves.

The optical detection of shear acoustic waves is not as straightforward as that for longitudinal waves. It is not possible to detect shear acoustic waves propagating perpendicular to the surface of a transparent isotropic medium using normally incident probe light [136], for example, because of the high symmetry of this configuration. One needs to exploit sample anisotropy or low-symmetry optical configurations, such as the use of obliquely incident probe light. Here, we consider the generation and detection of shear acoustic waves in transparent isotropic media using deposited metallic grating structures [103].

Figure 4.15 shows how shear acoustic waves can be generated by a metallic grating. In this case the *xyz* axes are defined with respect to the sample. As before, the *z*-axis is defined

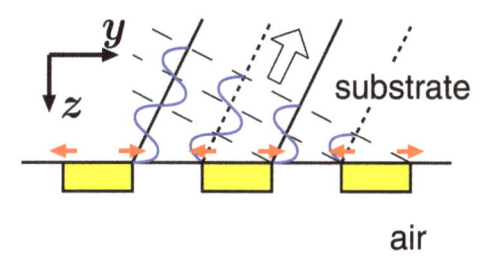

Figure 4.15. Shear-acoustic-wave generation using deposited grating bars: a cross section perpendicular to the grating bars (yellow rectangles). The grating edges exert forces along the surface in opposite directions for neighboring edges (red arrows). The shear acoustic waves (blue sinusoids) propagate in the direction of the first-order diffracted acoustic waves (white thick arrow). Adapted with permission from [103], Copyright (2020) by the American Physical Society.

as being in the thickness direction of the sample as viewed from the rear surface (without a grating) toward the front surface (with grating). The y axis is perpendicular to the grating bars. (This is different from the definition x in the previous section for convenience in the experimental description.) The x-axis is defined to be parallel to the grating bars. When a pump-light pulse is absorbed by the grating bars, they are heated and exhibit thermal expansion. In addition to pushing the substrate in the $-z$ direction, they also exert lateral forces, as shown by the red arrows in figure 4.15. This array of oppositely directed forces cancel each other out for acoustic wave propagation perpendicular to the surface, but contribute constructively for shear acoustic waves propagating in the first-order (or any odd-order) acoustic diffraction direction, as depicted by the blue sinusoids. As in the previous section for longitudinal acoustic wave generation using grating bars, here we must also consider the effect of acoustic diffraction. Because of the translational symmetry of the system in the x direction, the polarization of the generated shear acoustic waves is parallel to the y–z plane perpendicular to the grating bars.

The conditions for the optical detection of shear acoustic waves in an isotropic medium can now be derived. Consider a hypothetical scattering process with light wave vectors $\mathbf{k}_i$ before scattering, $\mathbf{k}_s$ after scattering, and an acoustic wave vector $\mathbf{k}_B$ which is associated with the light scattering (for brevity, only considered here for the case of phonon absorption). The condition for momentum conservation becomes

$$\mathbf{k}_s = \mathbf{k}_i + \mathbf{k}_B. \tag{4.24}$$

We define a right-angled coordinate system based on x_1, x_2, x_3 axes, that has x_3 parallel to $\mathbf{k}_B$ and the x_1-x_3 plane parallel to $\mathbf{k}_i$, $\mathbf{k}_s$ and $\mathbf{k}_B$. The permittivity modulation caused by the propagating acoustic strain due to the photoelastic effect is given by

$$\Delta\varepsilon_{ij} = P_{ijkl}\eta_{kl}, \tag{4.25}$$

where $\Delta\varepsilon$ is the modulation of the permittivity tensor, η is the strain tensor, and P_{ijkl} is the photoelastic tensor of the substrate. The light scattering caused by the acoustic wave can be described as light emission from the electric polarization, i.e., proportional to the product of the permittivity modulation and the electric field of the light, $\Delta\varepsilon_{ij}E_j$. Thus, by looking at the induced electric polarization, one may find the selection rules for the scattering. In the scattering process, there are four combinations of incident light polarization: p (the electric field $\mathbf{E}$ parallel to the x_1–x_3 plane) or s (the electric field $\mathbf{E}$ perpendicular to the x_1–x_3 plane), together with shear acoustic wave polarization along x_2 (strain component $\eta_{23} \neq 0$) or x_1 ($\eta_{13} \neq 0$), as schematically depicted in figure 4.16.

The matrix representing the photoelastic tensor of an isotropic medium in Voigt notation is given by [137]:

$$P_{IJ} = \begin{pmatrix} P_{11} & P_{12} & P_{12} & 0 & 0 & 0 \\ P_{12} & P_{11} & P_{12} & 0 & 0 & 0 \\ P_{12} & P_{12} & P_{11} & 0 & 0 & 0 \\ 0 & 0 & 0 & P_{44} & 0 & 0 \\ 0 & 0 & 0 & 0 & P_{44} & 0 \\ 0 & 0 & 0 & 0 & 0 & P_{44} \end{pmatrix}, \tag{4.26}$$

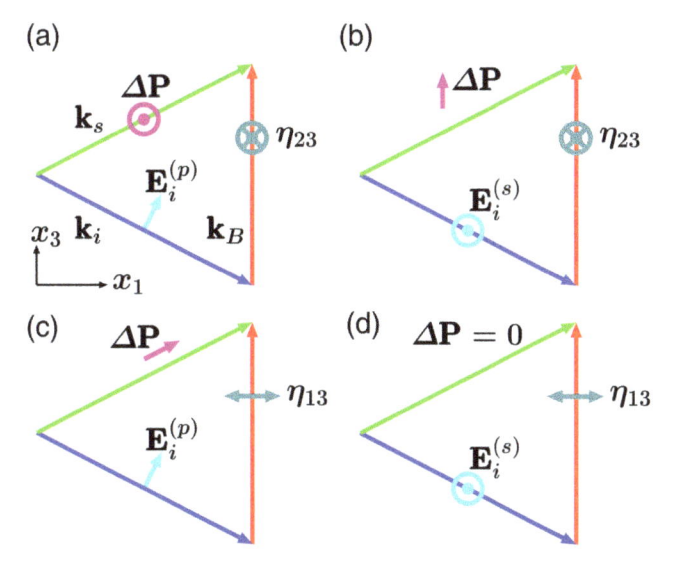

Figure 4.16. Selection rules for shear-wave detection. The blue arrows indicate the light wave vector before scattering. The green arrows indicate the light wave vector after scattering. The red arrows indicate the acoustic wave vector. The purple arrows indicate the polarization induced by the photoelastic effect. (a) p-polarized incident light and x_2-polarized shear wave. (b) s-polarized incident light and x_2-polarized shear wave. (c) p-polarized incident light and x_1-polarized shear wave. (d) s-polarized incident light and x_1-polarized shear wave. Acoustic wave detection is allowed in (a) and (b) but inhibited in (c) and (d). Adapted with permission from [103], Copyright (2020) by the American Physical Society.

where $I, J = 1, \ldots, 6$ represent 11, 22, 33, 23(32), 31(13), 12(21), respectively, for ij or kl of tensor P_{ijkl} in equation (4.25). The electric polarization $\Delta \boldsymbol{P}$ induced by the shear acoustic waves is given by

$$\Delta \boldsymbol{P} \propto \Delta \varepsilon \boldsymbol{E} = \begin{pmatrix} 0 & 0 & P_{44}\eta_{13} \\ 0 & 0 & P_{44}\eta_{23} \\ P_{44}\eta_{13} & P_{44}\eta_{23} & 0 \end{pmatrix} \begin{pmatrix} E_{i1} \\ E_{i2} \\ E_{i3} \end{pmatrix}, \tag{4.27}$$

where E_{ij} is the jth component of $\boldsymbol{E}_i$. For p-polarized light,

$$\boldsymbol{E}_i^{(p)} \propto \begin{pmatrix} -k_{i3} \\ 0 \\ k_{i1} \end{pmatrix}, \tag{4.28}$$

where k_{ij} is the jth component of $\mathbf{k}_i$, whereas for s-polarized light

$$\boldsymbol{E}_i^{(s)} \propto \begin{pmatrix} 0 \\ 1 \\ 0 \end{pmatrix}. \tag{4.29}$$

These expressions can be used to identify the selection rules for shear acoustic wave detection. For p-polarized light and x_2-polarized acoustic waves (figure 4.16(a)), $\Delta \boldsymbol{P}$

is directed along x_2 and is perpendicular to $\mathbf{k}_s$. This is favorable for shear-wave detection. For s-polarized light and x_2-polarized acoustic waves (figure 4.16(b)), $\Delta\mathbf{P}$ is directed along x_3, and may have a non-zero component perpendicular to $\mathbf{k}_s$. Shear-wave detection is still possible. For p-polarized light and x_1-polarized acoustic waves (figure 4.16(c)), $\Delta\mathbf{P}$ is directed along $\mathbf{k}_s$, and thus no light is emitted along $\mathbf{k}_s$. In this case shear-wave detection is prohibited. For s-polarized light and x_1-polarized acoustic waves (figure 4.16(d)), $\Delta\mathbf{P}$ is zero, and thus no light is emitted at all. Here, shear-wave detection is also prohibited. In either of the cases for which $\mathbf{k}_i$ is along x_3, i.e., $\mathbf{E}$ is perpendicular to x_3, equation (4.27) implies that $\Delta\mathbf{P}$ is parallel to $\mathbf{k}_s$. Thus, shear-wave detection is once again prohibited. In summary, the conditions for shear-wave detection are: (1) $\mathbf{k}_i$ must not be parallel to $\mathbf{k}_B$, and (2) the shear-wave polarization must not be parallel to the plane defined by $\mathbf{k}_i$ and $\mathbf{k}_s$. As shown in figure 4.15, the shear waves generated by the grating have both their polarization and wave vector $\mathbf{k}_B$ in the yz plane. Considering the above conditions for shear-wave detection, the light wave vector should not be in the yz plane.

Based on these considerations, shear-acoustic-wave generation and detection in grating samples becomes possible with picosecond laser ultrasonics. Here, we discuss the case of a sample based on a fused silica substrate that has a thickness of 1 mm and a deposited Al grating structure fabricated by the electron-beam lithography and lift-off techniques [103]. The grating pitch is $p = 380$ nm and the thickness is 40 nm. The nominal width of each grating bar is 190 nm. Measurements are performed with a standard picosecond laser ultrasonics setup similar to that shown in figure 4.4 at pump- and probe-light wavelengths of 830 and 415 nm, respectively, The sample orientation and optical configuration should fulfill one of the conditions for shear-wave detection discussed above (figure 4.17). To describe the sample orientation, we make use of the sample xyz axes and the laboratory XYZ axes. The probe light directed toward the sample is oriented along the Z-axis with light wave vector $\mathbf{k}_{\text{in}}$, which is expressed as $(0, 0, k)$ in the XYZ coordinate system. The sample is first placed so that the xyz axes coincide with XYZ. The sample is then rotated with respect to the $Y = y$ axis by an angle α. The rotated xyz axes are denoted by $x'yz'$. The sample is further rotated with respect to the x' axis by an angle β. The rotated xyz axes in this case are denoted by $x'y''z''$ (see figure 4.17), but hereafter we make use of the notation xyz for the sample coordinate axes, as previously mentioned. The probe light heading toward the sample is expressed in the xyz coordinate system through the wave vector

$$(k_x, k_y, k_z) = k(-\sin\alpha, \cos\alpha\sin\beta, \cos\alpha\cos\beta). \tag{4.30}$$

The condition for shear-wave detection requires both $\alpha \neq 0$ and $\beta \neq 0$. The first-order diffracted probe-light beam is fed to a photodetector, and the transient reflectivity variation is recorded. Figure 4.18 shows raw data for the transient reflectivity change measured at several different sample rotation angles: (1) $\alpha = 0°$, $\beta = 33.1°$, (2) $\alpha = 36.4°$, $\beta = 40.0°$, (3) $\alpha = 26.0°$, $\beta = 40.0°$. According to the above theoretical considerations, shear acoustic waves should be observed in cases (2) and (3), but not in case (1). The moduli of the Fourier amplitudes of these data are shown

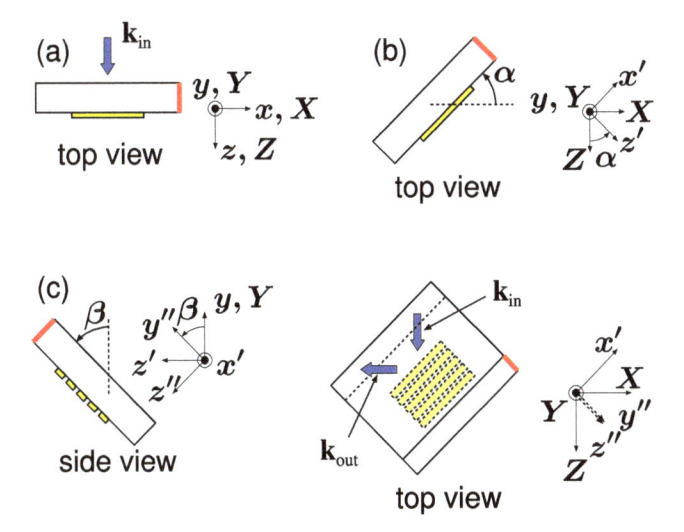

Figure 4.17. Geometries for sample orientation and optical configuration. (a) Sample orientation such that the xyz axes agree with the lab XYZ axes. The probe light incident from the rear surface of the sample (wave vector $\mathbf{k}_{in}$) is directed in the Z direction. (b) The sample is rotated with respect to the Y axis by an angle α. The rotated sample axes are denoted by $x'yz'$. (c) The sample is further rotated with respect to the x' axis by an angle β. The rotated sample axes are denoted by $x'y''z''$. The diffracted light (wave vector $\mathbf{k}_{out}$) is also shown. One of the edges in each case is marked in red to clarify the sample rotations. Adapted with permission from [103], Copyright (2020) by the American Physical Society.

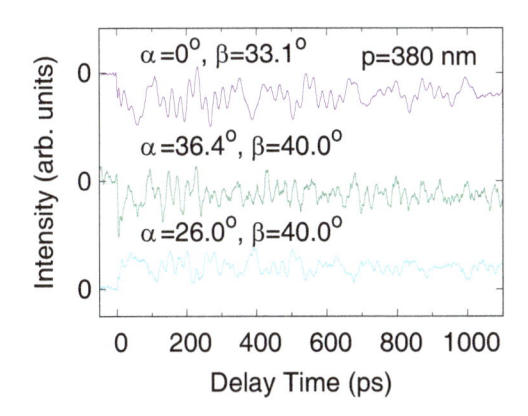

Figure 4.18. Experimental transient reflectivity changes versus delay time at several different sample rotations for shear acoustic wave generation and detection using deposited grating bars of pitch $p = 380$ nm. Adapted with permission from [103], Copyright (2020) by the American Physical Society.

in figure 4.19. The frequency resolution is about 0.9 GHz here. Some peak widths are broader than this, indicating that the corresponding (apparent) oscillation lifetime is shorter than the measured maximum delay time of around 1100 ps. This may result in part from the high-angle obliquely incident probe beam.

To understand these spectra, the possible Brillouin oscillation frequencies are formulated using an extension of equation (4.23):

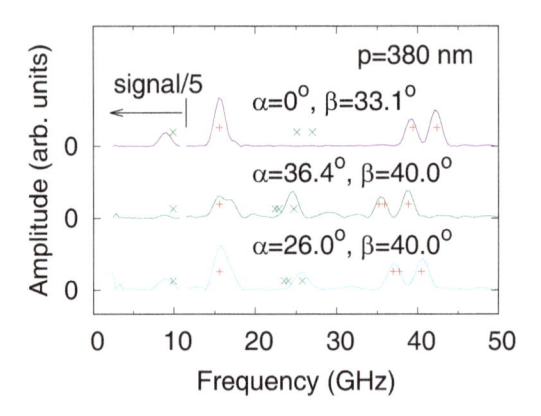

Figure 4.19. Moduli of the Fourier amplitudes of the transient reflectivity changes versus frequency at several different sample rotations for shear-wave generation and detection using deposited grating bars of pitch $p = 380$ nm. The red + symbols represent calculated frequencies for longitudinal acoustic waves. The green × symbols represent those for shear acoustic waves. The vertical scale to the left of the vertical black line has been changed to reduce the signal in the region <10 GHz by a factor of five. Adapted with permission from [103], Copyright (2020) by the American Physical Society.

$$f_B = \frac{v}{2\pi}\left\{[(m_s - m_i)q]^2 + \left[d_s\sqrt{k_l^2 - k_x^2 - (k_y + m_s q)^2} - d_i\sqrt{k_l^2 - k_x^2 - (k_y + m_i q)^2}\right]^2\right\}^{1/2}, \quad (4.31)$$

where v is the longitudinal or shear sound velocity, and k_x, k_y are as given in equation (4.30). The longitudinal sound velocity and the refractive index are determined by considering the least-square residuals, as described in the previous section, to be $v_l = 5.922 \times 10^3$ m s^{-1} and $n = 1.484$ at a wavelength of 415 nm, which agree well with the values given in the literature, $v_l = 5.968 \times 10^3$ m s^{-1} and $n = 1.470$ at this wavelength for fused silica at room temperature [128]. Predictions are marked as red + symbols in figure 4.19, and show good agreement with the experimental peaks. The shear sound velocity is also similarly estimated for $\alpha = 36.4°$, $\beta = 40.0°$ and $\alpha = 26.0°$, $\beta = 40.0°$ using the highest frequency peaks near 24.6 and 25.8 GHz to be $v_s = 3.772 \times 10^3$ m s^{-1}, which agrees well with the value given in the literature, 3.764×10^3 m s^{-1} [128]. The peak positions calculated using the derived v_s are marked by green × symbols, which show good agreement with the experimental peaks. As expected, there is no shear-wave peak at the frequencies around 25–27 GHz in the spectra for $\alpha = 0°$, $\beta = 33.1°$ in figure 4.19. The peak at around 9 GHz is observed in all spectra around the lowest expected shear-wave frequency. This peak, however, appears to arise from Rayleigh-like surface waves, and thus is observed even for $\alpha = 0°$. The second- and third-highest frequency peaks expected for the shear acoustic waves are missing for $\alpha \neq 0°$. These modes are calculated to correspond to shear waves propagating perpendicular to the surface, and so they cannot be excited by the grating structure, as explained above.

One can see that shear acoustic waves traveling in oblique directions can be generated by the grating structure and detected by careful choice of the optical detection configuration. It should be possible to extend this general method to study the elastic properties of anisotropic or inhomogeneous media.

4.4 Summary

In conclusion, we have described the basics of picosecond laser ultrasonics and some of its applications. Standard optical pump–probe techniques can be used to generate gigahertz to terahertz acoustic waves in samples and record their propagation through transient optical reflectivity. Using an extension of optical interferometric detection, one can also detect the optical phase variation with a sensitivity that reaches the picometer scale for surface/interface displacements. This allows the technique to be extended to a wider range of samples, such as those exhibiting negligible photoelastic response at the chosen optical probe wavelength and optical incidence angle. Some recent studies that made use of nanoscale metallic grating structures on transparent substrates were also described. This grating method allows the longitudinal sound velocity and refractive index of a transparent medium to be obtained using a single measurement. We show how this grating method can be extended to the generation and detection of shear acoustic waves. These studies should be applicable to the investigation of a range of elastic constants and refractive indices in anisotropic or graded media. Extension to more general types of grating, such as two-dimensional nanostructure arrays, should lead to further information being gleaned for the case of anisotropic samples.

References

[1] Thomsen C, Strait J, Vardeny Z, Maris H J, Tauc J and Hauser J J 1984 *Phys. Rev. Lett.* **53** 989–92
[2] Thomsen C, Grahn H T, Maris H J and Tauc J 1986 *Phys. Rev.* B **34** 4129–38
[3] Wright O B 1992 *J. Appl. Phys.* **71** 1617–29
[4] Tas G and Maris H J 1994 *Phys. Rev.* B **49** 15046–54
[5] Wright O B 1994 *Phys. Rev.* B **49** 9985–8
[6] Perrin B, Bonello B, Jeannet J-C and Romatet E 1996 Interferometric detection of hypersound waves in modulated structures *Prog. Nat. Sci.* **S6** S444–48
[7] Hurley D H and Wright O B 1999 *Opt. Lett.* **24** 1305–7
[8] Richardson C J K, Ehrlich M J and Wagner J W 1999 *J. Opt. Soc. Am.* B **16** 1007–15
[9] Nikoonahad M, Lee S and Wang H 2000 *Appl. Phys. Lett.* **76** 514–6
[10] Hurley D H, Wright O B, Matsuda O, Gusev V E and Kolosov O V 2000 *Ultrasonics* **38** 470–4
[11] Devos A and Lerouge C 2001 *Phys. Rev. Lett.* **86** 2669–72
[12] Matsuda Y, Richardson C J K and Spicer J B 2002 *IEEE Trans. Ultrason. Ferroelectr. Freq. Control* **49** 915–21
[13] Saito T, Matsuda O and Wright O B 2003 *Phys. Rev.* B **67** 205421
[14] Matsuda O, Wright O B, Hurley D H, Gusev V E and Shimizu K 2004 *Phys. Rev. Lett.* **93** 095501
[15] Hébert H, Vidal F, Martin F, Kieffer J C, Nadeau A, Johnston T W, Blouin A, Moreau A and Monchalin J P 2005 *J. Appl. Phys.* **98** 033104

[16] Rossignol C, Rampnoux J M, Perton M, Audoin B and Dilhaire S 2005 *Phys. Rev. Lett.* **94** 166106
[17] Dehoux T, Perton M, Chigarev N, Rossignol C, Rampnoux J M and Audoin B 2006 *J. Appl. Phys.* **100** 064318
[18] Chigarev N, Rossignol C and Audoin B 2006 *Rev. Sci. Instrum.* **77** 114901
[19] Vollmann J, Profunser D M, Bryner J and Dual J 2006 *Ultrasonics* **44** e1215–21
[20] Pezeril T, Chigarev N, Ruello P, Gougeon S, Mounier D, Breteau J M, Picart P and Gusev V 2006 *Phys. Rev.* B **73** 132301
[21] Bryner J, Profunser D M, Vollmann J, Mueller E and Dual J 2006 *Ultrasonics* **44** e1269–75
[22] Audoin B, Perton M, Chigarev N and Rossignol C 2007 *J. Phys.: Conf. Ser.* **92** 012028
[23] Dehoux T, Chigarev N, Rossignol C and Audoin B 2007 *Phys. Rev.* B **76** 024311
[24] Ogi H, Fujii M, Nakamura N, Yasui T and Hirao M 2007 *Phys. Rev. Lett.* **98** 195503
[25] Pezeril T, Ruello P, Gougeon S, Chigarev N, Mounier D, Breteau J M, Picart P and Gusev V 2007 *Phys. Rev.* B **75** 174307
[26] Nakamura N, Ogi H, Shagawa T and Hirao M 2008 *Appl. Phys. Lett.* **92** 141901
[27] Matsuda O, Wright O B, Hurley D H, Gusev V and Shimizu K 2008 *Phys. Rev.* B **77** 224110
[28] Mounier D, Morozov E, Ruello P, Breteau J M, Picart P and Gusev V 2008 *Eur. Phys. J. Spec. Top.* **153** 243–6
[29] Harata A and Sawada T 1993 *Jpn. J. Appl. Phys.* **32** 2188–91
[30] Sun C K, Liang J C and Yu X Y 2000 *Phys. Rev. Lett.* **84** 179–82
[31] Chigarev N V, Paraschuk D Y, Pan X Y and Gusev V E 2000 *Phys. Rev.* B **61** 15837–40
[32] Wright O B, Perrin B, Matsuda O and Gusev V E 2001 *Phys. Rev.* B **64** 081202(R)
[33] Hurley D H and Telschow K L 2002 *Phys. Rev.* B **66** 153301
[34] Holme N C R, Daly B C, Myaing M T and Norris T B 2003 *Appl. Phys. Lett.* **83** 392–4
[35] Côte R and Devos A 2005 *Rev. Sci. Instrum.* **76** 053906
[36] Wu S, Geiser P, Jun J, Karpinski J, Park J R and Sobolewski R 2006 *Appl. Phys. Lett.* **88** 041917
[37] Wen Y C, Ko T S, Lu T C, Kuo H C, Chyi J I and Sun C K 2009 *Phys. Rev.* B **80** 195201
[38] Babilotte P, Ruello P, Vaudel G, Pezeril T, Mounier D, Breteau J M and Gusev V 2010 *Appl. Phys. Lett.* **97** 174103
[39] Ishioka K, Rustagi A, Beyer A, Stolz W, Volz K, Höfer U, Petek H and Stanton C J 2017 *Appl. Phys. Lett.* **111** 062105
[40] Vialla F and Fatti N D 2020 *Nanomaterials* **10** 2543
[41] Lin H N, Stoner R J, Maris H J and Tauc J 1991 *J. Appl. Phys.* **69** 3816–22
[42] Wright O B 1995 *Opt. Lett.* **20** 632–4
[43] Gusev V E 1996 Laser hypersonics in fundamental and applied research *Acust. Acta Acust.* **82** S37–45 (Proc. of Forum Acusticum 1996)
[44] Morath C J and Maris H J 1996 *Phys. Rev.* B **54** 203–13
[45] Lee Y C, Bretz K C, Wise F W and Sachse W 1996 *Appl. Phys. Lett.* **69** 1692–4
[46] Matsuda O and Wright O B 2002 *J. Opt. Soc. Am.* B **19** 3028–41
[47] Rossignol C, Perrin B, Laborde S, Vandenbulcke L, Barros M I D and Djemia P 2004 *J. Appl. Phys.* **95** 4157–62
[48] Lee T, Ohmori K, Shin C S, Cahill D G, Petrov I and Greene J E 2005 *Phys. Rev.* B **71** 144106
[49] Mechri C, Ruello P, Breteau J M, Baklanov M R, Verdonck P and Gusev V 2009 *Appl. Phys. Lett.* **95** 091907

[50] Walker P M, Sharp J S, Akimov A V and Kent A J 2010 *Appl. Phys. Lett.* **97** 073106
[51] Nagakubo A, Arita M, Yokoyama T, Matsuda S, Ueda M, Ogi H and Hirao M 2015 *Jpn. J. Appl. Phys.* **54** 07HD01
[52] Lee H J *et al* 2021 *Phys. Rev. X* **11** 031031
[53] Fukuda H, Nagakubo A and Ogi H 2021 *Jpn. J. Appl. Phys.* **60** SDDA05
[54] Bonello B, Ajinou A, Richard V, Djemia P and Chérif S M 2001 *J. Acoust. Soc. Am.* **110** 1943–9
[55] Antonelli G A, Maris H J, Malhotra S G and Harper J M E 2002 *J. Appl. Phys.* **91** 3261–7
[56] Profunser D M, Vollmann J and Dual J 2002 *Ultrasonics* **40** 747–52
[57] van Dijk M A, Lippitz M and Orrit M 2005 *Phys. Rev. Lett.* **95** 267406
[58] Devos A, Poinsotte F, Groenen J, Dehaese O, Bertru N and Ponchet A 2007 *Phys. Rev. Lett.* **98** 207402
[59] Ayrinhac S, Devos A, Louarn A L, Mante P A and Emery P 2010 *Opt. Lett.* **35** 3510–2
[60] Bruchhausen A *et al* 2011 *Phys. Rev. Lett.* **106** 077401
[61] Ruello P, Ayouch A, Vaudel G, Pezeril T, Delorme N, Sato S, Kimura K and Gusev V E 2015 *Phys. Rev. B* **92** 174304
[62] Matsuda O, Pezeril T, Chaban I, Fujita K and Gusev V 2018 *Phys. Rev. B* **97** 064301
[63] Ortiz O *et al* 2020 *Appl. Phys. Lett.* **117** 183102
[64] Tas G, Loomis J J, Maris H J, Bailes III A A and Seiberling L E 1998 *Appl. Phys. Lett.* **72** 2235–7
[65] Grossmann M, Schubert M, He C, Brick D, Scheer E, Hettich M, Gusev V and Dekorsy T 2017 *New. J. Phys.* **19** 053019
[66] Devos A and Emery P 2018 *Surf. Coat. Technol.* **352** 406–10
[67] Yamamoto A, Mishina T, Masumoto Y and Nakayama M 1994 *Phys. Rev. Lett.* **73** 740–3
[68] Baumberg J J, Williams D A and Köhler K 1997 *Phys. Rev. Lett.* **78** 3358–61
[69] Mizoguchi K, Hase M, Nakashima S and Nakayama M 1999 *Phys. Rev. B* **60** 8262–6
[70] Özgür Ü, Lee C W and Everitt H O 2001 *Phys. Rev. Lett.* **86** 5604–7
[71] Lin K H, Chern G W, Huang Y K and Sun C K 2004 *Phys. Rev. B* **70** 073307
[72] Pu N W 2005 *Phys. Rev. B* **72** 115428
[73] Lin K H, Chern G W, Yu C T, Liu T M, Pan C C, Chen G T, Chyi J I, Huang S W, Li P C and Sun C K 2005 *IEEE Trans. Ultrason. Ferroelectr. Freq. Control* **52** 1404–14
[74] Martinez C E, Stanton N M, Walker P M, Kent A J, Novikov S V and Foxon C T 2005 *Appl. Phys. Lett.* **86** 221915
[75] Liu R, Sanders G D, Stanton C J, Kim C S, Yahng J S, Jho Y D, Yee K J, Oh E and Kim D S 2005 *Phys. Rev. B* **72** 195335
[76] Matsuda O, Tachizaki T, Fukui T, Baumberg J J and Wright O B 2005 *Phys. Rev. B* **71** 115330
[77] Kini R N, Kent A J, Stanton N M and Henini M 2006 *Appl. Phys. Lett.* **88** 134112
[78] Lanzillotti-Kimura N D, Fainstein A, Huynh A, Perrin B, Jusserand B, Miard A and Lemaître A 2007 *Phys. Rev. Lett.* **99** 217405
[79] Kuo W I, Pan E Y and Pu N W 2008 *J. Appl. Phys.* **103** 093533
[80] Reed E J, Armstrong M R, Kim K Y and Glownia J H 2008 *Phys. Rev. Lett.* **101** 014302
[81] Wang Y, Liebig C, Xu X and Venkatasubramanian R 2010 *Appl. Phys. Lett.* **97** 083103
[82] Czerniuk T, Ehrlich T, Wecker T, As D J, Yakovlev D R, Akimov A V and Bayer M 2017 *Phys. Rev. Appl* **7** 014006
[83] Maznev A A *et al* 2018 *Appl. Phys. Lett.* **112** 061903

[84] Rossignol C, Chigarev N, Ducousso M, Audoin B, Forget G, Guillemot F and Durrieu M C 2008 *Appl. Phys. Lett.* **93** 123901

[85] Audoin B, Rossignol C, Chigarev N, Ducousso M, Forget G, Guillemot F and Durrieu M C 2010 *Ultrasonics* **50** 202–7

[86] Danworaphong S, Tomoda M, Matsumoto Y, Matsuda O, Ohashi T, Watanabe H, Nagayama M, Gohara K, Otsuka P H and Wright O B 2015 *Appl. Phys. Lett.* **106** 163701

[87] Pérez-Cota F *et al* 2020 *J. Appl. Phys.* **128** 160902

[88] Hamraoui A, Sénépart O, Schneider M, Malaquin S, Becerra E P L, Semprez F, Legay C and Belliard L 2021 *Biophys. J.* **120** 402–8

[89] Decremps F, Belliard L, Perrin B and Gauthier M 2008 *Phys. Rev. Lett.* **100** 035502

[90] Lim D, Averitt R D, Demsar J, Taylor A J, Hur N and Cheong S W 2003 *Appl. Phys. Lett.* **83** 4800–2

[91] Rossignol C, Perrin B, Bonello B, Djemia P, Moch P and Hurdequint H 2004 *Phys. Rev. B* **70** 094102

[92] Ren Y H, Trigo M, Merlin R, Adyam V and Li Q 2007 *Appl. Phys. Lett.* **90** 251918

[93] Wang D, Cross A, Guarino G, Wu S, Sobolewski R and Mycielski A 2007 *Appl. Phys. Lett.* **90** 211905

[94] Scherbakov A V, Salasyuk A S, Akimov A V, Liu X, Bombeck M, Brüggemann C, Yakovlev D R, Sapega V F, Furdyna J K and Bayer M 2010 *Phys. Rev. Lett.* **105** 117204

[95] Kim J W, Vomir M and Bigot J Y 2012 *Phys. Rev. Lett.* **109** 166601

[96] Lejman M, Paillard C, Juvé V, Vaudel G, Guiblin N, Bellaiche L, Viret M, Gusev V E, Dkhil B and Ruello P 2019 *Phys. Rev. B* **99** 104103

[97] Raetz S *et al* 2019 *Appl. Sci.* **9** 736

[98] Li C, Harley R T, Lagoudakis P G, Wright O B and Matsuda O 2021 *Phys. Rev. B* **103** L241201

[99] Nikitin S M, Chigarev N, Tournat V, Bulou A, Gasteau D, Castagnede B, Zerr A and Gusev V E 2015 *Sci. Rep.* **5** 09352

[100] Kuriakose M *et al* 2017 *Phys. Rev. B* **96** 134122

[101] Zhao B, Xu F, Belliard L, Huang H, Perrin B, Djemia P and Zerr A 2019 *Phys. Status Solidi* **13** 1900173

[102] Mante P A, Stoumpos C C, Kanatzidis M G and Yartsev A 2018 *J. Phys Chem. Lett.* **9** 3161–6

[103] Matsuda O, Tsutsui K, Vaudel G, Pezeril T, Fujita K and Gusev V 2020 *Phys. Rev. B* **101** 224307

[104] Tomoda M, Matsuda O and Wright O B 2007 *Appl. Phys. Lett.* **90** 041114

[105] Lomonosov A M, Ayouch A, Ruello P, Vaudel G, Baklanov M R, Verdonck P, Zhao L and Gusev V E 2012 *ACS Nano* **6** 1410–5

[106] Nakamura N, Maehara A and Ogi H 2020 *Jpn. J. Appl. Phys.* **59** SKKB04

[107] Shelton L J, Yang F, Ford W K and Maris H J 2005 *Phys. Status Solidi* b **242** 1379–82

[108] Tas G and Maris H J 1997 *Phys. Rev. B* **55** 1852–7

[109] Msall M E, Wright O B and Matsuda O 2007 *J. Phys.: Conf. Ser.* **92** 012026

[110] Wright O B, Perrin B, Matsuda O and Gusev V E 2008 *Phys. Rev. B* **78** 024303

[111] Pezeril T, Klieber C, Andrieu S and Nelson K A 2009 *Phys. Rev. Lett.* **102** 107402

[112] Ogi H, Matsumoto K, Fujita Y, Nakamura T K N and Hirao M 2010 *Appl. Phys. Express* **3** 017001

[113] Ogi H, Kawamoto T, Nakamura N, Hirao M and Nishiyama M 2010 *Biosens. Bioelectron* **26** 1273–7

[114] Ogi H, Iwagami S, Nagakubo A, Taniguchi T and Ono T 2019 *Sensors Actuators* B **278** 15–20
[115] Tachizaki T, Muroya T, Matsuda O, Sugawara Y, Hurley D H and Wright O B 2006 *Rev. Sci. Instrum.* **77** 043713
[116] Chandezon J, Rampnoux J M, Dilhaire S, Audoin B and Guillet1 Y 2015 *Opt. Express* **23** 27011–9
[117] Liu L, Guillet Y and Audoin B 2018 *J. Appl. Phys.* **123** 173103
[118] Wright O B and Kawashima K 1992 *Phys. Rev. Lett.* **69** 1668–71
[119] Matsuda O, Larciprete M C, Voti R L and Wright O B 2015 *Ultrasonics* **56** 3–20
[120] Ruello P and Gusev V E 2015 *Ultrasonics* **56** 21–35
[121] Kouyaté M, Pezeril T, Gusev V and Matsuda O 2016 *J. Opt. Soc. Am.* B **33** 2634–48
[122] Anisimov S I, Kapeliovich B L and Perel'man T L 1974 *Sov. Phys. JETP* **39** 375–7
[123] Matsuda O and Wright O B 2014 Generation and observation of GHz–THz acoustic waves in thin films and microstructures using optical methods *Frontiers in Optical Methods* ed K Shudo, I Katayama and S Ohno (Heidelberg: Springer) pp 129–51
[124] Special Section: Ultrafast Acoustics 2015 *Ultrasonics* **56** 1–171
[125] Lin H N, Maris H J, Freund L B, Lee K Y, Luhn H and Kem D P 1993 *J. Appl. Phys.* **73** 37–45
[126] Colletta M, Gachuhi W, Gartenstein S A, James M M, Szwed E A, Daly B C, Cui W and Antonelli G A 2018 *Ultrasonics* **87** 126–32
[127] Edward S, Zhang H, Setija I, Verrina V, Antoncecchi A, Witte S and Planken P 2020 *Phys. Rev. Appl* **14** 014015
[128] Lide D R (ed) 2004 *CRC Handbook of Chemistry and Physics* 85th ed (Boca Raton, FL: CRC Press)
[129] Bienville T and Perrin B 2003 Generation and detection of quasi transverse waves in an anisotropic crystal by picosecond ultrasonics *Proc. of the World Congress on Ultrasonics: WCU 2003, Paris, France, 7–10 September 2003* (Paris: Société française d'acoustique) 813–6
[130] Pezeril T, Gusev V, Mounier D, Chigarev N and Ruello P 2005 *J. Phys. D: Appl. Phys.* **38** 1421–8
[131] Lejman M, Vaudel G, Infante I C, Gusev V E, Dkhil B and Ruello P 2014 *Nat. Commun.* **5** 4301
[132] Pezeril T 2016 *Opt. Laser Technol.* **83** 177–88
[133] Lejman M et al 2016 *Nat. Commun.* **7** 12345
[134] Kouyate M, Pezeril T, Mounier D and Gusev V 2011 *J. Appl. Phys.* **110** 123526
[135] Gusev V 2009 *Appl. Phys. Lett.* **94** 164105
[136] Matsuda O and Wright O B 2001 *Anal. Sci.* **17** S216–8
[137] Nye J F 1957 *Physical Properties of Crystals* (Oxford: Oxford University Press)

Part II

Industrial applications

IOP Publishing

Ultrasonics
Physics and applications
Mami Matsukawa, Pak-Kon Choi, Kentaro Nakamura, Hirotsugu Ogi and Hideyuki Hasegawa

Chapter 5

Ball surface acoustic wave sensor and its application to trace gas analysis

Kazushi Yamanaka, Takamitsu Iwaya and Shingo Akao

A thin beam of waves usually diverges owing to diffraction, which is a limitation of any device using such waves. However, a surface acoustic wave (SAW) on a sphere with an appropriate aperture does not diverge, but is naturally collimated and makes diffraction-free ultramultiple turns along the equator of a sphere. This effect has been utilized to realize high-performance ball SAW sensors. One application of ball SAW sensors, an extremely fast and sensitive trace moisture analyzer, has been developed and applied in the natural gas and semiconductor industries. In addition, a portable gas chromatograph has been developed to analyze food flavors and hazardous gases.

5.1 Introduction

Sensors that use chemical reactions, optical phenomena, field-effect transistors (FETs), and other electrical sensors have been developed and are used in a wide range of fields. In the case of hydrogen gas sensors, which are the focus of much interest owing to their application in fuel cells, catalytic combustion sensors that catalyze the oxidation reaction of hydrogen have been used from the start. FET-type sensors are also available that measure the changes in current caused by the work function change due to the accumulation of hydrogen atoms in the palladium electrode or other alloy gate electrodes [1].

However, on the basis of given chemical or physical phenomena, these sensors can only operate within a particular gas concentration range. For instance, a catalytic combustion-type hydrogen gas sensor [2] cannot be employed at hydrogen concentrations above the lowest explosion limit (LEL), because hydrogen is burned and may even explode because of the sensor itself. Moreover, FET-type sensors become saturated at gas concentrations above 1%–10%, which include the LEL. However, in hydrogen stations and fuel cell automobiles, not only small leaks but also intense jets or bursts may occur owing to the high pressure of the hydrogen. As a result, different emergency measures must be taken depending on whether the hydrogen concentration is below or above the LEL. Thus, hydrogen sensors that can work over a very wide range of concentrations have been desired but are unfortunately not yet realized.

As another example, the measurement of trace moisture in natural gas mixtures is important for the quality management of pipeline systems for natural gases. Various types of trace moisture analyzer (TMA) [3] are used to monitor moisture in different types of gas. Cavity ring-down spectroscopy (CRDS) has the lowest detection limit [4], but has mostly been applied for the detection of trace moisture in high-purity gases, whereas a natural gas mix typically consists of methane, ethane, propane, some heavier hydrocarbons, carbon dioxide, and nitrogen. A chilled mirror hygrometer [5] has good long-term stability and reproducibility, and often high resolution, but its response time is long for trace gases; therefore, it is suitable for calibration purposes but not for online measurement.

In contrast, elastic waves are dependent on elastic modulus, viscosity, conductivity, and other physical properties, and as a result, an elastic wave sensor operates on the basis of several mechanisms; hence, it can cover a wide range of concentrations. Surface acoustic wave (SAW) devices have successful applications in signal processing [6] and SAW sensors [7–9] have already been studied. The changes in oscillation frequency or delay time due to the mass loading are used to measure gas concentration. However, measuring the attenuation caused by gas concentration is not easy using SAW sensors due to the limited propagation length of SAW caused by diffraction loss [10]. SAWs are attenuated by the diffraction after propagating over the Fresnel distance $x = d^2/\lambda$, where d is the aperture of the source and λ is the wavelength. As a result, the potential performance of SAW sensors has not been fully exploited.

Overcoming these restrictions, our group developed a ball SAW hydrogen sensor with a wider sensing concentration range (of 10 parts per million volume (ppmv) to 100%) than previous SAW sensors [7, 8] and a ball SAW TMA with sub-parts per billion volume (ppbv) sensitivity higher than those of previous SAW TMAs [9]. Our sensor is the first to realize a background gas analysis capability using attenuation measurement at two frequencies. These features are based on a spherical substrate and use a novel phenomenon in which an SAW naturally forms a collimated beam that can circumnavigate the sphere more than 100 times. In this chapter, the authors review the fundamentals of SAW propagation on a sphere, the diffraction-free collimated beam, as well as future applications of ball SAW sensors in various fields.

5.2 SAWs on a sphere

Sato investigated elastic waves on a sphere in detail from the standpoint of geophysics [11] and Viktrov described a Rayleigh-mode SAW solution on a sphere [12]. Since the surface of a sphere is continuous and unbounded, there is no reflection loss. These characteristics are attractive for the long-distance propagation of SAWs.

Using this approach, we observed collimated SAWs during our studies of ball bearings [13–15]. When the frequency is sufficiently high and the wavelength is sufficiently smaller than the diameter of the ball, the radial component of particle displacement at a position Q (θ_1, φ_1) is given by [16]

$$u(\theta_1, \varphi_1, t) = u_0 \, \mathrm{Re}\left[\exp ika\left(-\frac{V_R t}{a}\right)\left[\int_{-\theta_A}^{\theta_A} \frac{1}{\sqrt{\sin\theta}} \exp(ika\theta) d\theta_0\right]\right], \quad (5.1)$$

where u_0 is the amplitude, i is the imaginary unit, k is the wave number, V_R is the phase velocity of the SAW, a is the radius of the sphere, and θ is the central angle between a point within the line source and the observation point Q. Using the geometric consideration of the coordinate system shown in figure 5.1(a), θ is given by

$$\theta = \cos^{-1}(\cos\theta_0 \cos\phi_1 \sin\theta_1 + \sin\theta_0 \cos\theta_1). \quad (5.2)$$

The sound field at point Q results from the arc-shaped sound source, where the apertural angle as seen from the center O is $2\theta_A$, can be obtained by integrating u in equation (5.1) from $\theta_1 - \theta_A$ to θ_A and using the angle θ_1 included in equation (5.1) as an independent variable. The spatial distribution of the sound field obtained is represented as a function of the angle of elevation θ_1 of point Q.

Figures 5.1(b)–(d) show the calculated intensity distribution of the SAW on a sphere [16]. In summary, (b) shows the focusing beam, (c) the collimated beam, and (d) the diverging beam.

Figure 5.1(b) shows the surface of a sphere in three dimensions with the SAW energy distribution emitted from an arc-shaped sound source where the wave number parameter $ka = 600$. The height of the spherical surface is proportional to the SAW energy. When the apertural angle is large ($2\theta_A = 60°$) and the propagation angle ϕ_1 increases, the width of the sound field decreases. After reaching a minimum at the focal point $\phi_1 = 90°$, the width increases again, and the same distribution is reproduced in the sound field at the opposite pole where $\phi_1 = 180°$.

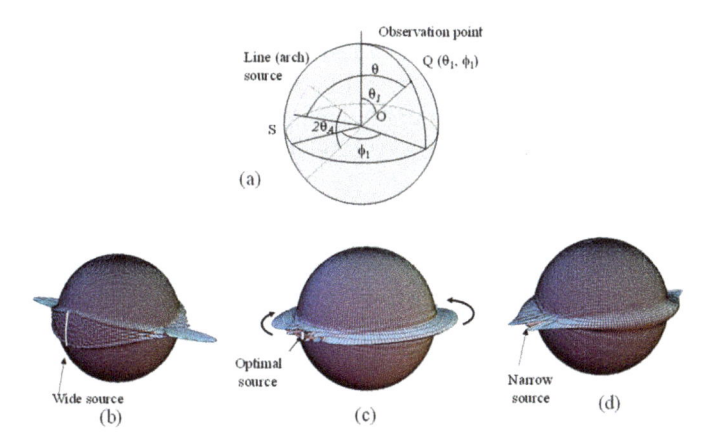

Figure 5.1. SAWs on a sphere. (a) Coordinate system, (b) focusing beam, (c) collimated beam, and (d) divergent beam. Reprinted with permission from [16]. Copyright 2006 Institute of Electrical and Electronics Engineers.

This is the focusing beam. After this, the change is repeated every 180° and does not vary regardless of the number of round trips. In this instance, the spread of the sound field due to the width of the sound source (aperture angle $2\theta_A = 60°$) is ignored. As a result, the SAW energy does not scatter where $\theta_1 > \theta_A$.

When the apertural angle is small ($\theta_A = 2°$), a diverging beam similar to that in the case of a point source is produced, as seen in figure 5.1(d). When the propagation angle ϕ_1 increases, the width of the sound field increases, and after reaching a maximum at $\phi_1 = 90°$, it decreases again, and a distribution identical to that of the sound source is reproduced at the opposite pole where $\phi_1 = 180°$. In contrast to the focusing beam, the SAW energy is not trapped within the band defined by $\theta_1 < \theta_A$. At $\phi_1 = 90°$, the beam spreads until it reaches a position far from the equator. When the support or other contact points are hit, the SAW is scattered. For this reason, this condition is undesirable for multiple round trips.

Finally, when the apertural angle $2\theta_A$ is approximately 7°, as shown in figure 5.1(c), the width of the sound field due to propagation remains virtually unchanged, and a naturally collimated beam is formed that propagates at a width of about $\theta_1 = \theta_A$. The apertural angle of this beam is referred to as the collimation angle θ_{COL}. A comparison of figures 5.1(b)–(d) shows that when the apertural angle $2\theta_A$ is almost the same as the collimation angle θ_{COL}, the SAW energy is trapped within the narrowest band. Even when there are distortions or irregularities at other points on the sphere, the propagation of the SAW is not disturbed. Even when there is a support or other contact points, the SAW is not scattered. Thus, the collimated beam can be expected to have the lowest possible attenuation and make the largest number of round trips.

The collimation angle is dependent on the wave number parameter ka. Consequently, mathematical analysis similar to that in figure 5.5 is performed for various ka, and the results are shown in table 5.1.

When the SAW is a pulse with a finite bandwidth, its displacement must be integrated for the wave number parameter. The origin of the naturally collimated beam can be thought of as the result of effective suppression of the spread of the SAW toward the periphery due to the diffraction effect of the geometrical focusing of the SAW toward the equator. Equation (5.1) does not have characteristics limited to an elastic wave, and as a result, the naturally collimated beam on a sphere is a general phenomenon that occurs for any surface wave, and possibly not just with SAWs.

Table 5.1. Wave number parameters and collimation angles (approximate values based on numerical calculation).

Wave number parameter ka	Collimation angle θ_{COL} (radians)
50	0.28
160	0.15
320	0.10
530	0.075
790	0.065

The collimation angle θ_{COL} is defined as the apertural angle $2\theta_A$ that realizes the collimated beam shown in (c). The numerical relation in table 5.1 is approximately expressed by [17]

$$\theta_{COL} = \sqrt{\frac{\pi}{ka}} = \sqrt{\frac{\lambda}{2a}}, \qquad (5.3)$$

where λ is the SAW wavelength. Note that the collimation width $2a\theta_{COL}$ that produces the collimated beam can be expressed by the remarkably simple relation $w_{COL} = \sqrt{2a\lambda}$, which is the geometrical mean of the diameter of the sphere and the wavelength [17]. This relation has been confirmed by numerical calculation and experiment.

Techniques are available that support the development of SAW devices using a naturally collimated beam on a ball. These include a method for sending and receiving an SAW by forming an electrode on a piezoelectric single-crystal ball and a method for forming a piezoelectric thin film on a ball made from a non-piezoelectric material. Multiple characteristics of round trips on crystal balls have been clarified experimentally [18]. For instance, on a $LiNbO_3$ ball, there are several round-trip routes [19]. In contrast, on quartz or langasite balls, the round-trip characteristics are best for the route along the equator perpendicular to the Z axis (Z cylinder). The effect of crystal anisotropy on SAWs on balls has not yet been fully understood, such as the case of the meandering collimated beam on a trigonal crystal ball [20].

5.3 Principles of the ball SAW sensor

In an SAW sensor, the SAW excited by a high-frequency pulse changes in amplitude and phase when passing through a sensitive film whose elastic properties change depending on the absorption of gas molecules (figure 5.2(a)). However, because of diffraction loss on a plane surface, the propagation distance is limited. Even in a planar SAW sensor with a resonator configuration, the propagation distance is limited because of diffraction loss. Thus, precise attenuation measurements are not possible. Consequently, the measurement precision of viscoelastic loss or leaky attenuation due to the environment is limited. Hydrogen gas sensors have been developed using planar SAW sensors [6, 7], but sensitivities sufficient for low-concentration hydrogen have not been achieved. The sensitive film must be made thick to improve the sensitivity, but the shortest response time is 100 s [7].

In the ball SAW sensor shown in figure 5.2(b), the naturally collimated beam passes through a region with a finite width along the equator, and it undergoes numerous circumnavigations without any diffraction loss. The changes in the SAW propagation characteristics resulting from the absorption of molecules into the sensitive film accumulate with each turn. As a result, if the change in delay time or amplitude is small at low gas concentrations, the change is multiplied 100 times after 100 circumnavigations (figures 5.2(c) and (d)). Thus, sensitivity is significantly increased. If the attenuation coefficient variation multiplied by the circumference of the sphere is $\Delta\alpha L = 10^{-3}$, the relative amplitude after one circumnavigation is $\exp(-\Delta\alpha L) = \exp(-10^{-3}) = 0.999$, which is practically indistinguishable. However,

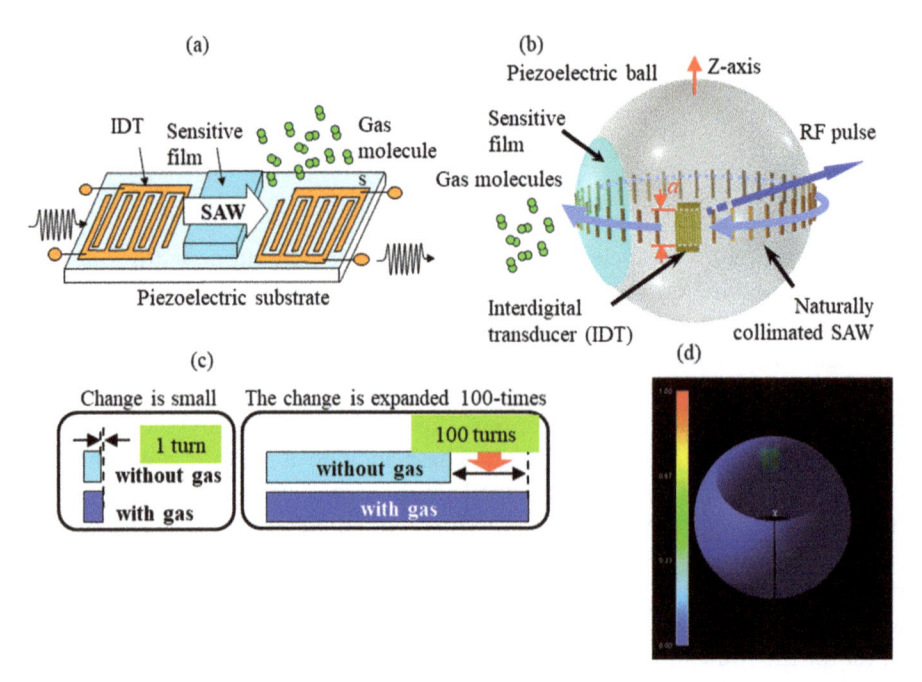

Figure 5.2. SAW sensors: (a) planar SAW sensor and (b) ball SAW sensor. (c) Operation of the ball SAW sensor. (d) Motion of an SAW on a quartz ball (video available at https://doi.org/10.1088/978-0-7503-4936-9).

the relative amplitude after 100 turns is $\exp(-100 \Delta\alpha L) = \exp(-0.1) = 0.905$, which is easily detected.

For this reason, the sensitive film of a ball SAW sensor can be made quite thin, and the response time is also shorter than that of a planar SAW sensor (one fiftieth in the case of a hydrogen gas sensor). Furthermore, the amplitude and phase vary due to different mechanisms resulting from various interactions between the elastic wave and molecules. As a result, a wide-concentration-range, highly sensitive sensor becomes feasible without saturation at high concentrations.

The design of a ball SAW sensor requires calculation of the waveform while considering the structure of an interdigitated transducer (IDT) and the properties and thickness of the sensitive film. Thus, we have developed a method [21] to predict the burst signal waveform generated by an IDT electrode after an arbitrary number n of circumnavigations:

$$s_O(t) = \frac{C}{2\pi} \sum_{n=1}^{N} \int_{k_0-\Delta k}^{k_0+\Delta k} A(k)^2 S[\omega(k)] \exp\left[i\omega(k)\left(t - \frac{nL}{V_P(k)}\right)\right] \exp[-\alpha(k)nL] \frac{\partial \omega}{\partial k} dk \quad (5.4)$$

for $nL/V_{G1} \leqslant t < (n+1)L/V_{G2}$, where $A(k)$ is an array factor of the IDT [22], C is a constant representing electromechanical coupling, k is the wave number, $k_0 = 2\pi/\lambda$ is the central wave number determined by the spatial period of the electrodes, Δk is the effective width of a wave number spectrum, $L = 2\pi a$ is the circumference of the ball with a radius of a, $V_P(k)$ is the phase velocity, $\omega = \omega(k)$ is the dispersion relation, and $\alpha(k)$ is the attenuation coefficient per unit length (1/m) of the SAW on the ball. V_{G1} and V_{G2} are respectively the smallest and largest group velocities of the SAW in the range of $k = k_0 \pm \Delta k$, which can be approximated by the Rayleigh wave velocity of the substrate V_R when the velocity dispersion is not very significant. Note that equation (5.4) is based on the ability of an SAW on a ball to eliminate the effects of diffraction and reflection, because the wave front is preserved even after multiple round trips.

If ball SAW sensors with thin sensitive films are operated with tone bursts that have different frequency components, the envelope of the tone burst is changed during SAW propagation, and a delayed peak may appear after multiple round trips due to frequency dispersion. This effect can be analyzed by approximating the dispersion relation as follows:

$$\omega = V_R k + \frac{c}{2}k^2, \qquad (5.5)$$

where c is a constant denoting dispersion.

The phase and group velocities are respectively given by $V_P = \omega/k = V_R + (c/2)k$ and $V_G = \partial\omega/\partial k = V_R + ck$. The group velocity changes from $V_G = V_R$ at zero frequency with $k = 0$ to $V_G = V_R + ck_0$ at the central frequency with $k = k_0$, and the magnitude of the change is $\Delta V = ck_0$. The attenuation per unit length (1/m) is given by $\alpha = \omega/(2QV_R)$, where $Q = \pi f/\alpha_t$ is the quality (Q) factor and α_t is the attenuation per unit time (1/s). If the Q factor is constant, the attenuation is proportional to the frequency. Substituting equation (5.5) into equation (5.2) gives the waveform. The parameters used in the following calculations are listed in table 5.2.

The waveform obtained at the 39th circumnavigation of a 10 mm-Φ 30 MHz ball SAW device is shown in figure 5.3(a). It has a double-electrode IDT that can generate harmonics at three times the fundamental frequency, and it is coated with a 40 nm-thick PdNi film. Note that a high-frequency signal at the third harmonic is observed with a delay due to the dispersion effect, and a second peak is formed at 403 μs. This behavior was precisely reproduced in the waveform shown in figure 5.3(b), which was calculated using equation (5.4) with the parameters in table 5.2. Hence, this theory is useful for the design analysis of ball SAW sensors with a sensitive film.

Table 5.2. Parameters used to simulate waveforms with bandwidth $\Delta\omega/2\pi = 30.0$ MHz, central wavelength $k_0/2\pi = 212.8$ μm, number of electrode pairs $N_P = 9$, circumference of the ball $L = 0.0314$ m, and SAW velocity at zero frequency $V_R = 3209$ m s^{-1}.

Sensitive film	Central frequency $\omega_0/2\pi$ (MHz)	Velocity dispersion parameter c (m^2 s^{-1})	Q factor
PdNi film	14.6	−169.3	4.4×10^4

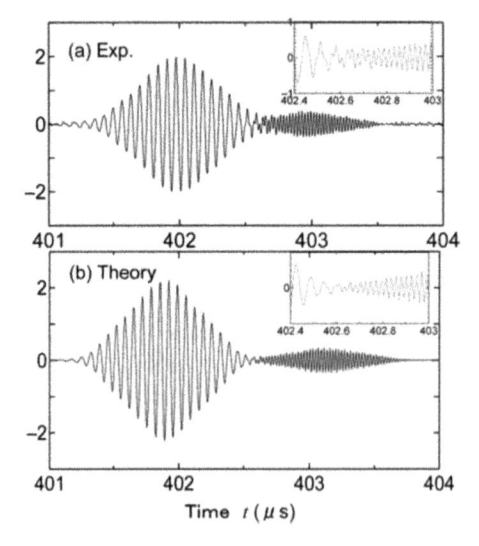

Figure 5.3. (a) Experimental and (b) calculated waveforms at the 39th circumnavigation of a ball SAW device coated with 40 nm-thick PdNi film. The parameters used for the calculation are given in table 5.2. Reprinted with permission from [21]. Copyright 2007 American Institute of Physics.

5.4 Hydrogen gas sensors

The authors developed a hydrogen gas sensor as the first application of the ball SAW sensor. For the sensitive film used to detect the hydrogen along the round-trip route, they developed a Pd or Pd alloy thin film that changes its conductivity [1] or elasticity when hydrogen is absorbed. In an experiment using a quartz ball that had a diameter of 10 mm, they fabricated an IDT (line width, 17.5 μm; length, 700 μm; number of pairs, 10) at the location where the SAW makes its round trip on the equator perpendicular to the crystal's Z axis. The Pd film was deposited at a thickness of 20 nm in the region corresponding to 80% of the SAW propagation route using a deposition mask, and a copper–constantan thermocouple thermometer was set up on the sensor surface to compensate for the effects of temperature variation on the SAW velocity. In an experiment using a quartz ball with a 1 mm diameter, an IDT with a line width of 5 μm was used, and a PdNi alloy thin film was deposited at a thickness of 40 nm on the area corresponding to 40% of the propagation route.

The hydrogen gas sensor was evaluated using a pulse-reflection-type ultrasonic transceiver in a cylindrical flow cell (40 mm in diameter) made of acrylic resin. H_2 gas and pure Ar or N (as carrier gases) were passed through the flow cell together, and the SAW waveform and temperature were measured at 2 to 10 s intervals. The concentration of hydrogen was adjusted using a mass flow controller, and the total gas flow rate was 5 L^{-1} min^{-1}.

Figure 5.4(a) shows the waveform received from the 10 mm sensor [16]. After Pd deposition, the SAW at the 51st circumnavigation could be clearly detected (central frequency: 44.8 MHz), and 100 round trips were observed. Note that the propagation distance was as long as 3142 mm, even though the width of the source was only 0.7 mm and the wavelength was 72 µm. At this propagation distance, SAW detection is impossible on a plane surface because of the diffraction loss. Figure 5.4(b) shows the waveform at the 51st turn in equilibrium with 3% H_2 in the Ar carrier gas. The SAW velocity was higher by 0.059 m s^{-1} in this gas than in the pure carrier gas, due to hydrogen absorption. Moreover, the amplitude was lower by 7% in the H_2 gas.

To evaluate the response time and sensitivity of the sensor, we then applied the wavelet transform using a Gabor function to the round-trip waveform at the 51st circumnavigation, and we found the delay time (propagation time) of a peak for the carrier gas between 506.070 µs and 506.085 µs. Moreover, the effect of temperature on the delay time was compensated for based on the measured temperature using a thermocouple in contact with the 10 mm sensor. The temperature coefficient of 12.5 ns °C^{-1} (= 25 ppm °C^{-1}) was separately evaluated and used for the temperature compensation.

Figure 5.5 shows the delay-time change (Δt) at various hydrogen concentrations. The delay-time changes were dependent on the concentration of hydrogen, and the

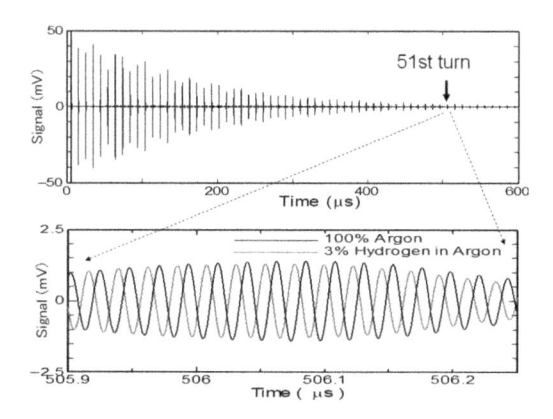

Figure 5.4. Waveforms produced by a ball SAW hydrogen gas sensor: (a) multiple round trips; (b) enlarged 51st circumnavigation signal. Reprinted with permission from [16]. Copyright 2006 Institute of Electrical and Electronics Engineers.

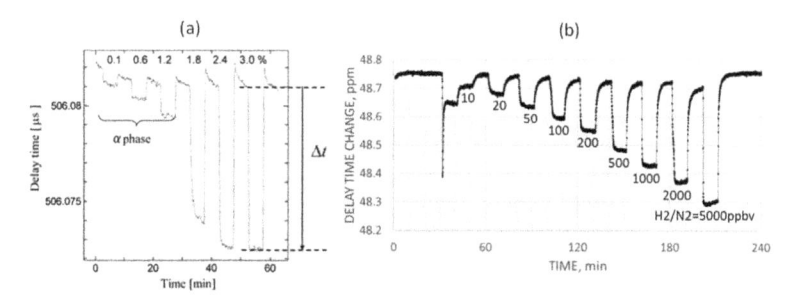

Figure 5.5. Delay-time responses of the hydrogen gas sensor: (a) high concentration range (reprinted with permission from [16]. Copyright 2006 Institute of Electrical and Electronics Engineers); (b) low concentration range.

delay time decreased with increasing hydrogen concentration. Moreover, the original reference values were restored on switching to the carrier gas.

Good detection sensitivity and reversibility were confirmed for hydrogen gas at a high concentration range from 0.1% (1000 ppmv) to 3% (30 000 ppmv), as shown in figure 5.5(a) for a 10 cm ball SAW sensor [16]. The temperature was approximately 22.5 °C. As a much lower concentration range from 5 ppmv (5000 ppbv) down to 10 ppbv, clear delay-time changes were observed at 60 °C as shown in figure 5.5(b). The result in figure 5.5(b) was achieved with a ϕ 3.3 mm quartz ball SAW sensor operated at 80 and 240 MHz coated with Pd–Pt alloy sensitive film. In this novel sensor, the temperature measurement performed for temperature compensation was realized by subtracting the response at 80 MHz from that at 240 MHz without touching the thermocouple to the sensor, as detailed later in section 5.5.1.

The measurement of 100% hydrogen was realized by the system shown in figure 5.6. In the driving circuit of the ball SAW sensor in figure 5.6(a) [23], a tone-burst RF signal at frequency 150 MHz with pulse width 1 μs is generated by a synthesizer and transmitted to the ball SAW sensor. An SAW is then received after multiple round trips.

The received signal is mixed in a heterodyne detection circuit with a reference signal at the local frequency $f_R + f_I$ generated by the synthesizer. The output of the mixer contains a signal,

$$V = V_0 \cos(2\pi f_R t + \phi) \cos\left[2\pi(f_R + f_I)t\right], \tag{5.6}$$

where V_0 and ϕ are the amplitude and phase of the RF signal, respectively, whose changes represent the response of the ball SAW sensor, and f_I is the intermediate frequency (IF). The multiplication in equation (5.6) gives a high-frequency signal at $2f_R + f_I$, which is filtered out by an IF filter and a signal downconverted to the IF

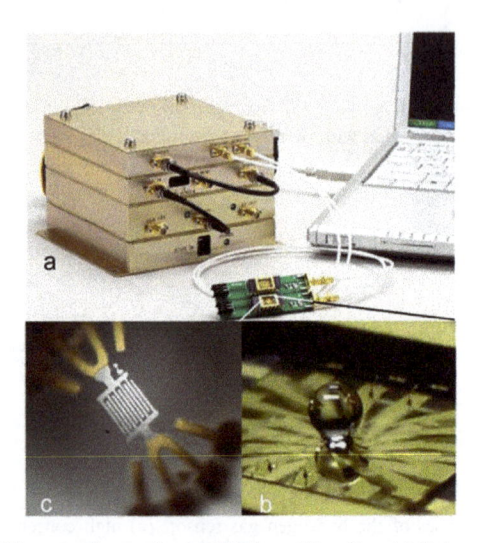

Figure 5.6. Quartz ball SAW sensor (1 mm ϕ) with PdNi sensitive film. (a) Driver circuit and sensor package. (b) Sensor element on a base plate. (c) IDT for 150 MHz.

signal, namely $V = (1/2)V_0 \cos(2\pi f_I t - \phi)$. Note that the phase ϕ of the RF signal is transferred to that of the IF signal.

In the digital quadrature detector (DQD) [23] shown in figure 5.6(a), the IF signal is digitized using an analog-to-digital (A/D) converter and Hadamard transformed to obtain the quadrature components $V_0 \cos \phi$ and $V_0 \sin \phi$ as an average in a specified time gate. The phase is obtained from $\phi = \tan^{-1}(\sin \phi / \cos \phi)$ and the delay time is obtained from $\Delta t = n_C/f_S - \phi/f_R$, where n_C is the number recorded by counters in the FPGA that accounts for the delay time of the signal and f_S is the system clock frequency. The amplitude V_0 is obtained either from the squared sum of $V_0 \cos \phi$ and $V_0 \sin \phi$ or from a separate power-detector signal. In the application of this approach to the ball SAW gas chromatograph described in section 5.6, an analog quadrature LSI detector is employed to realize a compact and low-cost sensor system.

Although a pure Pd film deteriorates because of the ß-phase transition at a hydrogen concentration of 3%, the phase transition in the film can be suppressed by adding Ni [1]. Thus, a stable film was obtained, even for 100% hydrogen, by alloying Pd with 30% Ni. We evaluated the variation in SAW velocity using the delay-time response of a ϕ 1 mm quartz ball SAW sensor operated at 156 MHz. The ϕ 1 mm sensor was installed in a package with an IDT fabricated on the bottom of the ball, as shown in figures 5.6(b) and (c). A 40 nm-thick PdNi film was deposited on top of the ball with 25% coverage of the whole equatorial path. SAW round trips consisting of as many as 200 circumnavigations were observed, but the signal at the 50th turn was used to obtain the response. Figure 5.7 (a) shows the delay-time response [16] over the range of hydrogen concentrations between 0.1% (1000 ppmv) and 100%. Because there were no signs of saturation even at a hydrogen concentration of 100%, measurement is not limited to 1 atm, and the sensor output for a hydrogen concentration under high pressure can be obtained even at pressures over 10 atm, such as those found in high-pressure hydrogen storage.

On the other hand, delay-time response at 15 °C to 75°C was observed for extremely low concentrations of less than 5 ppmv using a ϕ 3.3 mm quartz ball SAW

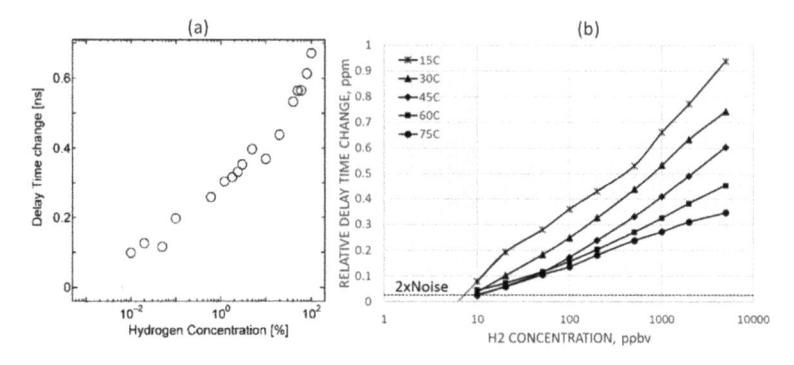

Figure 5.7. Delay-time response for a wide concentration range of hydrogen. (a) High concentration range of 0.01 to 100%. Reprinted with permission from [16]. Copyright 2006 Institute of Electrical and Electronics Engineers. (b) Low concentration range of 10 to 5000 ppbv.

sensor operated at 80 MHz and 240 MHz. As shown in figure 5.7(b), the limit of detection evaluated at twice the noise level was as low as 6 ppbv at 60 °C. These results clearly indicate that the ball SAW sensor is applicable to the detection of extremely high (100%) and low (10 ppbv) concentrations of hydrogen.

5.5 Trace moisture analyzer

5.5.1 Ball SAW TMA using phase signal for temperature compensation

In addition to the use of ball SAW in TMA as described in 5.1, measurement and control of trace moisture at a frost point (FP) as low as −100 °C (concentration of 14 ppbv) are also required to improve the yield of semiconductor devices and ensure their reliability. An SAW sensor with a metal–organic-framework coating [8] was developed for trace moisture analysis that had a sensitivity of 280 ppbv at −85 °C. However, its sensitivity does not fulfill the aforementioned requirements. Thus, our group developed a ball SAW TMA [23, 24], and a detection limit of 0.2 ppbv was realized [25].

A 3.3 mm-Φ quartz harmonic ball SAW device with a fundamental frequency of 80 MHz was coated with SiOx solution synthesized by a sol–gel reaction [26]. The ball SAW TMA was connected to a trace moisture generator (TMG) using a diffusion tube method [4], as shown in figure 5.8. It was capable of providing a N_2 flow of 0.1 l min^{-1} with moisture concentrations of up to 1000 nmol mol^{-1} (ppbv). A cavity ring-down spectroscope (Tiger Optics, HALO 3 H_2O) was connected downstream from the ball SAW TMA to measure the moisture concentration using SUS316L stainless-steel tubes that had 6.35 mm outer diameters and lengths of 300 mm. The gas pressure at the ball SAW TMA was regulated to 130 kPa by the built-in pressure regulator of the CRDS TMA.

In the earlier stage of ball SAW TMA development [26], an amorphous layer of polished quartz served as the layer sensitive to water molecules, but the reproducibility of such a layer has not been established. Thus, an amorphous sol–gel silica (SiOx) film was tested and proved to have a significantly high sensitivity to water.

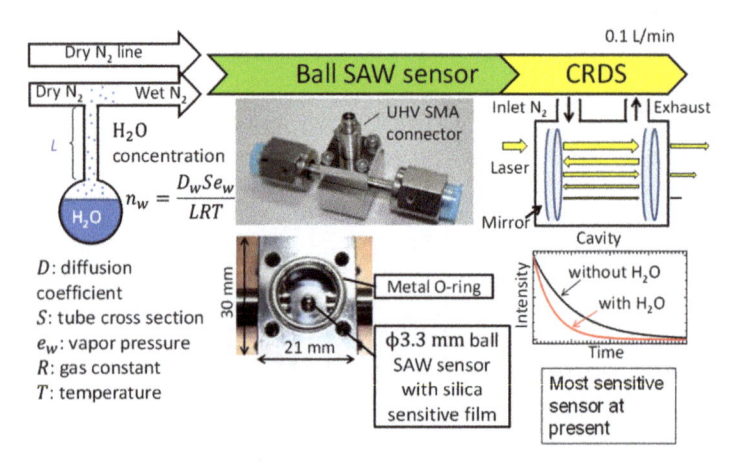

Figure 5.8. Evaluation of ball SAW TMA in comparison to CRDS. Reprinted with permission from [25]. Copyright 2014 The Japan Society of Applied Physics.

Tetraethoxysilane was hydrolyzed and polymerized with an acid as a catalyst to obtain SiOx [25]. A harmonic ball SAW sensor (quartz, ϕ 3.3 mm, 80 MHz, 240 MHz) was employed to compensate for the effects of temperature [25, 27].

The results of the trace moisture measurement are shown in figure 5.9, in which the concentration gradually increases and decreases every 3 h. Figure 5.9(a) shows the responses at 80 MHz and 240 MHz. Although the response at water concentrations of more than 80 ppbv was clear, it was disturbed by the temperature drift. Figure 5.9(b) shows the difference between the delay times at the two frequencies. The response was clear, even at 6 ppbv and 19 ppbv, as a result of the use of temperature compensation based on the frequency difference method [27, 28]. Figure 5.9(c) shows the response determined using CRDS, recognized as the most sensitive and accurate commercial TMA. It gave a total sequence of responses similar to that of the ball SAW TMA. Thus, the measurement of trace moisture at 10 ppbv by the ball SAW sensor was confirmed.

The response of the ball SAW TMA was faster than that of the CRDS and the 10%–90% response time was evaluated when the water concentration was changed from 400 ppbv to 810 ppbv. The response times of the ball SAW sensor and CRDS were 90 and 780 s, respectively. Since the response time of CRDS when it was connected before the ball SAW sensor was similar to this case, the response time of CRDS was not limited by the ball SAW sensor. The difference in the response time was probably caused by the difference between the cavity volume of the the cavity ring-down spectroscope (tens of mL) and that of the ball SAW sensor cell (0.3 mL).

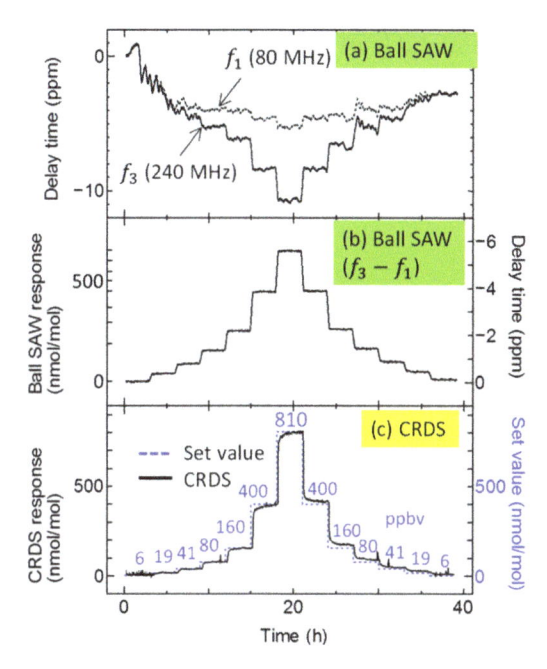

Figure 5.9. Trace moisture measurements: (a) raw signal obtained from the ball SAW TMA; (b) from the temperature-compensated ball SAW TMA; (c) from CRDS.

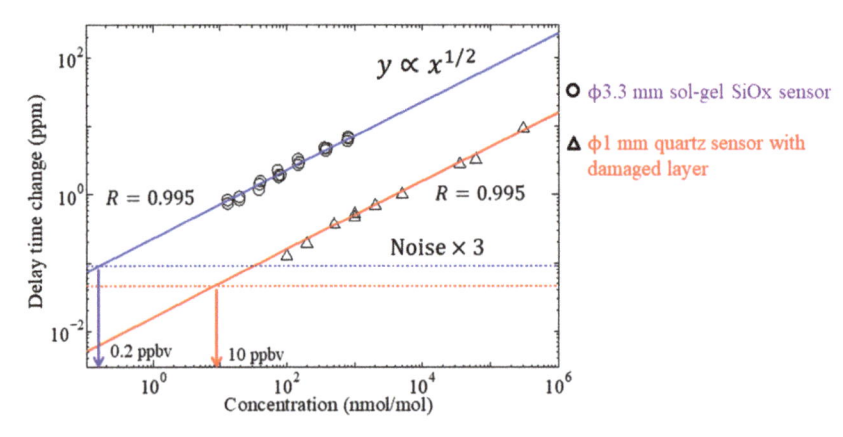

Figure 5.10. Calibration curve for delay time and sensitivity. Reprinted with permission from [25]. Copyright 2014 The Japan Society of Applied Physics.

The relationship between the delay-time change and the concentration is shown in figure 5.10. The open circles show the results for four replicates of the SiOx-film-coated ball SAW and the open triangles show the results for the quartz sensor with a damaged layer. The solid and dotted lines show the extrapolated lines with least-squares fitting to the experimental results and threefold values of rms noise, respectively. The intersections give a detection limit at a sound-to-noise ratio of three. The sensitivity was improved by one order of magnitude using the same measurement setup, resulting in a two-digit detection limit of 0.2 nmol mol^{-1} (ppbv), which is lower than that of the quartz sensor with the damaged layer. Note that the detection limit of the CRDS is on the order of 0.1 ppbv. From these results, it was demonstrated that the sensitivity of the ball SAW sensor can be comparable to that of the CRDS. Moreover, it was shown that the data for the SiOx-film-coated ball SAW sensor fit the square-root function down to the level of 10 ppbv. The square-root dependence is key to verifying the reaction model of the water molecules and the silica lattice [28].

5.5.2 Ball SAW TMA using amplitude signal for various background gases

In research into moisture analysis over a wide FP range from −100 °C to 0 °C [25], it has been found that the delay time Δt decreases (SAW velocity increases) as the moisture concentration increases or as the FP increases from −100 °C to −60 °C. However, Δt saturates at FPs of −50 °C to −40 °C, and then increases (SAW velocity decreases) at FPs of −40 °C to 0 °C. This behavior can be explained by the elastic stiffening due to siloxane bond formation on the quartz surface in the low moisture concentration range [28] and the mass loading due to the water molecule adsorption in the high moisture concentration range [25]. In contrast, the attenuation coefficient monotonically increases over the entire moisture concentration range. Although the amplitude signal is not sensitive at FPs below −70 °C, it can be used at FPs above −60 °C. Moreover, the attenuation coefficient has a significant advantage, since its frequency dependence varies depending on different mechanisms [29].

In TMA used in background gases (BGs), such as air, nitrogen (N_2), or natural gases (NGs), the composition of the BGs is not always constant but sometimes changes. For example, when H_2 is injected into NGs such as methane (CH_4) and ethane (C_2H_6) for the safe transport of H_2 or to improve the combustion performance of the NGs, the H_2 concentration should be measured and controlled to ensure the safety of the NG pipelines [30]. As another example, a glove box is filled with an inert gas such as Ar or He when Li-ion batteries are assembled [31] or three-dimensional (3D) metal printing takes place, in order to prevent the degradation of the products. After exposure to humid ambient air, the moisture in the glove box is purged using a dry inert gas flow. To optimize the purging process, the spatial distribution of not only the moisture concentration but also the inert gas concentration should be monitored, since an efficient exchange of air with the inert gas is required.

We have developed a ball SAW TMA that uses two-frequency measurement (TFM) of the delay time [31, 32] to compensate for the temperature variation shown in figure 5.10 as well as to measure the temperature itself [33]. In the FP range of $-60\ °C$ to $-10\ °C$, the attenuation of an SAW rather than its velocity is used to measure the moisture content. Since the attenuation is affected by BGs, the composition of the BGs should be determined and the variation in BG composition should be compensated for. To fulfill this requirement, TFM with attenuation measurement was attempted to determine the BG composition by considering the different frequency dependences of the SAW attenuation caused either by the moisture content or the BG composition [28]. We explain the principle and quantitative verification of this method.

For the SAW sensor that transmits a burst of two frequencies, $f = f_1$ and $f = f_2$, the attenuations α_1 and α_2 are respectively measured. The attenuations are given by

$$\alpha_1 = a_0 f_1 + a_1(w) f_1^2 + a_2 f_1^y, \quad \alpha_2 = a_0 f_2 + a_1(w) f_2^2 + a_2 f_2^y, \quad (5.7)$$

where

$$a_0 = \alpha_L l = \frac{Pl}{\rho_S V_S^2} \sqrt{\frac{\gamma M}{RT}} = \frac{Pl}{\rho_S V_S^2} \frac{G}{\sqrt{RT}} \quad (5.8)$$

is the loss due to the leaky attenuation of an SAW [29], $\alpha_L f$ is the attenuation coefficient due to gas loading, l the propagation length of an SAW, $G = \sqrt{\gamma M}$ the gas parameter, M the molecular weight, and γ the ratio of specific heat at a constant pressure to specific heat at a constant volume. ρ_S and V_S are the density and SAW velocity of the substrate, respectively. $a_1(w)f^2$ is the viscoelastic attenuation [34] caused by moisture, w is the moisture content, P is the pressure, R is the gas constant, and T is the temperature. The term a_2 is the device loss due to scattering or electromechanical conversion at the electrodes, and y is the frequency dependence index of the device loss.

Since the viscoelastic attenuation is proportional to f^2, it is canceled in a leakage factor defined as

$$\Delta \alpha_L \equiv \left[(f_2/f_1)^2 \alpha_1 - \alpha_2 \right]/l \quad (5.9)$$

and, from equation (5.7), it is given by

$$\Delta\alpha_L = \left[a_0(f_1^{-1}f_2^2 - f_2) + a_2(f_1^{y-2}f_2^2 - f_2^y)\right]/l \qquad (5.10)$$

Similarly, since the leaky attenuation is proportional to f, it is canceled in a viscoelastic factor defined as

$$\Delta\alpha_V \equiv \left[\alpha_2 - (f_2/f_1)\alpha_1\right]/l \qquad (5.11)$$

and, from equation (5.7), it is given by

$$\Delta\alpha_V = \left[a_1(w)(f_2^2 - f_1f_2) + a_2(f_2^y - f_1^{y-1}f_2)\right]/l \qquad (5.12)$$

In the special case of $f_2 = 3f_1$, where the second frequency is the third harmonic,

$$\Delta\alpha_L = [6a_0 + a_2(9 - 3^y)]/l \quad \text{and} \quad \Delta\alpha_V = [6a_1(w) + a_2(3^y - 3)]/l. \qquad (5.13)$$

Using equations (5.7) and (5.13), we can obtain a gas parameter given by

$$G = B(\Delta\alpha_L - d) \text{ with } B = \left(\rho_S V_S^2 \sqrt{RT}\right)/(6f_0 P) \text{ and } d = (a_2/l)(9 - 3^y). \qquad (5.14)$$

Since the device loss $a_2 f_2^y$ discretely increases as the number of circumnavigations increases, and the frequency dependence index of the device loss y is usually unknown, calibration is required at a specific number of circumnavigation for quantitative evaluation. We thus performed calibration to relate the viscoelastic factor calculated using equation (5.11) to the FP, a measure of water concentration. Figure 5.11 shows the calibration curve thus obtained with nitrogen as the BG [35].

To simulate a concentration variation of BG in a natural gas pipeline, the generated humidity was set to a certain value, for example, an FP of −60 °C, and the BG was switched in the following sequence: air, N_2, CH_4, 80% CH_4/20% C_2H_6, 50% CH_4/50% C_2H_6, CH_4, N_2, and then air. During this sequence, the attenuation coefficients of the ball SAW sensor were measured at 80 and 240 MHz at intervals of 12 s. Figure 5.12 shows the viscoelastic factor $\Delta\alpha_V$ and the leakage factor $\Delta\alpha_L$

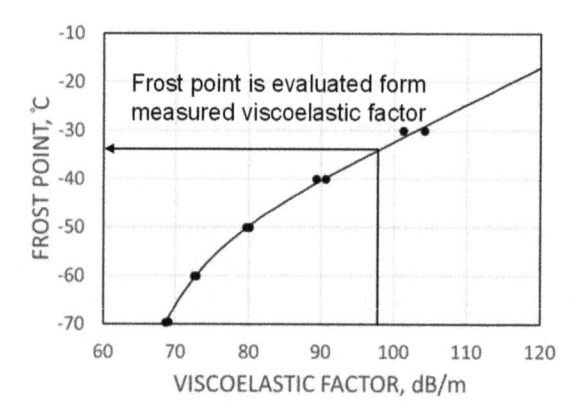

Figure 5.11. Calibration curve for amplitude.

calculated using equations (5.9) and (5.11). In figure 5.12(a), the viscoelastic factor remained almost constant, as expected. In figure 5.12(b), the leakage factor showed a clear change following the change in BG content. Since the gas parameter $G = \sqrt{\gamma M}$ of the BG can be estimated from the leakage factor, this measurement is useful for monitoring pipeline conditions [27].

The same procedure was repeated while the humidity generator produced nominal FPs of −70 °C to −30 °C at 10 °C intervals. The calibration curve was then applied to the other background gas mixtures and the resultant FPs of the trace moisture were compared with the reference FPs. Figure 5.13 shows the measurement error calculated using the resultant FP value minus the reference FP value as a function of nominal FP, for the different BGs and BG mixtures designated by symbols and lines. In this humidity range, the errors are within 1 °C for the FP.

Hence, these results verified that no additional calibrations are required for most practical applications, even when the combination of gas components in the background natural gas mixture is changed. This is clear evidence that the ball SAW TMA can measure the correct trace moisture concentration following a single

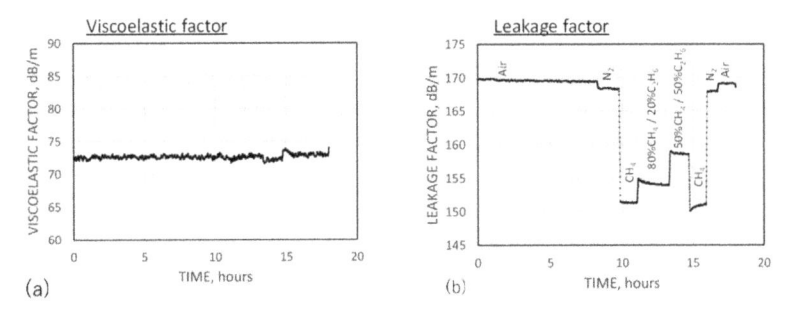

Figure 5.12. Variations of viscoelastic factor (a) and leakage factor (b).

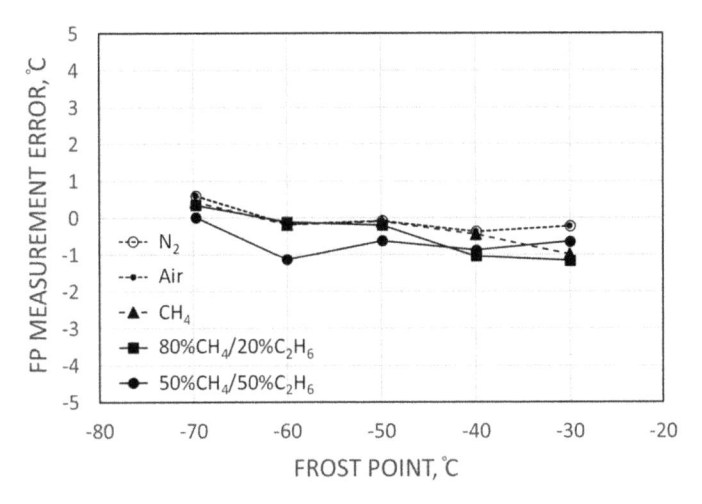

Figure 5.13. Evaluation of error.

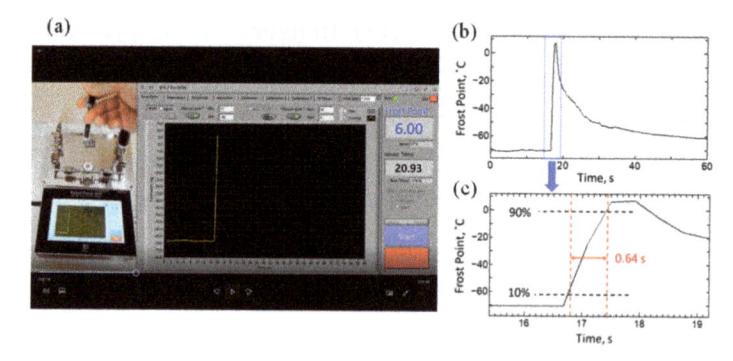

Figure 5.14. Quick response of the ball SAW trace moisture analyzer. (a) Experimental setup and display (video available at https://doi.org/10.1088/978-0-7503-4936-9). (b) Temporal variation of FP measured by ball SAW trace moisture analyzer. (c) Expanded view of the peak.

calibration for nitrogen background gas, even when the combination of the background gas components, such as methane, ethane, carbon dioxide, and nitrogen, changes in natural gas mixtures.

To evaluate the response time of the ball SAW TMA, we measured the FP after injecting saturated water vapor [36]. Figure 5.14(a) shows the experimental setup and the display of the ball SAW TMA. The injection volume was 1 mL and the flow rate of the background gas was 100 mL min^{-1}. Figure 5.14(b) shows the temporal variation of the FP after the injection of saturated water vapor. The FP immediately increased from −70 °C to 5 °C within 1 s and then gradually decreased in 10 min. The reason for the slow decrease is because the water adsorbed on the inner surface of the pipe was gradually desorbed. An expanded view of the peak is shown in figure 5.14(c). The response time taken for 10% to 90% of the FP to change from −70 °C to 10 °C was only 0.64 s. This is the shortest response time of a TMA reported so far.

5.6 Micro gas chromatography

5.6.1 Concept and problems of gas chromatography

As illustrated in the video of figure 5.15(a), in the food industry, it is sometimes necessary to judge the freshness of food using its emitted gas. In the fields of environmental measurement and security, hazardous or toxic gases of various types must be rapidly detected at high sensitivity. When a target gas is specified, a sensor that is highly sensitive to that gas can be prepared. However, when the target gas is unknown, the gas cannot in general be detected, even if various existing sensors are employed. In such cases, qualitative and quantitative analyses are performed by gas chromatography (GC) [37] in a laboratory after acquiring gas samples in the field.

However, in many cases, the gas cannot be identified unless the analysis is performed on site and in real time. For this reason, portable gas chromatographs have been developed, but they are usually larger than 20 cm per side and heavier than 5 kg, which makes it difficult to carry them to various sites. The development of a small gas sensor for individual use that can be used for practical on-site analysis has been problematic. This is one of the major issues in the realm of gas measurement technology today.

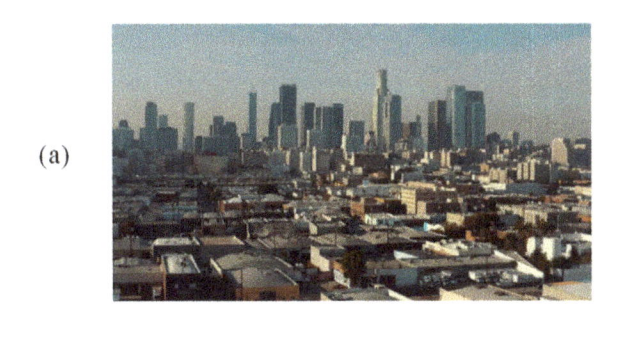

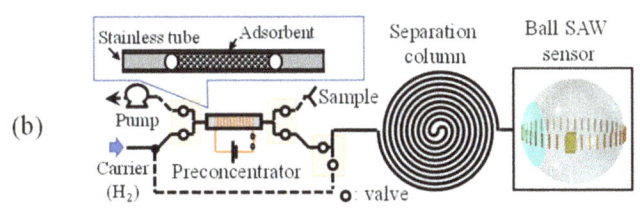

Figure 5.15. Concept of GC. (a) Monitored environment (video available at https://doi.org/10.1088/978-0-7503-4936-9); (b) schematic of the ball SAW gas chromatograph.

In this situation, we began research into the use of a ball SAW sensor and miniaturized GC components to develop a micro gas chromatograph smaller than a 20 cm cube and less than 2 kg in weight, which would solve the problems inherent in conventional GC. Figure 5.15(b) shows a schematic of the ball SAW gas chromatograph.

To start the GC analysis, sample gas in the atmosphere or in a gas bag is drawn in by a small pump and accumulated in an adsorbent inserted in the stainless-steel tube of a preconcentrator (PC) for a predetermined suction time. After the suction period is over, carrier gas is supplied by a hydrogen storage canister at a flow rate controlled by a pressure regulator. At the same time, the PC is heated by a Ni–Cr heater tightly wound around the stainless-steel tube at a rate of 35–40 °C s^{-1}. A band of the gas mixture is thus generated and injected into a gas separation column.

The sample gas is measured by separating it over time in the separation column. The time taken for a particular peak of the gas to appear at the output of the column (the retention time, t_R) can be approximated by

$$t_R = \frac{V_G + KV_L}{F}. \tag{5.15}$$

Here, V_G is the volume of the gas-phase component in the column, K is the partition coefficient for the sample gas in the liquid phase (coating the inner surface of the separation column), which corresponds to the solubility of the gas, V_L is the volume of the liquid phase (determined by the thickness of the liquid phase and the length of the column), and F is the flow rate of the carrier gas. Because t_R is different for each gas, the gases can be identified using peaks that occur at different times in the chromatogram.

5.6.2 Sensitive film used in the ball SAW gas chromatograph

In developing the gas chromatograph, we prepared a sensitive film for nonpolar gases and another for polar gases. For nonpolar gases, 0.5 wt% poly-dimethylsiloxane (PDMS) in toluene solvent was coated on a ball SAW sensor by the off-axis spin-coating method [38] and the solvent was purged by curing the film in an oven.

In the conventional spin-coating method, the flow of the solution of a sensitive film material is unstable, and abrupt emission might occur from the propagation route of SAW, since the direction of the centrifugal force is normal to the surface; thus, the film becomes thick and irregular. In contrast, in the off-axis spin-coating method, the solution flow is smooth along the propagation route, and excess solution is effectively removed since the direction of the centrifugal force is tangential to the surface; thus, the film becomes thin and uniform.

Three types of material were prepared: (poly-4-vinylpyridine (P4VP), poly-epichlorohydrin (PECH), and poly-N-vinylpyrrolidone (PNVP)); these are reported to be sensitive to polar gases when used in flat SAW sensors. The structural formulas of these materials are shown in figure 5.16. The P4VP was dissolved in tetrahydrofuran at 1 mg mL^{-1}, PECH at 2.5 mg mL^{-1} in chloroform, and PNVP at 0.5 wt% in 2-propanol, and films of these materials were formed on the ball SAW sensors by off-axis spin coating.

To evaluate the response of each sensitive film, we connected each ball SAW sensor to a desktop gas chromatograph and analyzed sample gas A, which was prepared by introducing four polar gases into the gas bag filled with nitrogen gas. The concentrations of the gas components are shown in table 5.3. The sample gas

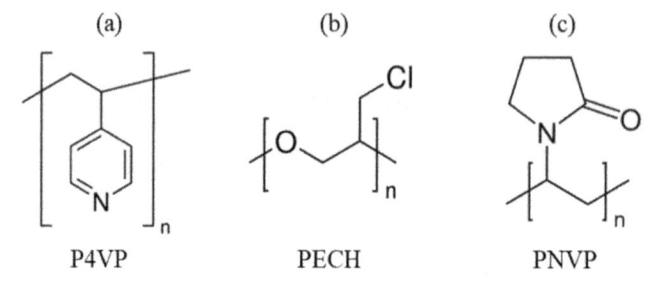

Figure 5.16. Structural formulas of the compounds for used to create films sensitive to polar gases: (a) poly-4-vinylpyridine, P4VP; (b) poly-epichlorohydrin, PECH; (c) poly-N-vinylpyrrolidone, PNVP.

Table 5.3. Components of sample gas A.

	Gas	Concentration of sample gas components (ppmv)
1	Acetaldehyde (CH$_3$CHO)	50
2	Acetone (ACE)	50
3	Methanol (MeOH)	50
4	2-Propanol (IPA)	50

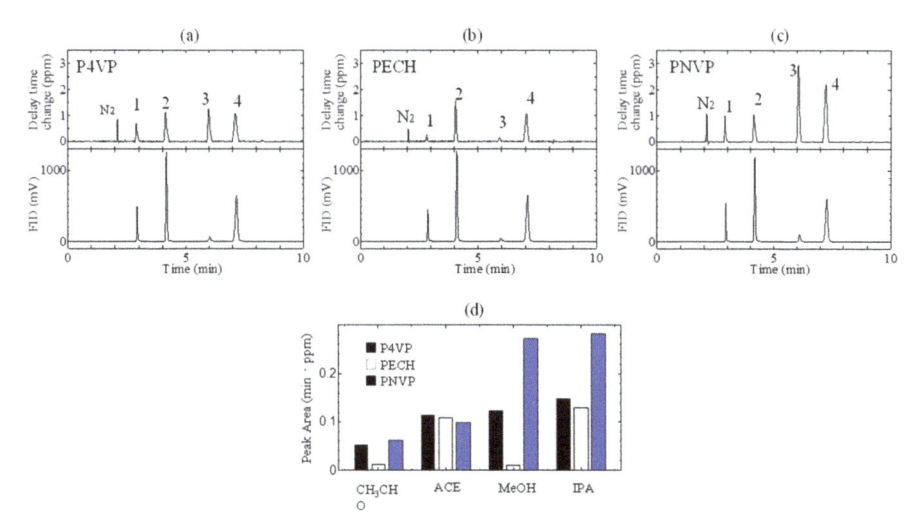

Figure 5.17. Chromatograms of sample gas A obtained using (a) P4VP, (b) PECH, and (c) PNVP. (d) Peak areas of the polar gases for each sensitive film material.

was collected at 17.3 mL min^{-1} for 0.5 min in a small PC filled with Tenax TA. We used a fused silica capillary column (Inert CAP® Elite-WAX, GL Science Inc.) that had a length of 30 m, an inner diameter of 0.32 mm, and a film thickness of 0.25 µm; the column was coated with polyethylene glycol (PEG) as the stationary phase. The column temperature was maintained at 40 °C by an oven of the desktop gas chromatograph. A ball SAW sensor was connected at the column outlet to confirm the response to each component. Furthermore, after the analysis, the gas was introduced into a flame ionization detector (FID) and measured at the same time.

Figures 5.17(a)–(c) show chromatograms obtained using the ball SAW sensors with three different sensitive films. The upper panels are chromatograms obtained from the delay-time change of the ball SAW sensor, and the lower panels are chromatograms obtained using the FID. Since the FID response was similar for the three measurements, it can be considered that the sample volume was the same for each measurement. Figure 5.17(d) shows a comparison of the peak areas of the responses of the ball SAW sensor to each component of sample gas A. It was found that PNVP was the most sensitive to all components. Therefore, PNVP was adopted as the sensitive film of the sensor for the polar gases.

5.6.3 Palm-sized ball SAW gas chromatograph as an example of micro GC

To study the feasibility of on-site GC analysis, we developed a palm-size ball SAW GC [39] with a 3 m long metal micro-electromechanical system (MEMS) column and a ball SAW sensor with an amplitude measurement circuit. To develop a portable GC applicable to space exploration (for example, to monitor the cabin atmosphere in spacecraft and for use in explorations for mineral resources and organic compounds on the Moon or other planets), we implemented a PC, a temperature controller for the column temperature programming, and a phase

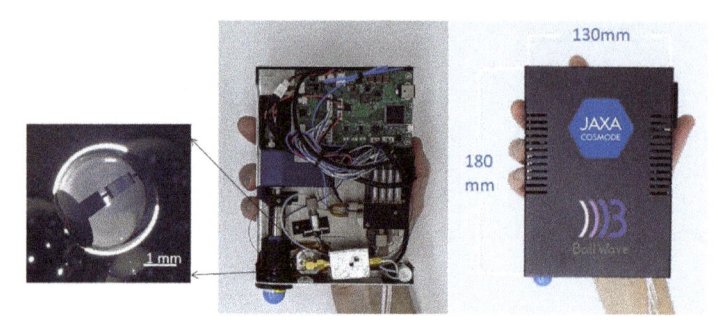

Figure 5.18. Palm-sized ball SAW GC.

measurement circuit into a ball SAW GC in collaboration with the Japan Aerospace Exploration Agency (JAXA) [40].

As an application of this technology to environmental monitoring and the terrestrial food industry, we developed a palm-sized ball SAW GC equipped with a 30 m long solenoid column [41] (figure 5.18). Its dimensions are 130 mm × 180 mm × 80 mm and its weight is 1.25 kg. This extremely small and light GC can easily be carried to any site. The carrier gas was supplied from a 6 L hydrogen storage canister at a flow rate precisely controlled by a pressure regulator. The PC was a stainless-steel tube with an outer diameter of 1.6 mm and a wall thickness of 0.18 mm. It was filled either with two types of adsorbent, Carboxen® 1000 (Sigma-Aldrich) and Tenax TA (GL Science) or with only Tenax TA. The solenoid column was fabricated by processing a commercially available metal capillary column Ultra ALLOY® (Frontier Laboratories Ltd) with a length of 30 m into a coil with a diameter of 27 mm and a length of 65 mm. The ball SAW sensor was coated with PDMS as the sensitive film.

To evaluate the precision of the GC, a retention index [42] is used to convert the retention times into system-independent constants. If a gas chromatograph provides a reliable retention index, it can be used to estimate unknown components by calculating the retention index and comparing it with the retention indices of known gases. To test it, we installed a 30 m long solenoid column coated with 5% diphenyl-PDMS as a stationary phase into the palm-sized gas chromatograph. We then analyzed sample gas B, in which linear alkanes C6 to C13 were mixed in a nitrogen atmosphere. The sample gas was collected at 26.5 mL min^{-1} for 10 s, and the column temperature was maintained at 50 °C for 2 min and then raised to 180 °C at 10 °C min^{-1}.

Next, hazardous gas components were mixed at the concentrations shown in table 5.4 in a nitrogen atmosphere to form sample gas C and analyzed under the same conditions. The results are shown in figure 5.19. The retention index [42] I_i of each component was calculated according to the following equation using the retention time t_i of each peak i and the retention times of the linear alkanes of sample B listed in table 5.5.

$$I_i = 100\left[n + \frac{t_i - t_n}{t_{n+1} - t_n}\right] \quad (5.16)$$

Table 5.4. Components of sample gas C.

	Gas	Concentration of sample gas components (ppmv)
1	Benzene (B)	50
2	Toluene (T)	30
3	Ethylbenzene (E)	20
4	m-Xylene (m-X)	20
5	o-Xylene (o-X)	20
6	Heptanal (C7O)	20
7	Nonanal (C9O)	10

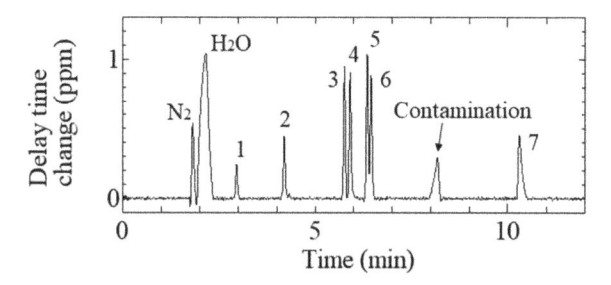

Figure 5.19. Chromatogram of sample gas C.

Table 5.5. Retention times of linear alkanes.

Gas	Retention time (min)
C6	2.51
C7	3.31
C8	4.69
C9	6.45
C10	8.36
C11	10.23
C12	12.03
C13	13.74

Here, n is the carbon number of the n-alkane leading peak i, and t_n and t_{n+1} are the retention times of the leading and trailing n-alkanes, respectively. Note that the retention index depends on the temperature program, gas velocity, and the column used in the analysis.

Table 5.6 summarizes the retention indices calculated from the chromatogram of sample gas C shown in figure 5.19 and the retention indices published by the column manufacturer [43]. The retention index for each component was within 1% of the published value. Therefore, if we did not know the components of sample gas C, this

Table 5.6. Retention time and calculated retention index of each component in the chromatogram in figure 5.20 and the published retention indices.

Gas	Retention time (min)	Calculated retention index	Published retention index [42]
B	2.95	655	659
T	4.19	764	767
E	5.76	861	864
m-X	5.91	869	871
o-X	6.35	894	897
C7O	6.45	900	
C9O	10.30	1004	

gas chromatograph could be used to identify the unknown components by calculating the retention indices and comparing them with a retention-time database. Thus, the palm-sized ball SAW GC is capable of monitoring hazardous gases in the atmosphere.

5.6.4 Analysis of the aroma components of sake — a crystal sommelier

We installed a solenoid column coated with PEG as a stationary phase into the palm-sized gas chromatograph and analyzed the aromatic components of sake, which is a brewed beverage, 'rice wine'. There are two types of sake, which differ in the polishing process used for the rice grains: Honjozo-shu has a rich aroma and Ginjo-shu has a fresh aroma. To evaluate the capability of the palm-sized GC to function as a sommelier of sake, Honjozo-shu samples A, B, and C and Ginjo-shu samples D, E, and F were prepared from different brands. The headspace gas of a vial of each sake was collected to the PC at 16 mL min^{-1} for 2 min. The column temperature was maintained at 40 °C for 5 min and then raised to 140 °C at 10 °C min^{-1}.

Figure 5.20 shows the chromatograms of the headspace gas of Honjozo-shu A and Ginjo-shu D [41]. The components corresponding to the peaks observed were identified as follows: 1, ethyl acetate; 2, ethanol; 3, water; 7, isoamyl alcohol; 9, ethyl caproate; and 10, ethyl caprylate. In addition, peak 5, which had a retention time of 8.6 min, was identified as corresponding to isoamyl acetate, but the components corresponding to peaks 4, 6, and 8 appearing before and after peak 5 are currently unidentified.

Figure 5.21 shows the peak areas of isoamyl acetate (*H*), a component that gives Honjozo-shu its banana-like aroma; ethyl caproate (*G1*), a component that gives Ginjo-shu its apple or melon-like aroma; and ethyl caprylate (*G2*), a component that gives Ginjo-shu its pineapple or apricot-like aroma. The symbol *H* stands for the Honjozo aroma, *G1* stands for the most typical Ginjo aroma and *G2* stands for a supplementary Ginjo aroma, respectively.

In the histograms in figure 5.21, Honjozo-shu's are mostly rich in *H* and Ginjo-shu's are mostly rich in *G1* and *G2*. Furthermore, the difference between the

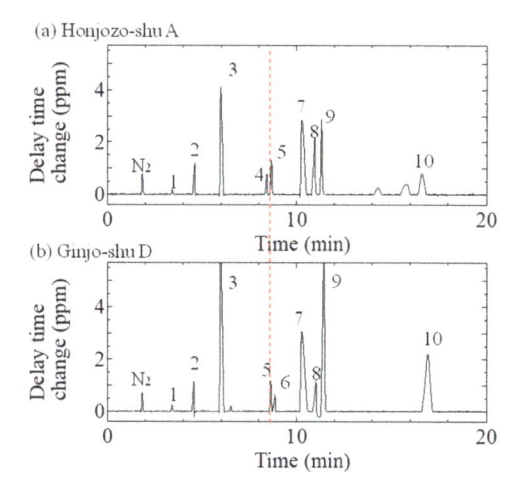

Figure 5.20. Chromatograms obtained by analysis of (a) Honjozo-shu A and (b) Ginjo-shu D.

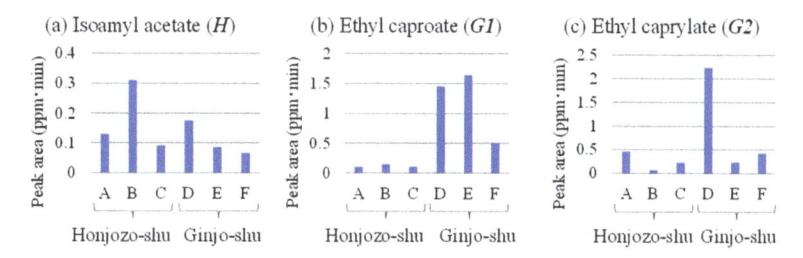

Figure 5.21. Peak areas of the aroma components of each brand: (a) isoamyl acetate; (b) ethyl caproate; (c) ethyl caprylate.

Honjozo-shu and Ginjo-shu histograms can be evaluated, and the character of each brewer becomes clear. Note that Honjozo-shu B differs from A and C in that it is rich in *H* but low in *G1* and *G2*. Similarly, Ginjo-shu E differs from D and F in that it is rich in *G1* but low in *G2* and *H*. Thus, brands B and E contain large amounts of a single typical aroma. It is known that they are brewed by the same brewer.

In contrast, Ginjo-shu D is different from E, F, and every other brand in that it contains several abundant aromas *G1*, *G2* and *H*. This significant character comes partly from the hybrid use of yeast for Honjozo-shu and yeast for Ginjo-shu. Ginjo-shu D has won a gold medal in the Ginjo-shu category in an international wine contest. It is presumed that the brewers of Honjozo-shu B, Ginjo-shu E, and Ginjo-shu D designed them to contain a characteristic combination of aromas.

In summary, we have developed a palm-sized portable gas chromatograph. This gas chromatograph is equipped with components comparable to those of a desktop GC, which include the sampler, PC, and column temperature controller. Using this gas chromatograph, we analyzed the headspace gas of six samples of sake and showed that the peak areas of the main components differed depending on the brand of sake. We also found a characteristic difference between Honjozo-shu and Ginjo-shu. Therefore, the ball SAW GC is expected to be useful not only for monitoring hazardous gases in the atmosphere but also in the food industry, for example, in quality control of the brewing process and on-site analysis of substances produced in yeast cultivation and development.

5.7 Conclusions

We discovered a collimated beam naturally forms from an SAW propagating on the surface of a sphere and then developed a ball SAW sensor. Very high sensitivity was achieved using the phenomenon of multiple round trips of the collimated beam. The applications of this phenomenon in hydrogen sensors, TMAs, and portable GC devices were discussed.

References

[1] Hughes R C and Schubert W K 1992 Thin films of Pd/Ni alloys for detection of high hydrogen concentrations *J. Appl. Phys.* **71** 542–4

[2] Yuasa M, Nagano T, Tachibana N, Kida T and Shimanoe K 2013 Catalytic combustion-type hydrogen sensor using $BaTiO_3$-based PTC thermistor *J. Am. Ceram. Soc.* **96** 1789–94

[3] Abe H 2009 A marked improvement in the reliability of the measurement of trace moisture in gases *Synthesiology* **2** 223–36

[4] Hashiguchi K, Lisak D, Cygan A, Ciuryło R and Abe H 2016 Wavelength-meter controlled cavity ring-down spectroscopy: high-sensitivity detection of trace moisture in N_2 at sub-ppb levels *Sens. Actuators* A **241** 152–60

[5] Wylie R G 1957 A new absolute method of hygrometry. I. The general principles of the method *Aust. J. Phys.* **10** 351–65

[6] Morgan D 1991 *Surface-wave devices for Signal Processing* (Amsterdam: Elsevier)

[7] D'Amico A, Palma A and Verona E 1982 Hydrogen sensor using a palladium coated surface acoustic wave delay-line *1982 IEEE Ultrasonics Symp.* (Piscataway, NJ: IEEE) pp 308–11

[8] Jakubik W, Urbancyzk M, Kochowski S and Bodzenta J 2002 Bilayer structure for hydrogen detection in a surface acoustic wave sensor system *Sens. Actuators* B **82** 265–71

[9] Robinson A, Stavila V, Zeitler T, White M, Thornberg S, Greathouse J and Allendorf M 2012 Ultrasensitive humidity detection using metal–organic framework-coated microsensors *Anal. Chem.* **84** 7043–51

[10] Palma F and Socino G 1984 Diffraction effects in surface acoustic wave harmonic generation *J. Acoust. Sec. Am.* **75** 376–81

[11] Sato Y 1947 Boundary conditions in the problem of generation of elastic waves *Bull. Earthq. Res. Inst.* **27** 1–9

[12] Viktrov I A 1967 *Rayleigh and Lamb Waves* (New York: Plenum Press) p 33

[13] Yamanaka K, Cho H and Tsukahara Y 2000 Precise velocity measurement of surface acoustic waves on a bearing ball *Appl. Phys. Lett.* **76** 2797–9

[14] Tsukahara Y, Nakaso H, Cho H and Yamanaka K 2000 Observation of diffraction-free propagation of surface acoustic waves around a homogeneous isotropic solid sphere *Appl. Phys. Lett.* **77** 2926–8

[15] Ishikawa S, Tsukahara Y, Nakaso N, Cho H and Yamanaka K 2001 Surface acoustic waves on a sphere-analysis of propagation using laser ultrasonics *Jpn. J. Appl. Phys.* **40** 3623–7

[16] Yamanaka K *et al* 2006 Ultramultiple roundtrips of surface acoustic wave on sphere realizing innovation of gas sensors *IEEE Trans. UFFC* **53** 793–801

[17] Ishikawa S, Nakaso N, Takeda N, Sim D Y, Mihara T, Tsukahara Y and Yamanaka K 2003 Surface acoustic waves on a sphere with divergent, focusing, and collimating beam shapes excited by an interdigital transducer *Appl. Phys. Lett.* **22** 4649–51

[18] Akao S, Nakaso N, Ohgi T and Yamanaka K 2004 Observation of the roundtrips of surface acoustic waves on a single crystal LiNbO$_3$ ball *Jpn. J. Appl. Phys.* **43** 3067–70

[19] Akao S, Nakaso N, Ohgi T and Yamanaka K 2004 Roundtrips of SAW along multiple routes on a single crystal LiNbO$_3$ ball *IEEE Ultrasonics Symp.* **2004** 1557–60

[20] Yanagisawa T, Ohgi T, Akao S, Nakaso N, Tsukahara Y, OharaY, Tsuji T and Yamanaka K Meandering collimated beam of surface acoustic waves on a trigonal crystal ball *Appl. Phys. Lett.* **98** 123508

[21] Yamanaka K, Singh K J, Iwata N, Abe T, Akao S, Tsukahara Y and Nakaso N 2007 Acoustic dispersion in a ball-shaped surface acoustic wave device *Appl. Phys. Lett.* **90** 214105

[22] Morgan D 1991 *Surface-wave devices for Signal Processing.* (Amsterdam: Elsevier) p 59

[23] Abe T *et al* 2007 Evaluation of response time in ball surface-acoustic-wave hydrogen sensor using digital quadrature detector *Jpn. J. Appl. Phys.* **46** 4726–8

[24] Takeda N and Motozawa M 2012 Extremely fast 1 μmol · mol^{-1} water-vapor measurement by a 1 mm diameter spherical SAW device *Int. J. Thermophys.* **33** 1642–9

[25] Hagihara S *et al* 2014 Highly sensitive trace moisture ball surface acoustic wave sensor using SiOx film *Jpn. J. Appl. Phys.* **53** 07KD08

[26] Takayanagi K, Akao S, Yanagisawa T, Nakaso N, Tsukahara Y, Hagihara S, Oizumi T, Takeda N, Tsuji T and Yamanaka K 2013 Detection of trace water vapor using SiO$_x$-coated ball saw sensor *Mater. Trans.* **55** 988–93

[27] Witkowski A, Rusin A, Majkut A and Stolecka K 2018 Analysis of compression and transport of the methane/hydrogen mixture in existing natural gas pipelines *Int. J. Press. Vessels Pip.* **166** 24–34

[28] Yamanaka K, Akao S, Takeda N, Tsuji T, Oizumi T, Fukushi H, Okano T and Tsukahara Y 2019 Background gas analysis with leaky attenuation in a trace moisture analyzer using a ball surface acoustic wave sensor *Jpn. J. Appl. Phys.* **58** SGGB04

[29] Slobodnik A J Jr 1971 Attenuation of microwave acoustic surface waves due to gas loading *J. Appl. Phys.* **43** 2565–3268

[30] Zhang L, Tarascon J-M, Sougrati M, Rousse G and Chen G 2015 Influence of relative humidity on the structure and electrochemical performance of sustainable LiFeSO$_4$F electrodes for Li-ion batteries *J. Mater. Chem.* A **3** 16988–97

[31] Tsuji T, Oizumi T, Takeda N, Akao S, Tsukahara Y and Yamanaka K 2015 Temperature compensation of ball surface acoustic wave sensor by two-frequency measurement using undersampling *Jpn. J. Appl. Phys.* **54** 07HD13

[32] Tsuji T, Oizumi T, Fukushi H, Takeda N, Akao S, Tsukahara Y and Yamanaka K 2018 Development of ball surface acoustic wave trace moisture analyzer using burst waveform undersampling circuit *Rev. Sci. Instrum.* **89** 055006

[33] Yamanaka K, Akao S, Takeda N, Tsuji T, Oizumi T and Tsukahara Y 2017 Simultaneous measurement of gas concentration and temperature by the ball surface acoustic wave sensor *Jpn. J. Appl. Phys.* **56** 07JC04

[34] Martin S J, Frye G C and Senturla S D 1994 Dynamics and response of polymer-coated surface acoustic wave devices: effect of viscoelastic properties and film resonance *Anal. Chem.* **66** 2201–19

[35] Takeda N, Carroll P, Tsukahara Y, Beardmore S, Bell S, Yamanaka K and Akao S 2020 Trace moisture measurement in natural gas mixtures with a single calibration for nitrogen background gas *Meas. Sci. Technol.* **31** 104007

[36] Iwaya T, Akao S, Okano T, Takeda N, Oizumi T, Tsuji T, Fukushi H, Sugawara M, Tsukahara Y and Yamanaka K 2020 Dynamic calibration method for trace moisture analyzer based on quick response of ball surface acoustic wave sensor *Meas. Sci. Technol.* **31** 094003

[37] Santos F and Galceran M 2002 The application of gas chromatography to environmental analysis *Trends Anal. Chem.* **21** 672–85

[38] Kobari K, Yamamoto Y, Sakuma M, Akao S, Tsuji T and Yamanaka K 2009 Fabrication of thin sensitive film of ball surface acoustic wave sensor by off-axis spin-coating method *Jpn. J. Appl. Phys.* **48** 07GG13

[39] Iwaya T, Akao S, Sakamoto T, Tsuji T, Nakaso N and Yamanaka K 2012 Development of high precision metal micro-electro-mechanical-systems column for portable surface acoustic wave gas chromatograph *Jpn. J. Appl. Phys.* **51** 07GC24

[40] Iwaya T *et al* 2020 Development of a portable ball SAW gas chromatograph using three-layered metal MEMS columns *Proc. 41st Symp. Ultrasonic Electronics* 3J3-1–3J3-2

[41] Akao S *et al* 2021 Odorant analysis of sake using a palm sized ball SAW gas chromatograph *Proc. 42nd Symp. Ultrasonic Electronics* 3Pb2–3-1–3Pb2–3-2

[42] IUPAC 1997 *Compendium of Chemical Terminology* 2nd edn (the 'Gold Book'). Compiled by A D McNaught and A Wilkinson (Oxford: Blackwell Scientific Publications)

[43] GL Sciences Inc. Analysis and retention indices of 61 organic solvent components by nitrogen carriers *GC Technical Note GT126* (https://glsciences.com/viewfile/?p=GT126 cited on 20/02/2022)

IOP Publishing

Ultrasonics
Physics and applications

Mami Matsukawa, Pak-Kon Choi, Kentaro Nakamura, Hirotsugu Ogi and Hideyuki Hasegawa

Chapter 6

Phase adjuster in a thermoacoustic system

Shin-ichi Sakamoto and Yoshiaki Watanabe

The introduction of a phase adjuster (PA) into a thermoacoustic system, resulting in a significant improvement in the conversion efficiency, is described herein. The operating principle of the PA is explained, with a focus on the temporal change of the sound field in the system during the period from heat injection into the system to self-excited oscillation, which is the final stable state. We then describe an experimental demonstration of the induction of a sound field in a tube by the insertion of a PA at an appropriate position, causing one-wavelength resonance that can realize superior conversion efficiency. The installation of a PA with a simple structure suppresses two-wavelength resonance, and the in-tube sound field is dominated by a highly efficient one-wavelength resonant sound field. Consequently, an approximately tenfold increase in the sound intensity in the system and a significant improvement in the heat-to-sound conversion efficiency are noted.

6.1 Introduction

The Rijke tube [1, 2], a simple device that has been known for a long time, essentially comprises a metal mesh in a glass tube. Interestingly, simply heating this mesh with a burner produces a loud tone with a pitch corresponding to the length of the tube. This energy conversion from heat to sound is the result of thermoacoustic phenomena [3–6]. The propagation of the sound waves we encounter daily is an adiabatic process; thus, there is no heat transfer. However, in sound wave propagation in a space narrower than the wavelength of sound, the sound wave propagates with heat transfer to and from the surrounding medium, such that the sound wave interacts with heat in this environment. This interaction is referred to as a thermoacoustic phenomenon [3–6].

The active use of the thermoacoustic phenomenon facilitates energy conversion from heat to sound or vice versa. This conversion has the potential to utilize waste heat, which is difficult to handle using conventional energy conversion techniques. Thus, the thermoacoustic phenomenon has garnered the attention of scientists seeking solutions for global warming and energy problems, and several studies have been conducted in this regard.

Since the introduction of the Rijke tube, researchers have been interested in the thermoacoustic phenomenon, have been particularly attracted by the potential of thermoacoustic systems, and have progressed to practical realization as described below.

Although the phenomenon whereby sound is generated by heat is well known from natural phenomena, such as lightning strikes, it was in the middle of the 18th century that the thermoacoustic phenomenon was first utilized in artificial mechanisms. In Europe, a phenomenon similar to the sound generated by the Rijke tube [1, 2] is known: during the construction or repair of pipe organs, a loud sound occurs when the pipe is heated. Furthermore, Sondhauss found that when the spherical part of a flask was heated to create a temperature gradient in the throat part, the inner gas vibrated and generated sound [7].

In addition, in Japan, the phenomenon of sound produced by a hot oven (a type of thermoacoustic phenomenon) was introduced in 'Kibitsu no Kama' in *Ugetsu Story* published in 1776 [8]. Although such thermoacoustic phenomena were previously known, as described, they began to receive attention as research objects in the 19th century. Lord Rayleigh, who founded the fundamentals of acoustics, also described them in his famous book '*The Theory of Sound*' [1]. However, the driving principle of the Rijke and Sondhauss tubes was not clarified in detail. In the 20th century, the phenomenon was observed in which one closed end of a tube was maintained at room temperature, whereas another open end was cooled by approaching liquid helium; the helium gas in the tube vibrated and generated sound, as reported by Taconis *et al* [9]. Subsequently, the thermoacoustic phenomenon started to attract attention again after the study conducted by Ceperley [10, 11]. He suggested the use of the mechanism, utilized in the Sterling engine, in which the pressure and particle velocity temporally change in phase, enabling the realization of a high-efficiency thermoacoustic engine. Subsequently, studies were actively conducted by Wheatley *et al* [12] and others including Swift [4, 6, 12, 13, 16] and Tominaga [3, 5, 14, 15]. Furthermore, a high-efficiency thermoacoustic system called a looped tube was proposed by Yazaki *et al* [14, 15] and Backhaus *et al* [16], and its usefulness as a prototype for a thermoacoustic engine was verified. Motivated by these accomplishments, the significant potential of thermoacoustic phenomena was recognized, and many researchers and engineers started working on research and development. Furthermore, in recognition of the current global warming situation, these studies have been accelerated. Ueda *et al* [17] and Hasegawa *et al* [18] proposed a cooling system that was assumed to have enhanced the practical realization of the thermoacoustic phenomenon, and Backhaus *et al* [16] and Biwa *et al* [19] proposed the use of a new engine. Furthermore, as exemplified by the proposals for electric generators by Backhaus *et al* [20] and Hamood *et al* [21], as well as the effective utilization of sunlight by Adeff *et al* [22] and of unused natural energy by Yu *et al* [23], various application systems have been proposed, and research and development into their practical realization have been progressing. Focusing on a stack configuration, Tijani *et al* [24] conducted a study of the improvement of the cooling performance of thermoacoustic cooling systems.

Furthermore, Ueda et al [25] investigated a stacked-screen regenerator, and Tsuda et al [26] and Kawashima et al [27] investigated a wet regenerator. Sakamoto et al [28] studied heat flow in a stack. Belcher [29] and Tijani et al [30] proposed an improvement in system efficiency, in which attention was focused on the properties of the working fluid. Furthermore, Raspet et al [31] and Noda et al [32] aimed to improve system efficiency by conducting an investigation using a working fluid containing vapor. Most of these methods were focused on the system components, such as the devices used in the system and constituents such as the working fluid.

In techniques that focus on the component devices of the system, there is a practical problem, because the working of the device must be designed according to each oscillating condition of the system in order to retain high efficiency. In addition, to generalize the system, the working fluid must primarily consist of atmospheric air instead of any expensive or high-pressure gas. Thus, a phase adjuster (PA) [33], an efficiency-improving technique that focuses on the sound field, which is a common approach in these devices, may be introduced.

In the thermoacoustic phenomenon, a temperature change occurs at the heated end of the stack provided that self-excited oscillation appears. This change influences the frequency of the self-excited oscillation. Furthermore, from the viewpoint of realizing high-efficiency conversion, it is desirable for the selected frequency to produce one-wavelength resonance within the tube length of the system [34, 35]. The PA ensures that the system oscillates stably and can simultaneously retain stable oscillation under the condition of one-wavelength resonance, which is suitable for high-efficiency conversion. In addition, this technique has an advantage of applicability, as it can be combined with other improvement techniques focused on the device because it is solely concerned with the sound field. The realization process is discussed in the following sections.

6.2 Thermoacoustic phenomenon leading to steady oscillation

6.2.1 Loop-tube-type thermoacoustic cooling system

In this study, a loop-tube-type thermoacoustic cooling system proposed by Yazaki et al [14, 15], which is expected to be a high-efficiency system, was investigated [34, 35]. A photograph and a schematic view of the entire system are shown in figures 6.1 and 6.2 [34, 35], respectively. The loop-tube-type thermoacoustic cooling system was constructed by connecting stainless steel tubes and elbows with flanges. The inner diameter of the tube was approximately 42 mm, and the total length was approximately 3.3 m. Atmospheric air was used as the working fluid enclosed in the system. A prime mover (PM) and a heat pump (HP) were installed in the looped tube. A PM converts heat to sound, and an HP does the reverse. The PM consisted of a stack sandwiched between an electric heater, which was the heat source at its hot end, and a heat exchanger made of copper. Water maintained at room temperature by passing through a constant-temperature bath was circulated in the heat exchanger. In the experiment, honeycomb ceramics originally used to depurate car exhaust, which have a structure that packs many narrow tubes in a bundle, were cannibalized for the PM stack. The honeycomb ceramics had a flow channel radius

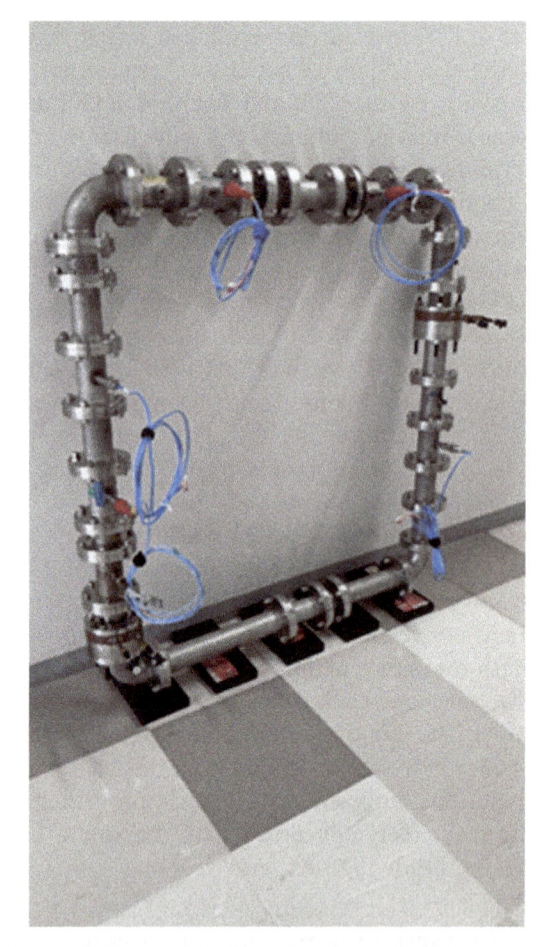

Figure 6.1. Photograph of the thermoacoustic cooling system.

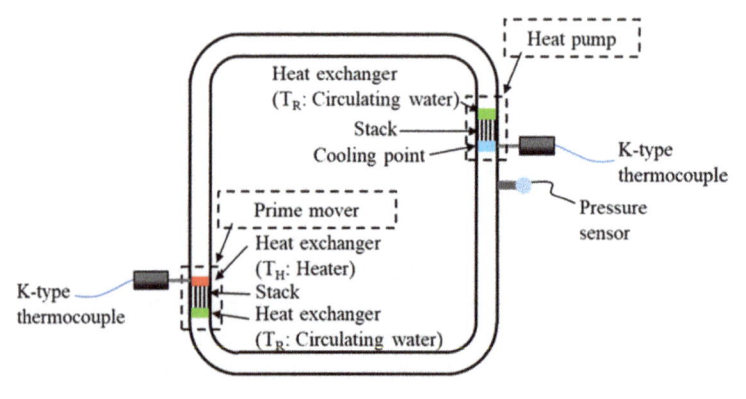

Figure 6.2. Schematic of the thermoacoustic cooling system and its experimental setup. Reproduced from [34], with the permission of AIP Publishing. Adapted from [35], with the permission of the Acoustic Society of Japan.

of 0.45 mm. The HP, consisting of a similar stack with a flow channel radius of 0.35 mm, was sandwiched between a heat exchanger and a thermocouple to measure the cooling temperature. In addition, by connecting the path of the water circulation through the heat exchanger for the HP and the heat exchanger for the PM in series, both heat exchangers were maintained at a constant temperature. The input to the electric heater was set to 330 W. A pressure sensor was installed beneath the HP to measure the sound generated in the system by thermoacoustic self-excited oscillation.

Using this thermoacoustic experimental system, various examinations were conducted to improve the conversion efficiency [33–35, 39–45]. Most of the investigations of techniques to enhance efficiency were conducted by targeting steady oscillation after the system was stabilized. However, the physics of the development process of the thermoacoustic phenomenon was deemed difficult to elucidate using such a method. Thus, an investigation was performed to focus on the fluctuation of the sound field and the temperature in the period from the point of heat injection to the point of stable steady oscillation in the system. Consequently, during the process of stable oscillation, the resonant frequency of the self-excited oscillation was observed to shift from the frequency of one-wavelength resonance to that of two-wavelength resonance under a specified condition. The temperature change in the cooling portion, i.e. the difference in cooling capacity, was also observed together with this frequency change [34, 35].

6.2.2 Mechanism of thermoacoustic cooling

To elucidate the change in resonant frequency before stable self-excited oscillation is reached, we first briefly explain the mechanism of the cooling effect of the thermoacoustic cooling system and the sound field in the cooling system at that time [3, 6, 33–35].

When the hot end of the PM is heated by an electric heater, a large temperature gradient is formed between both ends of the stack. Fluctuation of the working fluid in the system due to the temperature gradient becomes the seed which leads to self-excited oscillation, resonance through the total length of system, and the generation of sound. Conversely, a temperature gradient is formed in the HP stack by the excited sound, and accordingly, the temperature at the cooling point decreases.

A conceptual diagram of the sound field in the system at this moment is shown in figure 6.3 [33]. In this figure, the thermoacoustic cooling system is cut at the top of the PM and straightened. The top and bottom figures show the conditions of one-wavelength resonance and two-wavelength resonance, respectively, in which the red and blue curves represent the sound pressure and particle velocity, respectively. From the figures, it is evident that the vicinities of the positions where the PM and HP are installed become the antinodes of the sound pressure and the nodes of particle velocity. Furthermore, under the condition of two-wavelength resonance, the vicinities of the positions where the PM and HP are installed were observed to be the antinodes of the sound pressure and the nodes of the particle velocity, as in the case of one-wavelength resonance [33].

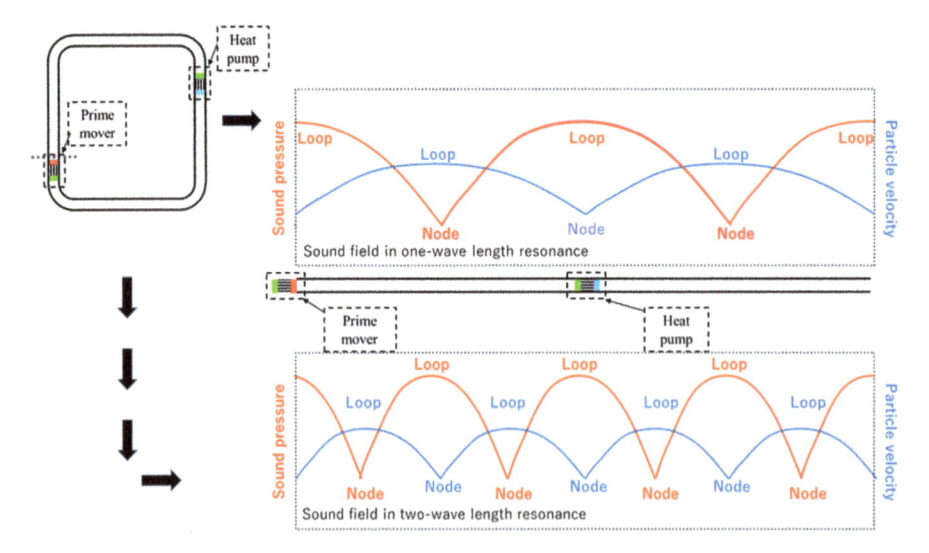

Figure 6.3. Conceptual diagram of the sound field in the thermoacoustic cooling system: comparison of sound pressure and particle velocity distributions in the cases of one-wavelength resonance and two-wavelength resonance. Adapted from [33], copyright the Acoustic Society of Japan.

Considering the fluctuation of the sound field and the temperature change before the system settles down into steady oscillation, their variation was circumstantially observed. In the next section, the observation results are discussed based on the sound fields shown in figure 6.3 [33].

6.2.3 Variation of resonant wavelength and cooling capacity

We first focused on the change in frequency that occurs in the period from the start of driving by heat injection to the point at which steady self-excited oscillation occurs. The description of the experimental method and the results is as follows [34]. The experiment was performed using a system similar to that shown in figure 6.2 [34, 35]. After injecting the 330 W input into the electric heater, the thermal input was stopped after 200 s. The temporal changes in temperatures at the cooling point of the HP and at the hot end of the PM are shown in figures 6.4 and 6.5 [34], respectively. As shown in figure 6.5 [34], the temperature at the hot end of the PM began rising immediately after the injection of the input to the heater and settled down at approximately 600 °C after 200 s when the input stopped. Conversely, as shown in figure 6.4 [34], the temperature at the cooling point began dropping at the same moment as the generation of thermoacoustic self-excited oscillation sound (after approximately 35 s). Subsequently, the temperature drop at the cooling point slowed down from approximately 60–80 s, and then the temperature gradually started rising, and continued to gently rise until approximately 200 s when the input stopped. Furthermore, the temperature continued to increase after the input was stopped and returned approximately to the temperature before the input. In addition, the timings of the signal observations used to analyze the

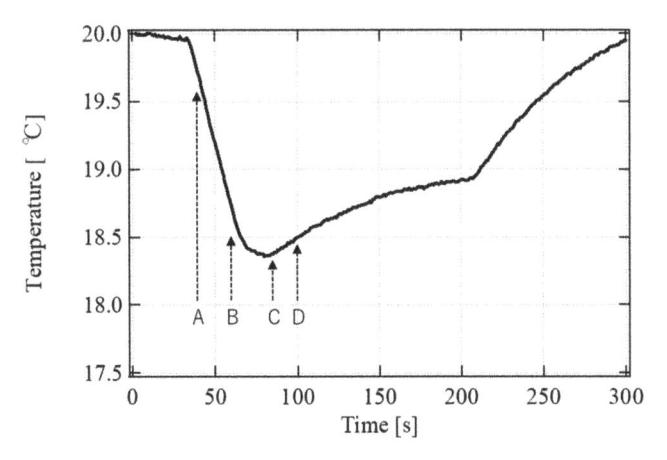

Figure 6.4. Temporal change in temperature at the cooling point of a thermoacoustic cooling system and FFT timings. Reproduced from [34], with the permission of AIP Publishing.

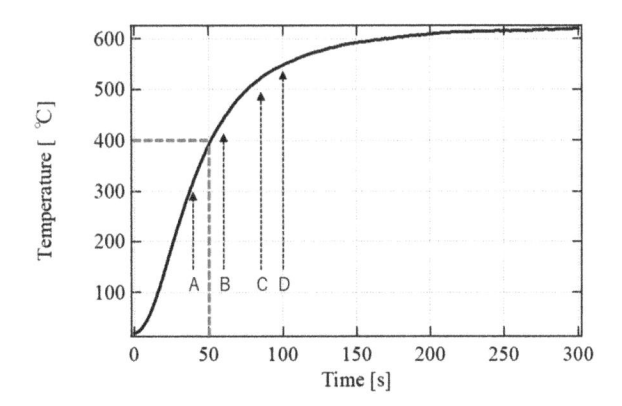

Figure 6.5. Temporal change in temperature at the upper end of the prime mover in the thermoacoustic cooling system and FFT timings. Reproduced from [34], with the permission of AIP Publishing.

oscillation frequency described later in figure 6.6 [34] are marked in figures 6.4 and 6.5 [34] with arrows from A to D.

The temporal variation of the sound field in the system was then considered. The results of the frequency analysis at each observation time from A to D are shown in figure 6.6 [34]. In the figure, panels (A)–(D) show the spectra after 40, 60, 80, and 100 s of heat injection, respectively [34]. This result indicates that the oscillation frequency shifts from 100 Hz of one-wavelength resonance to 200 Hz, i.e. a two-wavelength resonant frequency, in a short time after starting the system. Immediately after the start of the self-excited oscillation, when a 100 Hz one-wavelength resonant frequency is dominant, as shown in figure 6.6(A) [34] (after 40 s), the temperature at the cooling point monotonously drops. However, as shown in figure 6.6(B) [34] (after 60 s), where

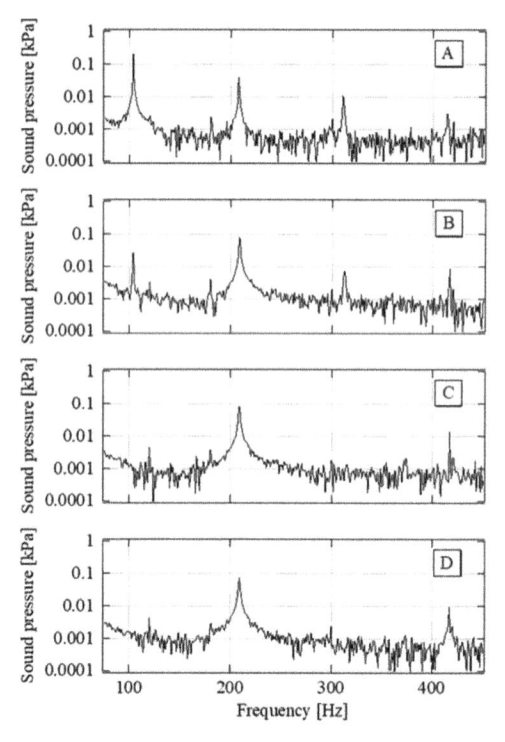

Figure 6.6. Frequency spectrum of sound generated by thermoacoustic self-excited oscillation in the thermoacoustic cooling system. (A): after 40 s, (B): after 60 s, (C): after 80 s, and (D): after 100 s. Reproduced from [34], with the permission of AIP Publishing.

the temperature at the cooling point stops decreasing, the 200 Hz of the two-wavelength resonant frequency began growing and coexisted with the 100 Hz one-wavelength resonant frequency. Subsequently, the results depicted in figures 6.6(C) (after 80 s) and (D) (after 100 s) [34] indicate that the 200 Hz two-wavelength resonant frequency became dominant. At this moment, the temperature at the cooling point increased, and the cooling capacity was degraded. Evidently, driving the system at one-wavelength resonance can better enhance the cooling capacity. Furthermore, focusing on the change in temperature at the cooling point, because the change in temperature from dropping to rising occurs almost simultaneously with the change in resonant wavelength, it is inferred that there is a close relationship between the temperature drop and the oscillation frequency. In the next section, this relation is explained by focusing on the thicknesses of the thermal boundary layer and the viscosity boundary layer in the narrow tubes of the stack [34, 35].

6.2.4 Resonant frequency before stable self-excited oscillation: changes in cooling capacity and resonant wavelength observed in the boundary layer

To understand the working principle of the stack in a thermoacoustic system, it is necessary to consider the influence of the thermal and viscosity boundary layers on the working fluid present in the narrow tubes of the stack [3, 6, 34, 35]. In the case of a temperature difference between the walls of the narrow tubes in the stack and the working fluid, the temperature of the fluid becomes equal to that of the contacting surface of the wall. However, the influence of the temperature difference decreases as the fluid is positioned away from the wall surface. Thermoacoustic phenomena appear according to the mutual heat exchange between the fluid and the wall surface, which is performed in the narrow tubes of the stack. The layer near the surface, where the heats of the materials influence each other in this manner, is called the thermal boundary layer. Because heat exchange is performed in this thermal boundary layer, the thickness of the thermal boundary layer significantly influences the heat exchange capacity. Thus, the cooling capacity of a thermoacoustic system depends on the heat exchange capacity of the HP stack. Furthermore, as a known rule of thumb, the heat exchange is determined by the relation between the thickness of the thermal boundary layer and the radius of the flow channel of the narrow tube in the stack. In addition, the ideal approach matches the flow channel radius of the narrow tube in the stack to the thickness of the thermal boundary layer [3, 6, 34, 35]. A viscosity boundary layer is another important boundary layer used to understand thermoacoustic phenomena; this is a layer near the stack wall where the particle velocity of the fluid decreases due to the action of the viscosity of the working fluid.

The thickness of the thermal boundary layer $\delta\alpha$ in the narrow tube of the stack is expressed as follows:

$$\delta\alpha = \sqrt{\frac{2\alpha}{\omega}}, \tag{6.1}$$

where α is the thermal diffusion coefficient, and ω is the angular frequency of the thermoacoustic self-excited oscillation sound [3, 6, 34–36]. Furthermore, the thickness of the viscosity boundary layer $\delta\nu$ is expressed as

$$\delta\nu = \sqrt{\frac{2\nu}{\omega}}, \tag{6.2}$$

where ν is the dynamic viscosity coefficient [3, 6, 34–36].

According to equation (6.1), $\delta\alpha$ decreases with sound frequency. Consequently, the heat exchange capacity in the thermal boundary layer also decreases. Therefore, as already shown in figure 6.4 [34], when the self-excited oscillation frequency shifts to the two-wavelength resonance, the conversion capacity from sound to heat decreases compared with the case of one-wavelength resonance, and consequently, the temperature at the cooling point increases. This aspect can also be inferred from figures 6.7(A) and (B) [34], which show the temperature dependence of $\delta\alpha$ and $\delta\nu$ for one-wavelength and two-wavelength resonances. In these figures, the radii of the flow channels of the HP and PM stacks are indicated with a thin dotted line (0.35 mm) and a thin solid line (0.45 mm), respectively. Focusing on the flow channel radius of the HP stack and the change in $\delta\alpha$ at each resonant frequency shown in figures 6.7(A) and (B) [34] by bold broken curves, it is evident that $\delta\alpha$ becomes small at two-wavelength resonance compared with one-wavelength

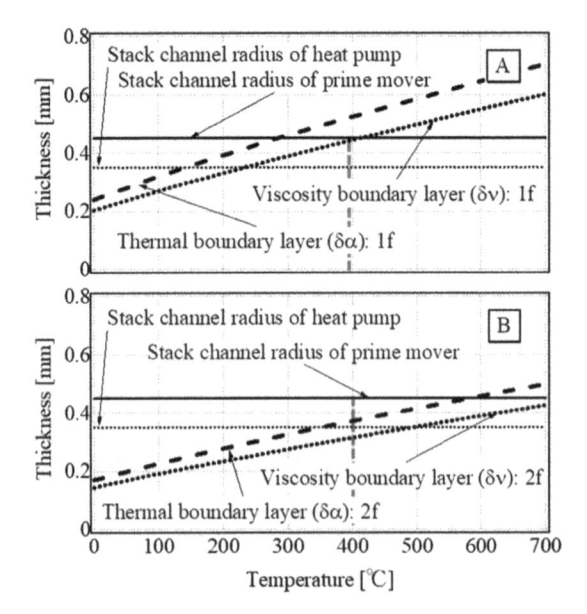

Figure 6.7. Thicknesses of the thermal and viscosity boundary layers formed in the stack of the thermoacoustic cooling system: (a) one-wavelength resonance, and (b) two-wavelength resonance. Reproduced from [34], with the permission of AIP Publishing.

resonance over the entire temperature range. Furthermore, as indicated by figure 6.4 [34], the cooling capacity decreases when the frequency shifts to that of two-wavelength resonance.

$\delta\alpha$ changes depending on the frequency of the sound entering the HP, and the cooling capacity decreases under the condition of two-wavelength resonance at a higher frequency than that of one-wavelength resonance. However, the mechanism responsible for the change in the self-excited oscillations is still unexplained. Thus, as the next step, the change in resonant wavelength that occurs with the time lapse after injection of the heat is considered.

To conclude, the oscillation frequency changes because of the change in $\delta\nu$ in the PM stack. In addition, the $\delta\nu$ required to start self-excited oscillation is smaller than the flow channel radius of the stack [34–36]. Focusing on $\delta\nu$, this conclusion can be explained as follows using figures 6.7(A) and (B) [34]: $\delta\nu$ increases as the temperature increases, as shown by the bold dotted curves in the figures. As shown in figure 6.5 [34], the temperature at the hot end of the PM rapidly increases immediately after the injection of the heat. Furthermore, as indicated by figure 6.6 [34], the oscillation frequency shifts from one- to two-wavelength resonance within approximately 40–60 s. As shown by the red dotted curve in figure 6.5 [34], the temperature at the hot end of the PM during this period reaches 400 °C in approximately 50 s from the start of the input. In contrast, from figure 6.7(A) [34] showing $\delta\nu$ at one-wavelength resonance, it is evident that $\delta\nu$ for a temperature of 400 °C at the hot end of PM becomes approximately 0.45 mm, which is almost the same as the 0.45 mm flow channel radius of the PM stack. Furthermore, when the temperature rises to over

400°C after 50 s, $\delta\nu$ at one-wavelength resonance becomes larger than the flow path radius of the stack, and the working fluid in the narrow tubes becomes unavailable for the thermoacoustic phenomenon. In addition, as shown in figure 6.6 [34], the oscillation frequency shifts from one- to two-wavelength resonance at this time. $\delta\nu$ at this two-wavelength resonant frequency is smaller than the flow channel radius of the PM stack in figure 6.7(B) [34]. Furthermore, it is observed that even at 600 °C, which is the temperature at the hot end of the PM before the input to the heater is stopped, $\delta\nu$ at the two-wavelength resonant frequency becomes smaller than the flow channel radius of the PM stack. When the temperature at the hot end of the PM increases and $\delta\nu$ at one wavelength becomes larger than the flow channel radius of the stack, the working fluid becomes immovable and is influenced by viscosity. Therefore, the thermoacoustic self-excited oscillation cannot be maintained at one-wavelength resonance. Under these conditions, the thermoacoustic system is assumed to retain the self-excited oscillation by changing the resonant wavelength to that of the two-wavelength resonance, at which $\delta\nu$ is smaller. In addition, if the hot end of the PM can be set at a temperature, such that $\delta\nu$ does not exceed the flow channel radius, the system can retain one-wavelength resonance. However, the temperature control for the thermal input is required separately in this case.

The changes in the cooling capacity and the change in the resonant wavelength is summarized below [3, 6, 34–36]. The change in cooling capacity shown in figure 6.4 [34] can be explained as follows: after injection of the heater, the system starts the excitation of the one-wavelength resonance that is easiest to oscillate. Owing to this one-wavelength resonance sound, a thermoacoustic phenomenon appears, and the temperature at the cooling point begins to decrease. Meanwhile, in parallel with this phenomenon, the temperature at the hot end of PM heated by the heater continues to rise; finally, the inside of the narrow tube of the PM stack is filled with the viscosity boundary layer. Consequently, the system is unable to maintain thermoacoustic self-excited oscillation at the one-wavelength resonant frequency and raises the frequency to the two-wavelength resonance, which can easily oscillate next to the one-wavelength resonance and maintains a stable self-excited oscillation. However, when the excited frequency increases, because $\delta\alpha$ in the stack decreases, as shown in equation (6.1) [3, 6, 34–36] compared with the case of the one-wavelength resonant frequency, the cooling capacity decreases and the temperature at the cooling point increases [34, 35].

6.2.5 Resonant frequency under conditions of stable self-excited oscillation: influence of total length of, and pressure in the tube

In the previous section, the process by which the thermoacoustic system reaches stable steady oscillation after heat injection to the PM was discussed by focusing on the changes in $\delta\alpha$ and $\delta\nu$ in the narrow tubes of the stack [34, 35]. Here, we discuss the change in each boundary layer in the narrow tubes of the stack after the oscillation is stabilized, focusing on the influence of the total system length and the pressure in the tube. The experiment was conducted using a thermoacoustic cooling system which had the same shape as that shown in figure 6.2 [34, 35], and the PM, HP, and each stack also had similar shapes. Argon, which can change the pressure, was used as the working fluid. Setting the argon pressure and the input to the electric heater to 0.1 MPa and 330 W, respectively, the frequency of the self-excited oscillation sound was measured for various total system lengths of 1900, 2600, 3270, and 3970 mm.

Figure 6.8 [35] shows the measurement results for the oscillation frequency after steady oscillation was stabilized. As shown in the figure, while sound at the frequency of the one-wavelength resonance was generated by the system with a total length of 1900 mm, sound at the two-wavelength frequency was generated for each of the remaining tube lengths (2600, 3200, or 3970 mm).

We consider these results by focusing on the thickness of the boundary layer. Figure 6.9 [35] shows the calculation results for $\delta\nu$ in the PM and the HP at the

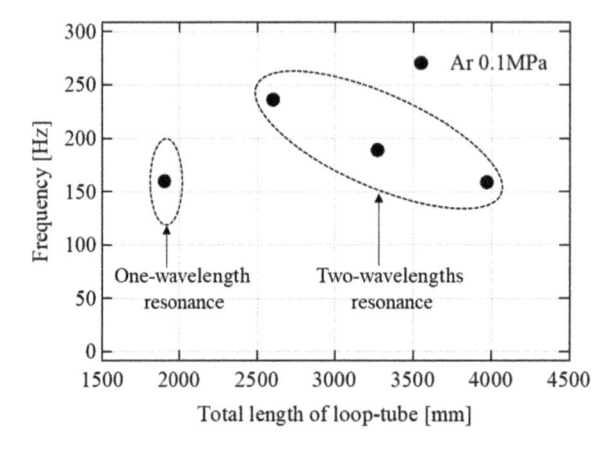

Figure 6.8. Frequency of thermoacoustic self-excited oscillations at different lengths of the thermoacoustic cooling system. Adapted from [35], with the permission of the Acoustical Society of Japan.

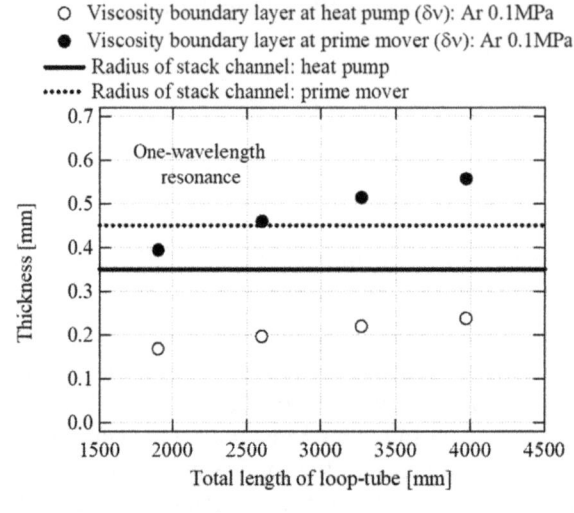

Figure 6.9. Comparison between the thickness of the viscosity boundary layer and flow channel radius in the stacks of the prime mover and heat pump for different lengths of the thermoacoustic cooling system at one-wavelength resonance. Adapted from [35], with the permission of the Acoustical Society of Japan.

one-wavelength resonant frequency for various total lengths of the thermoacoustic system. The flow channel radii in the stacks of the PM and the HP are indicated by dotted and solid lines, respectively. Attention was paid to the flow channel radius of the narrow tube in the stack of the PM and $\delta\nu$ in this figure. The figure indicates that $\delta\nu$ at the one-wavelength resonant frequency for a total length of 1900 mm is smaller than the flow channel radius of the PM stack. Meanwhile, because $\delta\nu$ is larger than the flow channel radius of the PM stack when the total length is 2600, 3270, or 3970 mm, the working fluid cannot enter a state of one-wavelength resonance in tubes of these lengths. In addition, for all total lengths, $\delta\nu$ in the HP is smaller than the flow channel radius of the HP stack [35].

Conversely, the sound excited in the tubes that had total lengths of 2600, 3270, or 3970 mm was not at the one-wavelength resonance but at the two-wavelength resonance for each tube length. Thus, the calculation results for $\delta\alpha$ and $\delta\nu$ at the two-wavelength resonant frequency are shown in figure 6.10 [35]. This result indicates that $\delta\nu$ in the narrow tube of the PM is smaller than the flow channel radius of the PM stack for any length. Furthermore, $\delta\nu$ is smaller than the flow channel radius in the HP stack. Thus, it is inferred that the resonant frequency for the self-excitation oscillation is selected in the PM such that $\delta\nu$ does not exceed the flow channel radius in the stack, even after the oscillation is stabilized [35].

Next, by changing the pressure of the working fluid and the total length of the system, we examined whether the pressure in the tube influences the selection of the self-excited oscillation frequency [35]. This was projected because it was considered that the oscillation at one-wavelength resonance can be expected to decrease under the increased pressure of the working fluid. The total length of the system was the same as that previously described. The self-excited oscillation frequency was measured when the pressure of the working fluid was increased from 0.2 to 0.5 MPa. Consequently, the system exhibited self-excitation at the

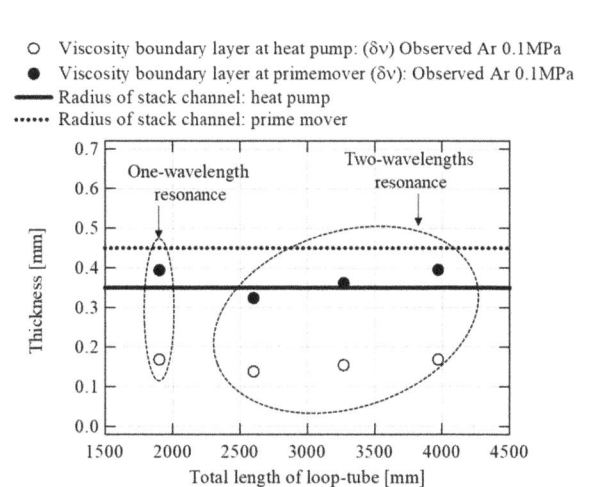

Figure 6.10. Comparison between the thickness of the viscosity boundary layer and the flow channel radius in the stacks of the prime mover and heat pump for different lengths of the thermoacoustic cooling system at the observed frequency. Adapted from [35], with the permission of the Acoustical Society of Japan.

one-wavelength resonant frequency under working fluid pressures of more than 0.2 MPa for all total lengths. Furthermore, it was confirmed that $\delta\nu$ at the PM did not exceed the flow channel radius of the PM stack. These results indicate that the thermoacoustic system generates self-excited oscillation by selecting the resonant frequency such that $\delta\nu$ does not exceed the flow channel radius of the PM stack [35].

6.3 Progression to phase adjuster

In the previous section, it was established that when the resonant frequency shifts from the frequency of one- to that of two-wavelength resonance, the capacity of the thermoacoustic cooling system significantly degrades [34, 35]. Therefore, to realize high conversion efficiency, a sound field that inhibits the transition of self-excited oscillation to the two-wavelength resonance and simultaneously maintains the one-wavelength resonance should be realized.

Hence, we discuss a method of controlling the sound field to maintain a stable one-wavelength resonance condition without losing the advantages of the thermoacoustic system, such as a simple structure and no moving parts. First, we focus on the difference in the particle velocity distributions of the intratubular sound fields of the one-wavelength resonance and two-wavelength resonance. The particle velocity taken from the conceptual diagram of figure 6.3 is shown in figure 6.11 [33]. Focusing on the vicinity of the intermediate position between the PM and the HP, which is the yellow area in the figure, the particle velocity distribution in this area is

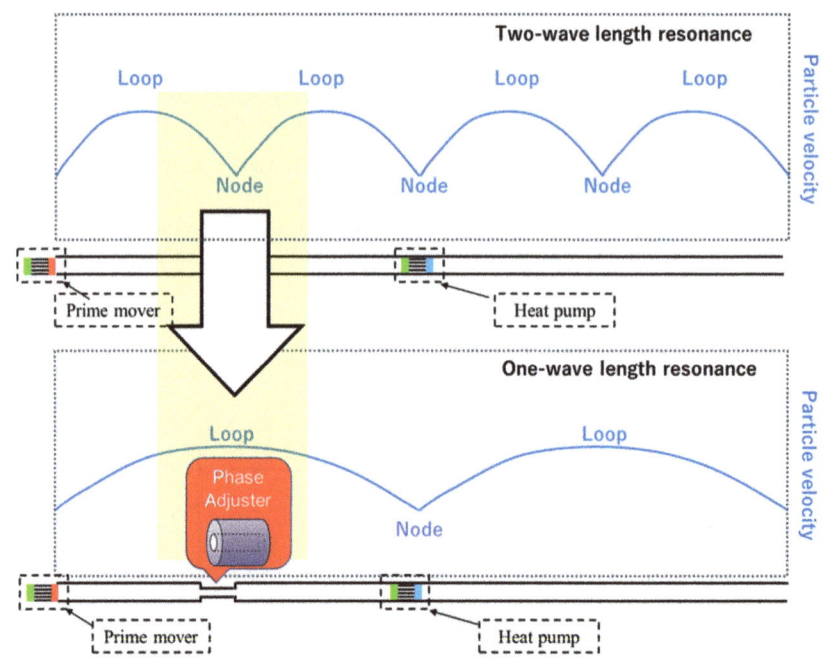

Figure 6.11. Conceptual diagram of the phase adjuster in the sound field in a thermoacoustic cooling system, inspired by a comparison of the particle velocity distribution for the case of one-wavelength resonance with that of two-wavelength resonance. Adapted from [33], copyright The Japan Society of Applied Physics.

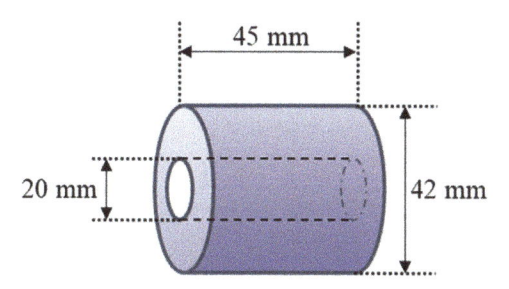

Figure 6.12. Conceptual diagram of the PA. Adapted from [33], copyright The Japan Society of Applied Physics.

located at the antinode for one-wavelength resonance and inversely located at the node for two-wavelength resonance. If the particle velocity distribution for two-wavelength resonance in this area can be forcibly set to the antinode, the two-wavelength resonance can be suppressed, and consequently, the resonant frequency of the system can be fixed to that of one-wavelength resonance. Hence, we propose a PA that can be realized with a simple structure according to Bernoulli's theorem as a mechanism to forcibly increase the particle velocity in this area [33].

A conceptual diagram of the PA is shown in figure 6.12 [33] and a conceptual diagram of the PA installed in the thermoacoustic cooling system is additionally shown in figure 6.11 [33]. As shown in the figures, the PA is installed in the area that is the antinode for one-wavelength resonance and the node for two-wavelength resonance, which is the intermediate position between the PM and the HP. Consequently, because the particle velocity increases as the cross-sectional area of the tube decreases in the area where the PA is located, the node of the sound field is less likely to form. Consequently, the two-wavelength resonance is suppressed, and the system only exhibits the self-excited oscillation of one-wavelength resonance.

To verify the effect of the PA, an experiment was conducted using the system shown in figure 6.13 [33], which was almost the same as the system used in a previous study. Using argon as the working fluid, pressure sensors were set at multiple positions to measure the sound field in the system. The two-sensor method was used to measure the sound field [36–38]. The PA is a cylindrical device with an inner diameter of 20 mm, an outer diameter of 42 mm, and a length of 45 mm. Installing this PA at a position of 0.925 m from the top end of the PM stack, a comparison between cases with and without the PA installation was performed for the generated sound pressure and cooling capacity.

The results of a frequency analysis of the sound of the thermoacoustic self-excited oscillation generated in the system are shown in figure 6.14 [33]; panels (A) and (B) are the results for the cases with and without the PA installation, respectively. When the PA is installed, a 100 Hz sound corresponding to one-wavelength resonance is strongly excited [33]. Meanwhile, in the case without installation of the PA, excitation at 200 Hz, i.e. the two-wavelength resonant frequency, can be confirmed. Consequently, if the described PA is installed, one-wavelength resonance with superior thermoacoustic conversion efficiency can easily be realized. This can also

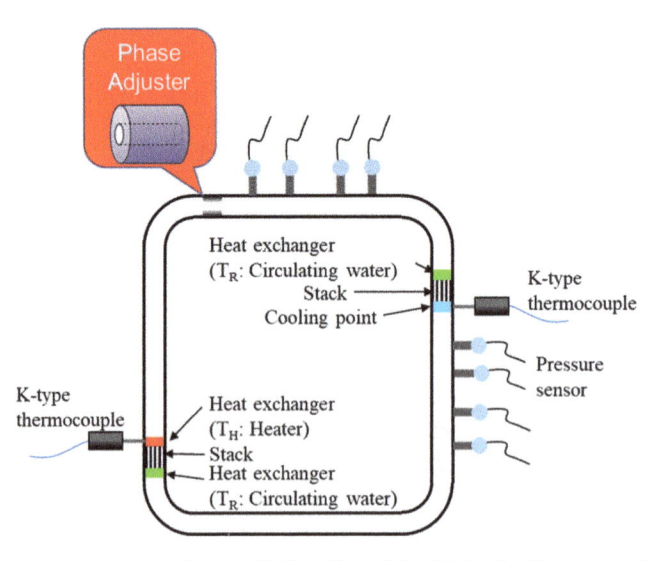

Figure 6.13. Experimental system used to verify the effect of the PA in the thermoacoustic cooling system. Adapted from [33], copyright The Japan Society of Applied Physics.

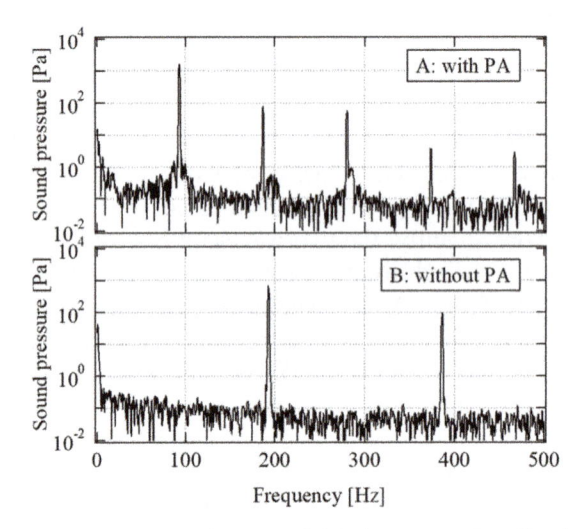

Figure 6.14. Frequency spectrum of sound generated by thermoacoustic self-excited oscillations in the thermoacoustic cooling systems with the PA (A) and without the PA (B). Adapted from [33], copyright The Japan Society of Applied Physics.

be inferred from the fact that a higher cooling capacity is observed when the PA is installed than when the PA is not installed in figure 6.15 [33], which shows the temporal change in cooling temperature at the HP.

Furthermore, based on the measurement results for the pressure, the results for the particle velocity distribution in the system obtained using the two-sensor method are shown in figure 6.16 [33], where the results for the cases with and without the PA

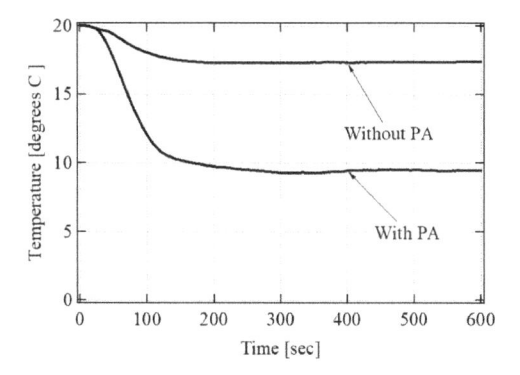

Figure 6.15. Temporal change in temperature at the cooling point of the thermoacoustic cooling systems for two cases with and without the PA. Adapted from [33], copyright The Japan Society of Applied Physics.

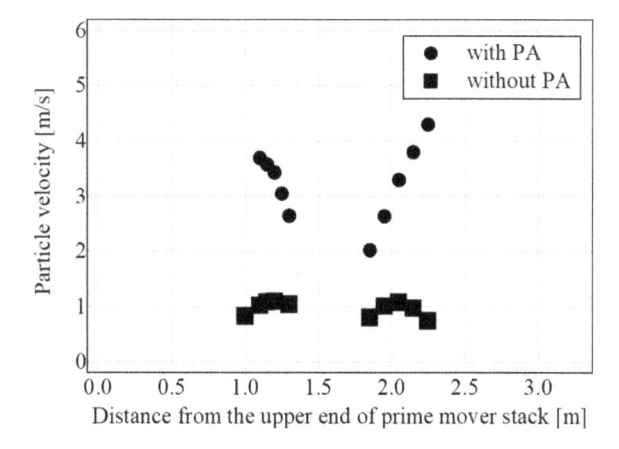

Figure 6.16. Distributions of particle velocities generated by thermoacoustic self-excited oscillations in the thermoacoustic cooling system. Adapted from [33], copyright The Japan Society of Applied Physics.

installation can be found [33]. In these figures, the particle velocity is smaller in the case without the PA installation. Conversely, in the case with the PA installation, the particle velocity is considerably enlarged and increases toward the vicinity of the PA. In addition, from the changing pattern of the particle velocity with respect to distance, the self-excited oscillation is one-wavelength resonance. These results confirm that when the two-wavelength resonance was suppressed, the system was driven by self-excited oscillation, and the PA worked as expected.

We consider these results from the viewpoint of sound intensity. The sound intensity I is a parameter that expresses the sound energy represented as

$$I = \frac{1}{2} |p||u| \cos \varphi, \tag{6.3}$$

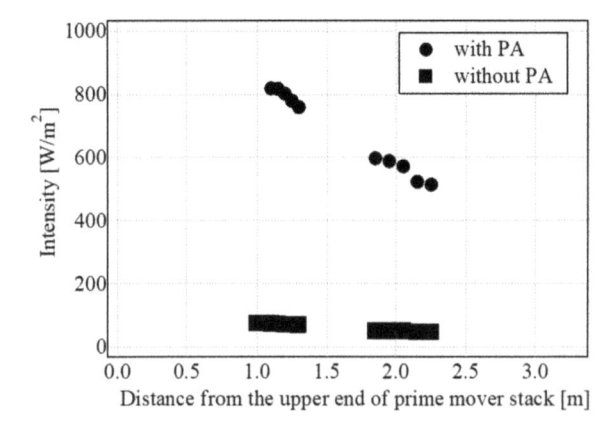

Figure 6.17. Distribution of sound intensity generated by thermoacoustic self-excited oscillation in a thermoacoustic cooling system. Adapted from [33], copyright The Japan Society of Applied Physics.

where p is the sound pressure, u is the particle velocity, and φ is the phase difference between p and u [3, 6, 37, 38]. Based on equation (6.3), the distribution of sound intensity in the system calculated from the measurement results of the pressure using the two-sensor method is shown in figure 6.17 [33], which includes the results for the cases with and without the PA installation. These figures confirm the increase in acoustic energy resulting from the installation of the PA. For example, the sound intensity at a position of 1 m from the upper end of the PM shows an enormous increase of approximately tenfold. This shows that the installed PA prevents the process that follows thermal input to the system, which is the main cause of the reduced efficiency, the temperature rise in the stack, the increase in $\delta \nu$, the rise of the resonant frequency, and the degradation of the cooling capacity. Furthermore, because the system structure has not been altered except for the installation of PA, the significant increase in the sound intensity is considered to result from the efficient conversion of thermal input to sound. This means that the conversion efficiency from heat to sound has increased significantly [33].

These results confirm that the PA significantly enhanced the cooling capacity and energy conversion efficiency of the thermoacoustic cooling system and played a role in realizing a significant improvement in the system. This is only possible if the PA is installed at the position of the node of particle velocity for two-wavelength resonance and the antinode of particle velocity for one-wavelength resonance; the sectional area of this portion was forcibly reduced and the particle velocity locally increased, such that the one-wavelength resonance was maintained whereas the two-wavelength resonance was suppressed. In addition, the PA is responsible for phase adjustment, which can realize a sound field in which the pressure and velocity are in phase, as proposed by Ceperley [10, 11]. Thus, by controlling the sound field in the system, particularly the phase relation between sound pressure and particle velocity in the PM, which converts heat to sound, the PA promotes high-efficiency energy conversion between heat and sound. Therefore, the PA 'adjusts' the 'phase' for energy conversion in a thermoacoustic system; hence the name phase adjuster [33, 39–41].

By increasing the energy conversion efficiency with the phase adjustment using the PA, low-temperature oscillation of the thermoacoustic system was also successfully observed [33, 39–41].

6.4 Beyond the PA

Using a PA, the phase difference between the sound pressure and particle velocity can be controlled such that the performance is significantly enhanced [33, 39–41]. Moreover, a PA realizes a performance improvement without negating the advantage of the thermoacoustic system, which is that it can be realized by a simple structure without moving parts. This concept of adjusting the phase by focusing on the sound field, which is the basic principle of PA performance, can be developed for various methods to improve the efficiency of the system [33, 39–45]. Here, two representative methods, the expanded phase adjuster (EPA) [42, 45] and the heat phase adjuster (HPA) [44], are briefly explained.

In contrast to the PA, the EPA adjusts the sound field by forcibly enlarging the cross-sectional area of a part of the thermoacoustic system tube. That is, by partially decreasing the particle velocity in the tube (in contrast to the PA), the EPA adjusts the phase of the sound field where the energy conversion between heat and sound is performed in the system [42, 45]. Figure 6.18(a) illustrates a conceptual diagram of the EPA. By installing an EPA, self-excited oscillations can be guided to a one-wavelength resonant frequency and the cooling capacity can be improved; that is, the energy conversion efficiency between sound and heat in the HP can be improved, as in the case of PA installation [42, 45].

The HPA is a based on a method that aims at an effect similar to that of PA by heating the objective part of the system tube and changing the specific acoustic impedance through its temperature rise. The realization is extremely simple: a sheath heater is wrapped around the objective part of the tube that forms the system [44]. A conceptual diagram is shown in figure 6.18(b). Similarly to the PA and the EPA, the application of an HPA to the system significantly contributes to improving its performance through control of the self-excited oscillation frequency. Furthermore, because it is possible to adjust the temperature setting of the HPA, unlike the PA and

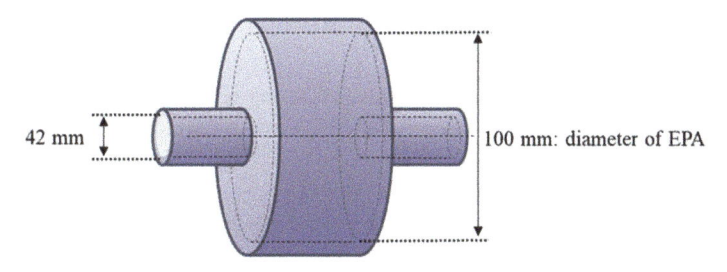

Figure 6.18(a). Conceptual diagram of the expanded phase adjuster.

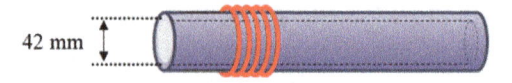

Figure 6.18(b). Conceptual diagram of the HPA.

the EPA, the HPA has the advantage that the sound field in the system can be flexibly adjusted [44].

In addition, there is a new device for enhancing the efficiency, the expansion prime mover (EPM), which has a structure that combines an EPA and a PM [41, 43, 45]. Enhancing heat absorption to the system by increasing the cross-sectional area of the PM, which is the heat injection part, this device can simultaneously adjust the sound field in a system in a similar way to the EPA. The EPM, which adopts these two concepts, also significantly contributes to improving the efficiency of the system and has the remarkable ability to enable oscillation even at a low temperature of approximately 70 °C [41, 43].

The EPA, HPA, and EPM, which were inspired by the PA, are introduced above. Similarly to the PA, by controlling the intratubular sound field of a thermoacoustic system, they significantly improve the performance of the system using the operating principle of adjusting the phase responsible for the energy conversion between heat and sound.

6.5 Conclusions

Considering the intratubular sound field formed during the thermoacoustic self-excited oscillation, the PA was introduced as an efficiency improvement method for practical use. The change in the sound field before the system finally settled into steady oscillation was observed in detail. Based on the results, we developed a PA capable of inducing the intratubular sound field to adopt one-wavelength resonance with higher conversion efficiency and demonstrated the capacity to realize a large breakthrough in the conversion from heat to sound. Furthermore, it was shown that the EPA, HPA, and EPM designs can be realized by developing the idea of the PA while focusing on the sound field.

The potential to solve global warming and energy-related problems using thermoacoustic technology is expected to increase in the future. The findings of our study may be remarkably helpful in this regard.

References

[1] Lord R 1945 *Theory of Sound* vol 2 2nd edn (Dover, NY: Dover Publications)
[2] Feldman K T Jr. 1968 Review of the literature on RIJKE thermoacoustic phenomena *J. Sound Vib.* **7** 83–9
[3] Tominaga A 1995 Thermodynamic aspects of thermoacoustic theory *Cryogenics* **35** 427–40
[4] Swift G W 1988 Thermoacoustic engines *J. Acoust. Soc. Am.* **84** 1145–80
[5] Tominaga A 1998 *Netsu Onkyo Kogaku no Kiso (Fundamental Thermoacoustics)* (Tokyo: Uchida Roukakuho) (in Japanese)

[6] Swift G W 2003 Thermoacoustics: a unifying perspective for some engines and refrigerators *J. Acoust. Soc. Am.* **113** 2379
[7] Feldman K T Jr. 1968 Review of the literature on sondhauss thermoacoustic phenomena *J. Sound Vib.* **7** 71–82
[8] Uzuki H 1969 *Ugetsu Monogatari Kaishaku (Ugetsu Story Interpretation)* (Tokyo: Kadokawa) (in Japanese)
[9] Taconis K W, Beenakker J M, Nier A O C and Aldrich L T 1949 Measurements concerning the vapor-liquid equilibrium of solutions of He^3 in He^4 below 2.19 K *Phys. Rev.* **75** 1966
[10] Ceperley P H 1979 A pistonless Stirling engine—the traveling wave heat engine *J. Acoust. Soc. Am.* **66** 1508–13
[11] Ceperley P H 1985 Gain and efficiency of a short traveling wave heat engine *J. Acoust. Soc. Am.* **77** 1239–44
[12] Wheatley J, Hofler T, Swift G W and Migliori A 1985 Understanding some simple phenomena in thermoacoustics with applications to acoustical heat engines *Am. J. Phys.* **53** 147
[13] Swift G W 1995 Thermoacoustic engines and refrigerators *Phys. Today* **48** 22–8
[14] Yazaki T, Iwata A, Maekawa T and Tominaga A 1998 Traveling wave thermoacoustic engine in a looped tube *Phys. Rev. Lett.* **81** 3128
[15] Yazaki T, Biwa T and Tominaga A 2002 A pistonless Stirling cooler *Appl. Phys. Lett.* **80** 157–9
[16] Backhaus S and Swift G 1999 A thermoacoustic Stirling heat engine *Nature* **399** 335–8
[17] Ueda Y, Biwa T, Mizutani U and Yazaki T 2004 Experimental studies of a thermoacoustic Stirling prime mover and its application to a cooler *J. Acoust. Soc. Am.* **115** 1134–41
[18] Hasegawa S, Yamaguchi T and Oshinoya Y 2013 A thermoacoustic refrigerator driven by a low temperature differential, high efficiency multistage thermoacoustic engine *Appl. Therm. Eng.* **58** 394–9
[19] Biwa T, Hasegawa D and Yazaki T 2010 Low temperature differential thermoacoustic Stirling engine *Appl. Phys. Lett.* **97** 034102
[20] Backhaus S, Tward E and Petach M 2004 Traveling-wave thermoacoustic electric generator *Appl. Phys. Lett.* **85** 1085–7
[21] Hamood A, Jaworski A J, Mao X and Simpson K 2018 Design and construction of a two-stage thermoacoustic electricity generator with push-pull linear alternator *Energy* **144** 61–72
[22] Adeff J A and Hofler T J 2000 Design and construction of a solar-powered, thermoacoustically driven, thermoacoustic refrigerator *J. Acoust. Soc. Am.* **107** L37
[23] Yu Z, Jaworski A J and Backhaus S 2012 Travelling-wave thermoacoustic electricity generator using an ultra-compliant alternator for utilization of low-grade thermal energy *Appl. Energy* **99** 135–45
[24] Tijani M E H, Zeegers J C H and de Waele A T A 2002 The optimal stack spacing for thermoacoustic refrigeration *J. Acoust. Soc. Am.* **112** 128–33
[25] Ueda Y, Kato T and Kato C 2009 Experimental evaluation of the acoustic properties of stacked-screen regenerators *J. Acoust. Soc. Am.* **125** 780–6
[26] Tsuda K and Ueda Y 2017 Critical temperature of traveling- and standing-wave thermoacoustic engines using a wet regenerator *Appl. Therm. Eng.* **196** 62–7
[27] Kawashima Y, Sakamoto S, Onishi R, Hiramatsu K and Watanabe Y 2021 Energy conversion in the thermoacoustic system using a stack wetted with water *Jpn. J. Appl. Phys.* **60** SDDD05

[28] Sakamoto S, Ise Y and Orino Y 2019 Measurement of heat flow caused by a standing-wave component generated by a thermoacoustic phenomenon *AIP Adv.* **9** 115006

[29] Belcher J R 1999 Working gases in thermoacoustic engines *J. Acoust. Soc. Am.* **105** 2677–84

[30] Tijani M E H, Zeegers J C H and de Waele A T A 2002 Prandtl number and thermoacoustic refrigerators *J. Acoust. Soc. Am.* **112** 134–43

[31] Raspet R, Slaton W V, Hickey C J and Hiller R A 2002 Theory of inert gas-condensing vapor thermoacoustics: propagation equation *J. Acoust. Soc. Am.* **112** 1414

[32] Noda D and Ueda Y 2013 A thermoacoustic oscillator powered by vaporized water and ethanol *Am. J. Phys.* **81** 124

[33] Sakamoto S, Imamura Y and Watanabe Y 2007 Improvement of cooling effect of loop-tube-type thermoacoustic cooling system applying phase adjuster *Jpn. J. Appl. Phys.* **46** 4951–5

[34] Sakamoto S, Shibata K, Kitadani Y, Inui Y and Watanabe Y 2012 One factor of resonant wavelength shift from onewavelength to two-wavelength resonance in loop-tube-type thermoacoustic cooling system *Int. Congress on Ultrasonics (Gdańsk, 2011) AIP Conf. Proc.* **1433** 628–31

[35] Sakamoto S and Watanabe Y 2006 Experimental study on resonance frequency of loop-tube-type thermoacoustic cooling system *Acoust. Sci. Tech.* **27** 361–5

[36] Vargaftik N B 1975 *Handbook of Physical Properties of Liquid and Gases* (New York: Hemisphere Publishing Corp.)

[37] Fusco A M, Ward W C and Swift G W 1992 Two-sensor power measurements in lossy ducts *J. Acoust. Soc. Am.* **91** 2229–35

[38] Biwa T, Tashiro Y, Nomura H, Ueda and Yazaki T 2008 Experimental verification of a two-sensor acoustic intensity measurement in lossy ducts *J. Acoust. Soc. Am.* **124** 1584

[39] Sakamoto S, Nishikawa M, Ishino T, Watanabe Y and Senda J 2008 Effect of inner diameter change of phase adjuster on heat-to-sound energy conversion efficiency in loop-tube-type thermoacoustic prime mover *Jpn. J. Appl. Phys.* **47** 4223–5

[40] Sakamoto S and Watanabe Y 2008 Reduction in temperature difference of prime mover stack in loop-tube-type thermoacoustic cooling system by applying phase adjuster *Jpn. J. Appl. Phys.* **47** 3776–80

[41] Orino Y, Sakamoto S, Inui Y, Ikenoue T and Watanabe Y 2014 Numerical analysis of the effect of local diameter reduction on the critical temperature of thermoacoustic oscillations in a looped tube *Jpn. J. Appl. Phys.* **53** 07KE13

[42] Inoue M, Sakamoto S, Nakano Y and Watanabe Y 2013 The effect of resonance mode control by expanding of cross-section area on cooling capacity in a loop-tube type thermoacoustic cooling system *21st Int. Congress on Acoustics* 19 *Proc. Mtgs. Acoust.* 030006

[43] Ishino T, Sakamoto S, Orino Y, Inui Y and Watanabe Y 2015 Effect of the relative installation position of two enlarged prime movers on the onset temperature in loop-tube-type multistage thermoacoustic system *Jpn. J. Appl. Phys.* **54** 07HE11

[44] Kido A, Sakamoto S, Taga K and Watanabe Y 2016 Control of self-excitation mode in thermoacoustic system using heat phase adjuster *Jpn. J. Appl. Phys.* **55** 07KE14

[45] Inui K, Sakamoto S, Egawa K, Wada T and Kataoka S 2018 Influence of local inner diameter changes on the onset temperature and the energy conversion efficiency of a loop-tube-type thermoacoustic system *Jpn. J. Appl. Phys.* **57** 07LE01

Part III

Biological and medical applications

IOP Publishing

Ultrasonics
Physics and applications
Mami Matsukawa, Pak-Kon Choi, Kentaro Nakamura, Hirotsugu Ogi and Hideyuki Hasegawa

Chapter 7

Ultrasonic characterization of bone

Mami Matsukawa

This chapter introduces the use of ultrasonic studies for bone evaluation. Ultrasonic studies of biological tissues are usually divided into two parts, evaluation (diagnosis) and therapy. In the evaluation stage, it is common to apply pulse techniques in the megahertz range to measure the wave properties of cortical and cancellous bones. From their interesting ultrasonic characteristics, it is possible to estimate bone shape, elasticity, and porosity in addition to elastic anisotropy. The application of a light-scattering measurement technique is another unique idea, which enables bone matrix elasticity to be evaluated without being affected by microstructures. Ultrasonic bone therapy is used in the field of orthopedic surgery; however, the precise mechanism of ultrasonic stimulation is still unknown. One of the possible physical mechanisms is piezoelectricity in bone.

7.1 Why should we study bone using ultrasound?

The skeleton is an important organ. There are more than 200 bones in the body. However, ultrasonic studies of bone are not as popular as soft-tissue studies. One reason for this is the complicated nature of bone. Bone is a hard and anisotropic solid tissue with high heterogeneity. The evaluation of bone *in vivo* is difficult because of its high acoustic impedance, which results in low ultrasound penetration [1, 2]. In addition, the two main types of bone, cortical (compact) bone and cancellous (trabecular) bone, differ in terms of shape and structure. Dense cortical (compact) bone forms the external envelope of all bones, and cancellous (trabecular) bone is found in the inner portion of bones [3]. Their complicated shapes and structures also prevent the precise evaluation of the wave velocity and attenuation of ultrasound.

In today's aging societies, however, bone health is an important factor in the quality of life (QOL) and the activities of daily living (ADL), because bones support the body load and enable walking, which ensures proper functioning of the circulatory system. In addition to their kinematic importance, they act as a reservoir of calcium and phosphorus and maintain electrolyte equilibrium in bodily fluids. They are living materials that adapt their shapes, properties, and structures according to their mechanical environments via continuous remodeling. Wolff's law [4] tells us that mechanical stress is a principal factor that influences bone health.

Considering these characteristics of bones, ultrasonic studies have focused on both types of bone, namely, cortical and cancellous. In order to perform a mechanical and ultrasonic characterization of cortical bone, the hierarchical structural organization should be carefully considered (figure 7.1) [5]. Bone is a composite material containing approximately 70% mineral (calcium phosphate), 22% proteins (type I collagen), and 8% [6] water by weight. The mineral and collagens are present in approximately the same volumes. The basic matrices of bone consist mainly of collagen fibrils accompanied by hydroxyapatite (HAp), which form a 'twisted plywood' structure with cylindrical osteons [7]. The osteons consist of several concentric lamellae surrounding the Haversian canals, including blood vessels and nerves. The microscopic structures at the sub-millimeter level depend on the species; for example, large animals, such as bovines, have plexiform structures to support their heavy body loads [3]. Figure 7.2 shows scanning acoustic microscopy (SAM) images of human cortical bone cross-sections from a femoral mid-diaphysis [8, 9]. Numerous Haversian canals and osteocyte lacunae are present. The former

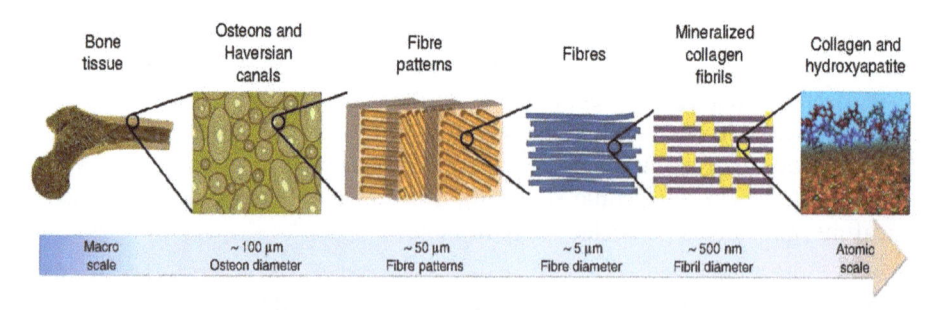

Figure 7.1. Hierarchical structure of bone ranging from the macroscale to the nano scale. Reproduced from [5] with permission of Springer.

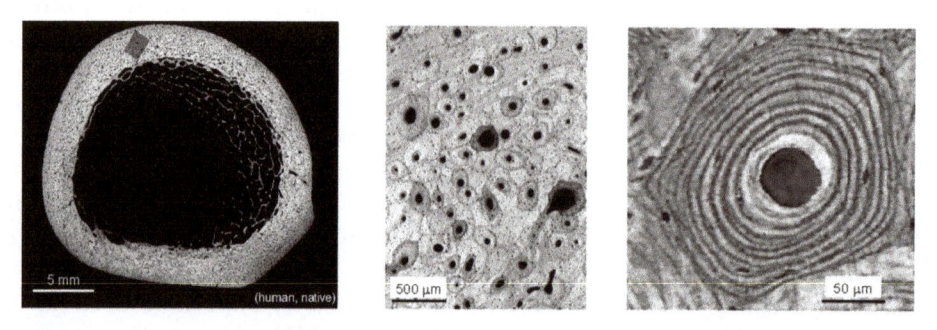

Figure 7.2. Acoustic impedance images of human cortical bone cross-sections from the femoral mid-diaphysis. The large dark spots in the center are Haversian canals and the small spots are osteocyte lacunae. Reproduced from [8, 9], with permission of IEEE.

are typically in the range of several microns in size, which is smaller than the ultrasonic wavelength of a medical diagnostic system. However, they affect the measurements of anisotropic elastic properties and cause scattering of ultrasound in the megahertz range.

The cancellous bone (highly porous spongy bone), which has a complicated 3D structure composed of connected bone plates and/or rods, called trabeculae, is located inside an envelope of cortical bone. This trabecular network is filled with viscous bone marrow [10–12]. The trabecular structure also depends on the body load, and the network structure shows strong anisotropy. The thickness and average interval of trabeculae in cancellous bone (trabecular separation: Tb. Sp) [13] are typically in the range of 100–300 μm, which is comparable to the wavelength of the ultrasound used for medical diagnosis. Cancellous bone also functions as a scatterer of ultrasound. As a result of its characteristic structure, most ultrasonic studies of cancellous bone have focused on a structural evaluation of cancellous bone using transmitted and scattered ultrasound, rather than material evaluation. This is important because early symptoms of osteoporosis appear in the structure of cancellous bone [14].

Clinical ultrasonic studies of bone primarily aim to evaluate osteoporosis using ultrasonic transmission measurements of the cortical and cancellous bone and signals backscattered by cancellous bone [14–18]. Because the diagnostic criteria of bone still depend on the bone mineral density (BMD) measured using x-ray techniques, ultrasonic data are often discussed in relation to BMD data [19, 20]. However, ultrasonic wave properties reflect the macroscopic viscoelastic properties of the bone, including its collagen, which cannot be evaluated via x-ray mineral evaluation. For endocrine diseases, such as diabetes, the bone fracture risk cannot be evaluated by measuring the mineral amount [21, 22]. Detailed ultrasonic investigations of bone quality, including its structural and material changes, are required.

In this chapter, recent topics of bone studies are introduced using the keyword 'ultrasound,' focusing on the properties that cannot be evaluated using x-ray techniques. Studies of ultrasonic wave velocity and attenuation, which are related to the viscoelasticity of bone, are discussed. The anisotropic elasticity and piezoelectricity are also discussed as related properties. The quality of collagen in bone is the second most important topic in this chapter, because it is a property that cannot be evaluated using x-ray evaluation.

7.2 Ultrasonic wave properties in bone tissues

7.2.1 Conventional ultrasonic characterization in the megahertz range

As mentioned above, the elastic properties of bone depend on the multiplicity of the material and structural properties at several hierarchical length scales. The bone tissue matrix predominantly consists of the following elementary constituents: organic and mineral components with water. The ultrasonic wave properties change depending on the composition of this compound material. However, even in dense cortical bone, the wave properties are affected by the complicated microstructure of the bone. As shown in figure 7.2, there are various pores present in the cortical bone that are smaller than the wavelength of the ultrasound used for conventional ultrasonic pulse techniques (around 0.8 mm for 5 MHz). These pores, referred to as Haversian canals, encompass the blood vessels and nerves [23]. Their distribution is heterogeneous, and their shape is anisotropic, which affects wave propagation. However, because of its comparatively low porosity, wave properties in cortical bone may reflect the material properties of the bone matrix and microstructures [24–27].

Cortical bone in large animals can be classified based on two main specific microstructures: plexiform and Haversian. The former rarely exists in human cortical bone. The effects of these microstructures on wave properties have been reported using conventional ultrasonic techniques and acoustic microscopy [26–29]. The bone matrix is composed of organic components (type I collagen and polysaccharides) and mineral components (calcium phosphate). As mentioned above, calcium phosphate constitutes 70% of the total bone matrix mass, mainly in the form of hydroxyapatite (HAp) crystals, $Ca_{10}(PO_4)_6(OH)_2$. HAp crystals have a hexagonal system with uniaxial anisotropy, whose elasticity is the greatest in the c-axis direction [30, 31].

Most cortical bone studies in the megahertz range have reported wave properties such as the speed of sound (SOS) [32–36] and attenuation [37–40] by measuring *ex vivo* bone samples in water. The wave properties dynamically change depending on the heterogeneity, anisotropy, temperature, species, position in the body, etc. Figure 7.3 shows the velocity anisotropy of the cortical bone in the mid shafts of two left bovine femora measured using a conventional ultrasonic pulse immersion technique at 10 MHz [27]. In the ring-shaped mid shaft of the cortical femur, the observed velocity is strongly dependent on the propagation direction (axial (body weight direction), tangential (circumferential), or radial). We can also determine the effects of the microstructure (plexiform or Haversian) on the velocity. In addition, although the measurement area was comparatively large (diameter of the transmitter

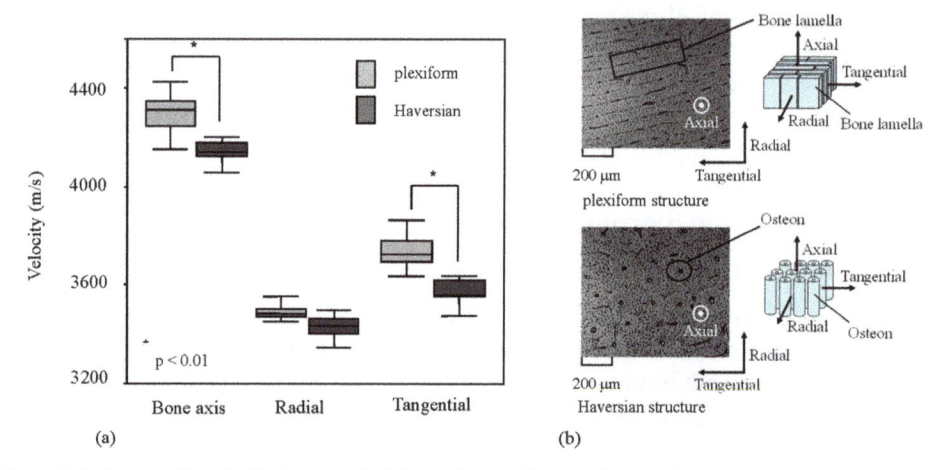

Figure 7.3. Range of longitudinal wave velocities in the plexiform and Haversian structures. The cortical bone sample was obtained from a mid shaft of a bovine femur. Reproduced from [27], with permission of Springer.

and receiver: 8 mm), the velocities showed large dispersions due to heterogeneity. The results were in good agreement with the studies of Katz *et al*, which showed that cortical bone has a quasi-hexagonal or axisymmetric character and five independent elastic constants [26]. In the mid shaft of a bovine femur, however, the velocities in the tangential direction are slightly higher than those in the radial direction. Nakatsuji's study of the cortical bone ball provided angle-dependent longitudinal wave velocities and showed that the elastic properties of bone are not perfectly axisymmetric (figure 7.4) [41]. The cortical bone should be considered an orthotropic material with nine independent elastic constants. Xu and Bernard *et al* also succeeded in obtaining the elastic constants of cortical bone using a resonant ultrasound spectroscopy technique [42]. These studies of wave velocity in the megahertz range have become the basis of clinical studies of cortical bone, which typically measure the SOS *in vivo*.

The velocity distribution due to the site often reaches 20% in the axial direction in the cortical mid shaft of a large animal's femur. Figure 7.5 shows the velocity distribution of longitudinal waves in the axial direction of the third equine metacarpal bone at 5 MHz. Measurements were also performed using the pulse

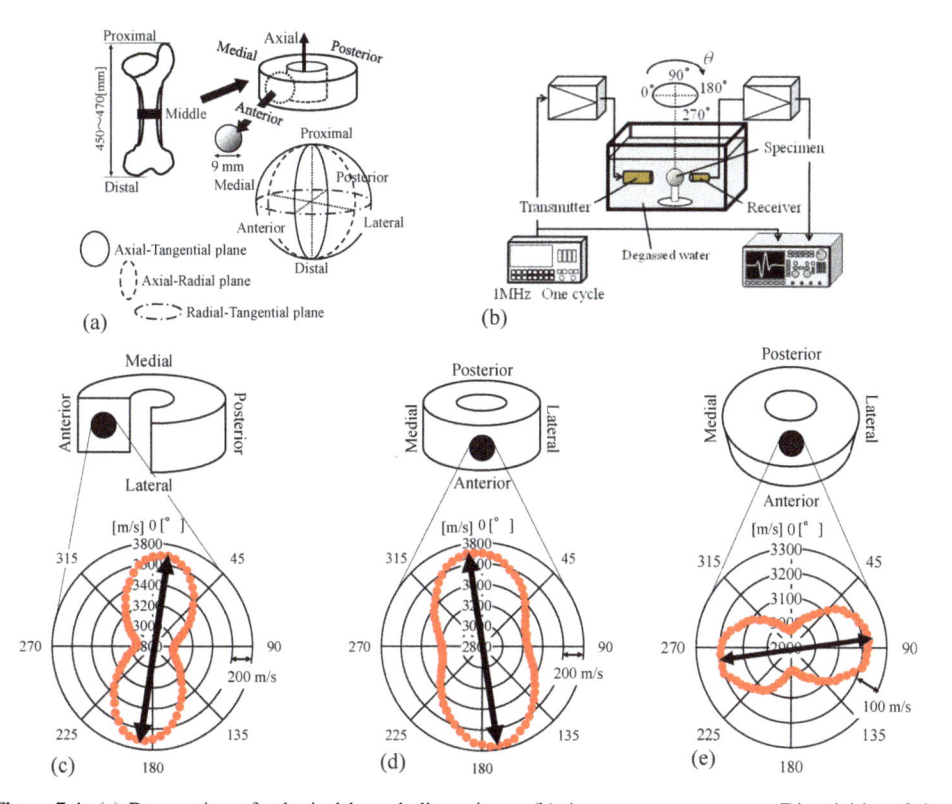

Figure 7.4. (a) Preparation of spherical bone ball specimen. (b) A measurement system. Directivities of the measured wave velocity in the specimen (c) in the axial–radial plane, (d) in the axial–tangential plane, and (e) in the radial–tangential plane. Reproduced from [41]. All rights reserved.

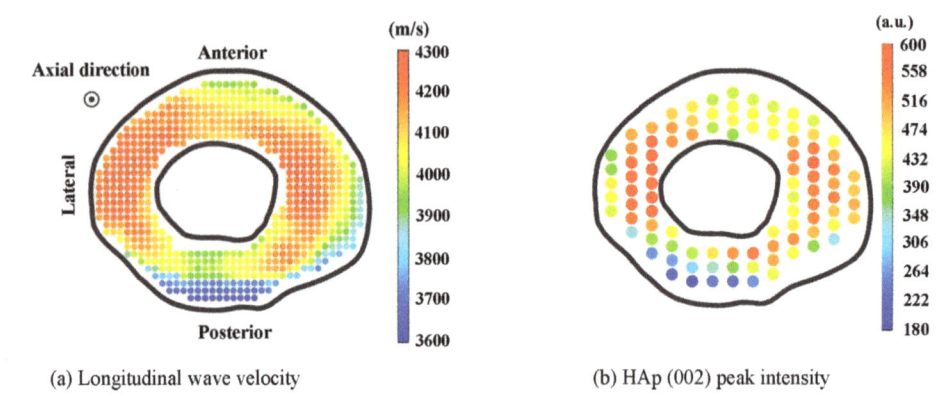

Figure 7.5. Measured data of an equine third metacarpal bone. Distributions of (a) the longitudinal wave velocity in the axial direction measured by a pulse immersion technique at 5 MHz and (b) HAp (002) peak intensity obtained from $2\theta-\omega$ scan x-ray diffraction (XRD) patterns are shown. The peak intensities reflect the number of HAp crystallites aligned in the bone-axis direction.

immersion technique. The spatial resolution of each measurement was 1 mm. As shown, the maximum velocity difference was approximately 700 m s^{-1}, depending on the site at the specimen surface. The velocity distribution may originate from the BMD, bone mass density, and microstructure. Interestingly, in large animals (cows and horses), the posterior part of the mid shaft of the leg bone often shows lower longitudinal wave velocities [27, 28]. The bone properties change in response to functional forces on the bone, in accordance with Wolff's law [4]. The velocity distribution in the cortical bone may show adaptation of the bone resulting from daily stress distribution in the legs.

In the bone matrix, the minerals align with collagen fibers and are located in interfibrillar spaces. As mentioned above, the minerals in bone are mostly HAp with a hexagonal structure, whose alignment directions can be evaluated via small-angle x-ray scattering (SAXS) and x-ray diffraction (XRD) [30, 43–47]. Since the initial studies, strong alignment of HAp crystallites in the axial direction has been observed in mature bone. Yamato *et al* discussed the relationship between HAp crystallite alignment and longitudinal wave velocity in three directions (the tangential, radial, and body weight (axial) directions) of the cortical bone in the mid shaft of the bovine femur [27, 28]. In the axial direction, the effects of the alignment strongly affect the velocity. This can be observed in the bones of large animals. Figure 7.5 shows the distribution of the (002) peak intensities of HAp crystallites in equine cortical bone measured by $2\theta-\omega$ scan XRD patterns. This reflects the *c*-axis alignment of HAp crystallites in the bone-axis direction. We found a similar relationship between velocity and HAp alignment. The correlation between the values of the (002) peak intensity and velocity was larger than that between the values of BMD and velocity, indicating that the axial velocities depended on the alignment of HAp crystallites rather than the BMD. The cortical bones of large animals are dense, and the ultrasonic wave velocities may reflect the microscopic material properties of the bone matrix.

7.2.2 Microscopic bone evaluation by Brillouin scattering

As mentioned above, from the microscopic to the macroscopic level, bone has a complex structure. Litniewski and Raum investigated the microscopic and hierarchical structures of bone samples using scanning acoustic microscopy (SAM) [8, 9, 48]. SAM can measure the elastic properties of a local area at a specific acoustic impedance. A series of studies conducted by Raum reported the elastic constants of bone derived from the measured acoustic impedance [49–52]. The studies described heterogeneous and hierarchical structures at each level over three orders of magnitude, that is, from the millimeter to the micrometer range, together with the imaging approaches used. He also evaluated the anisotropy using a small cylindrical cortical bone specimen for SAM measurements. This study of SAM in the gigahertz range showed typical alterations of the elastic coefficient in the osteonal lamellae [53].

One trial evaluated ultrasonic wave properties in bone using the non-contact measurement of wave velocity via Brillouin scattering (BS). BS is a well-known interaction between light and thermally excited phonons, which was first reported by Brillouin and independently by Mandelstam [54, 55]. In BS techniques, incident light is scattered, and the spectral shifts of the scattered light are typically measured using a high-performance Fabry-Pérot interferometer [56]. Such non-contact and non-destructive measurements can measure wave velocities in the gigahertz range. The most important requirement for BS measurements is the transparency of the sample, because the incident light interacts with the bulk phonons in the material. Therefore, the first challenge of BS measurement for bone characterization was late, compared to several studies of soft tissues and collagen [57–60]. This was a study by Lees et al [61]. They reported longitudinal wave velocities of 4.06×10^3 m s^{-1} (wet) and 4.86×10^3 m s^{-1} (dry) at around 11 GHz in the axial direction of a dried cow tibia. The velocity measured in the dry specimen was higher than that of the conventional wet specimen measurement data in the megahertz range [25]. This velocity difference seems to originate from the air-drying condition. Theoretically, shear waves can be measured using BS techniques simultaneously; however, it is difficult to observe shear phonons because of the weak scattering produced by semi-transparent thin bone specimens.

The optical geometric conditions are important for BS measurements of anisotropic materials. In this technique, the target wavelength of the ultrasound is kept constant by selecting the optical geometry, and the frequency shift is measured. In backscattering geometry (180°), strong light scattering can be obtained; however, the frequency shift of the Brillouin component includes the effects of the refractive index n in obtaining the wave velocity. One technique used to avoid these effects is the 45° −45° scattering geometry (referred to as the 90A geometry), as shown in figure 7.6 [62]. The modified 90A scattering geometry is the reflection-induced Θ angle (RIΘA) geometry reported by Krüger et al [63]. This geometry does not require complicated adjustment of the incident and scattered light, such as that required by the 90A scattering geometry. The simple procedure of the RIΘA geometry enables highly accurate incident angle setting, which improves the accuracy of the wave velocity measurements. In this geometry, the specimen is placed on a mirror, which may reduce the effects of the laser heat via thermal conduction. In the case of thin bone

$$\lambda^{180} = \frac{\lambda_0}{2n}$$

(a) Back (180° scattering)

$$\lambda^{90A} = \frac{\lambda_0}{\sqrt{2}}$$

(b) 90A scattering

$$\lambda^{\Theta A} = \frac{\lambda_0}{\sqrt{2}}$$

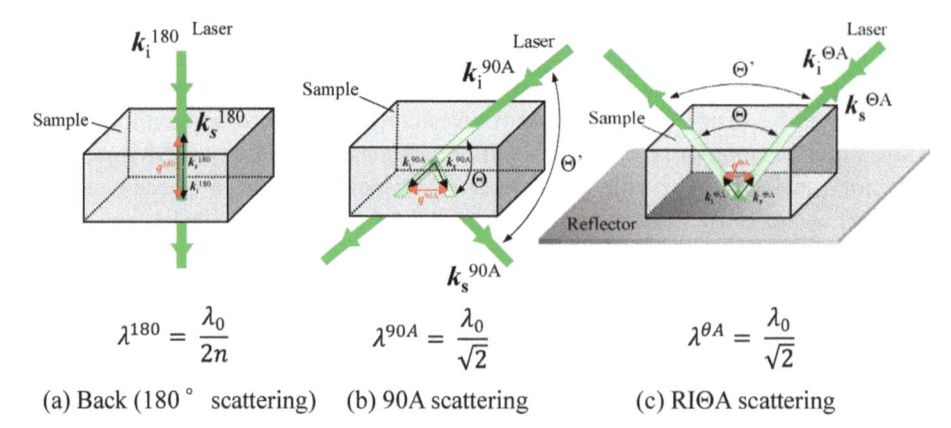

(c) RIΘA scattering

Figure 7.6. Scattering geometries used in the Brillouin scattering measurements. In the case of RIΘA scattering measurements, the samples are usually thin films. Here, k_i and k_r are the wave vectors of the incident and scattered light, respectively; q is the wave vector of the phonons; λ_0 is the wavelength of light; and λ^{180}, λ^{90A} and $\lambda^{\Theta A}$ are phonon wavelengths.

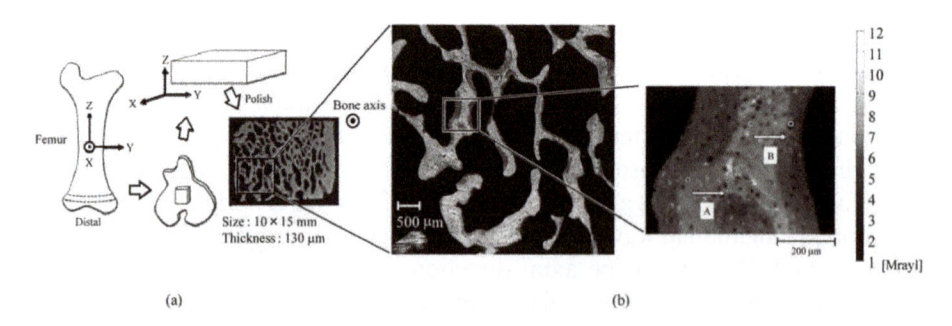

Figure 7.7. (a) Thin trabecular specimen and (b) acoustic impedance mapping image in trabecula. Micro-Brillouin measurements were performed for two lines (marked A and B) across the trabecula shown in the square region. Reproduced from [66], with permission of AIP publishing.

specimens measured by this geometry, the velocity changes caused by the heat were less than 0.5% [64, 65] for measurements of more than 1.5 h, which was smaller than the measurement errors of the Brillouin frequency shift (approximately 1%) of weak scattered light. Because the thin specimens used for the RIΘA scattering geometry dry quickly during long-term measurements, most bone studies were performed using perfectly dry specimens.

Integrating a microscope with the BS technique (μ-Brillouin scattering: μ-BS), Kawabe reported a site-matched comparative study of bone elasticity using μ-BS and reflection SAM techniques. These techniques have similar spatial resolutions (spot diameters of 10 and 8 μm, respectively). As shown in figure 7.7 [66], a transverse cross-sectional specimen of the trabecula at the distal end of a 30-month old bovine femur was sliced across the long-axis direction. The specimen's surface (x–y) plane was polished, and the acoustic impedance on the specimen's surface was measured using a 200 MHz SAM. After the SAM measurements, the thickness of the specimen was reduced by polishing the opposite surface of the specimen. The final thickness of the specimen used for the μ-BS technique was 130 μm, which was thin enough to achieve sufficient transparency. The SAM measurement surface was set on the surface of the mirror for the μ-BS measurements, because the scattering volume of the RIΘA geometry was near the mirror surface. By considering the refractive index of bone (1.2–1.3) [64] and the sample thickness, the position of the laser incidence was carefully determined for site matching. Figure 7.7 shows the SAM image (acoustic impedance) and the lines measured by BS. Although the measured properties were different (out-of-plane acoustic impedance (SAM) and the velocity of in-plane longitudinal waves propagating perpendicular to the trabecular axis (BS)), the data in figure 7.8 show a good correlation between the lines (line A: $R^2 = 0.63$ ($P < .01$), line B: $R^2 = 0.67$ ($P < .01$)). The average velocity in the dried trabecula was similar to that of the cortical bone in the bovine femora [64].

In spite of the comparison of different properties, the correlation shows that μ-BS may be a good tool with which to evaluate the wave velocity of bone matrices at the micrometer scale. However, the heterogeneity and anisotropy of the bone need to be considered. Kawabe *et al* examined the 3D alignment of wave velocities in trabeculae in the cancellous bone at the distal end of the bovine femur. Based on the velocity measurements and considering their spatial distribution, the average longitudinal

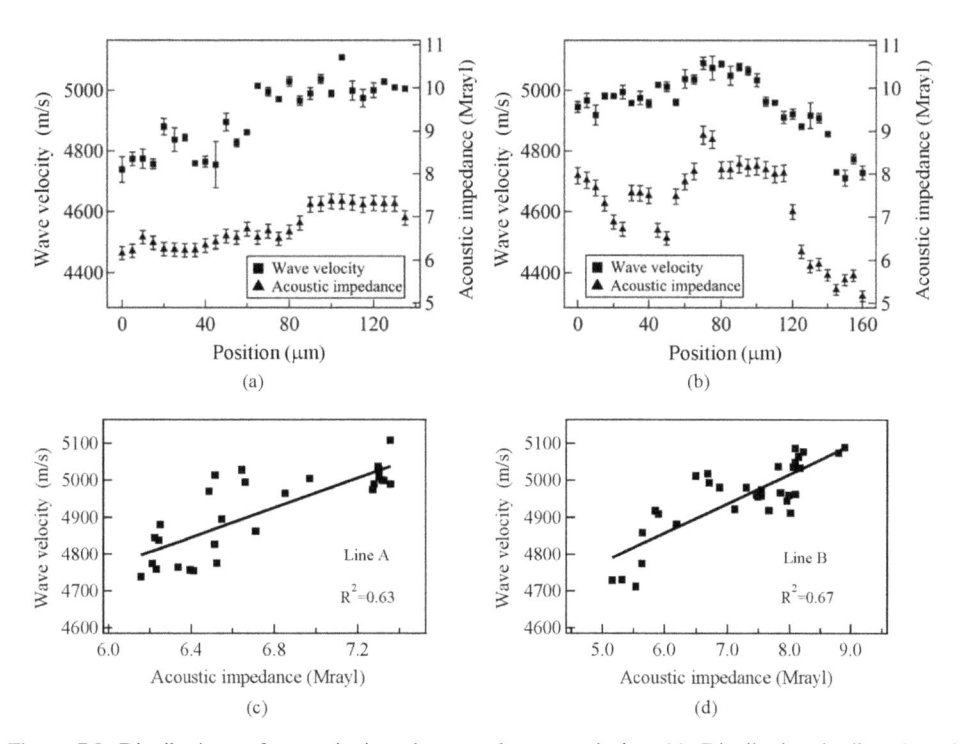

Figure 7.8. Distributions of acoustic impedance and wave velocity. (a) Distribution in line A and (b) distribution in line B. Graphs (c) and (d) show the site-matched correlations between the SAM and μ-BS data at lines A and B, respectively. Reproduced from [66], with permission of AIP publishing.

wave velocities in the trabeculae aligned in the bone-axis and the anterior–posterior (A–P) directions were similar [65]. At the distal end of the bovine femur, the cancellous bone forms a plate-like structure along the bone-axis and A–P directions. The results indicated that the velocity in the cancellous plate was approximately isotropic.

The μ-BS technique with the RIΘA geometry can be used to measure the velocity in all in-plane directions by simply rotating the specimen on the mirror, whereas for a given specimen (cut in a specific direction with respect to the bone anatomical direction) SAM and nanoindentation measure properties only in the thickness direction. Therefore, the in-plane anisotropy of the bone sample can be evaluated as the velocity changes. Fukui *et al* attempted to evaluate the anisotropy of the trabecula at the distal end of the bovine femur. A weak anisotropy of the longitudinal wave velocity was found in the trabecula, indicating that each trabecula seemed approximately isotropic (figure 7.9) [67–69].

Figure 7.10 shows the relationship between the trabecular length and velocity in the cancellous bone at the distal end of the bovine femur [70]. In this cancellous bone, the dispersion of trabecular widths was small; therefore, the aspect ratios of the trabeculae depend on the trabecular length. Figure 7.10 shows that the velocity tended to decrease in the longer trabeculae, approaching a minimum value (approximately 4.75×10^3 m s^{-1}). Small values were found in the trabeculae aligned in the A–P and bone-axis directions. As mentioned above, the porous plate-like trabeculae in the A–P and axial directions were supported by rod-like trabeculae in the mediolateral (ML) direction of the cancellous bone. Therefore, the results show that the wave velocity (elasticity) in the trabecula depends on the cancellous structure. In plate-like trabeculae, the elasticity may be smaller than that in

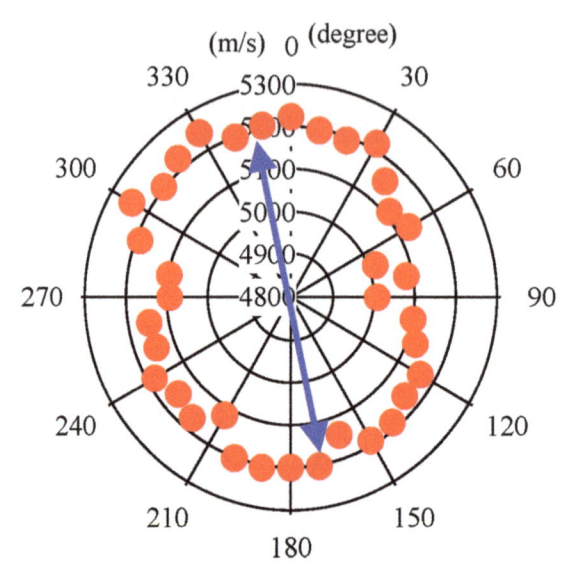

Figure 7.9. Anisotropy of the longitudinal wave velocity in a trabecula in the distal end of a bovine femur. The arrow indicates the maximum velocity direction. Trabecular alignment direction: 0 to 180 degrees. Reproduced from [68], with permission of Elsevier.

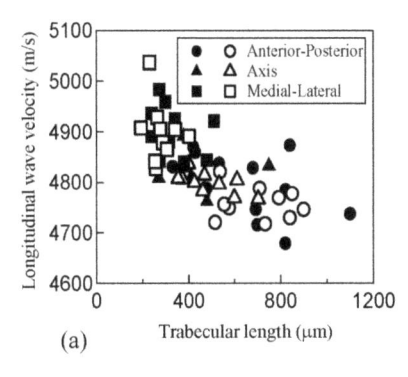

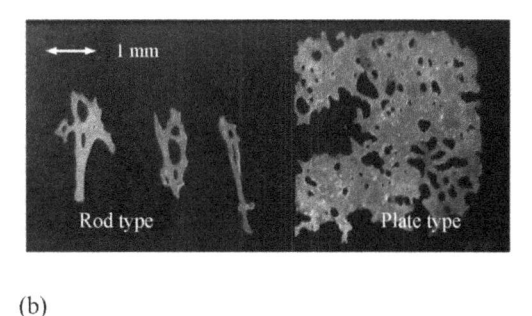

Figure 7.10. (a) Longitudinal wave velocities and trabecular lengths (filled markers indicate data for a 29-month-old specimen; other markers indicate data for a 31-month-old specimen) of the distal end of bovine femora. (b) Examples of rod- and plate-type trabeculae. Reproduced from [70], with permission of AIP publishing.

rod-like short trabeculae. The elasticity of the bone trabeculae and trabecular structure may be optimized for complementary support of body weight.

Since the μ-BS technique enables in-plane velocity measurements in a minute area, it can evaluate the elasticity changes of the bone matrix. For example, the effects of compression load were investigated [71] and the human femoral head [72] was evaluated. One example is the elasticity changes caused by bone growth [73, 74]. Fraulob et al studied the osseointegration phenomena near titanium implants in rabbit tibiae [75]. The results, which combined nanoindentation, μ-BS and histology showed the spatiotemporal evolution of newly formed bone properties by considering different regions of interest. The wave velocities were higher close to the implant surface, as well as after longer healing times, suggesting a higher degree of mineralization consistent with bone tissue maturation. Another example of this application is the evaluation of diabetic bone, in which abnormal collagen crosslinks are known as advanced glycation end-product (AGE) crosslinks. A typical AGE crosslink is pentosidine, formed by nonenzymatic glycation or oxidation reactions [76]. AGE crosslinks may deteriorate the collagen in bone, which cannot be evaluated using x-ray techniques. The BMD often remains normal in bones [77]. A μ-BS study of an artificially glycated bone specimen showed a velocity decrease owing to the formation of AGE crosslinks [78]. A comparative study of young bones from spontaneously diabetic torii (SDT) rats (an animal model of type 2 diabetes) and healthy Sprague Dawley (SD) rats also showed a longitudinal wave velocity decrease (2%–4%) caused by diabetes in the cortical and cancellous bones [79]. A velocity decrease was found in the early stages of hyperglycemia, and reduced bone elasticity was indicated. Yano measured the effects of glycation in type I collagen films and reported a decrease in wave velocity. The study confirmed that the small velocity decrease in bone was due to glycation in the collagen [80].

7.2.3 Piezoelectricity in bone in the megahertz range

The first study of bone piezoelectricity was reported by Fukada and Yasuda in 1957, based on the measurement of electrical potentials in dry bone induced by mechanical stress [81]. Because electricity injected into bone through electrodes induces callus formation [82], mechanical stress might stimulate bone metabolism through piezoelectricity. Several studies have shown mechanically induced electrical potentials in wet and dry bones, even in bone with dissolved hydroxyapatite crystallites [81]. Thus, the origin of piezoelectricity is possibly the collagen which occupies half of the bone volume. In addition, the induced potentials found in dry bone imply that the main mechanism is piezoelectricity rather than the streaming potential [83]. Despite the long history of bone piezoelectricity, there have been few discussions of piezoelectricity in the ultrasonic frequency range. Most research has focused on mechanical studies, evaluating the anisotropic character using long bones at low frequencies [84].

In addition, piezoelectricity in the megahertz range could be used to understand the mechanism of bone fracture healing by low-intensity pulsed ultrasound (LIPUS) [85, 86]. As mentioned above, Yasuda and Fukada reported that mechanical stress might stimulate bone metabolism through piezoelectricity [81, 82]. If this is applicable in the megahertz range, piezoelectricity in bones should be evaluated in this range. An initial *in vivo* study of the electromechanical response in cortical bone at 1.27 MHz was reported by Behari and Singh [87], who implanted electrodes inside a rabbit femur and tibia. They reported small electrical signals were detected in the bone as a result of ultrasonic irradiation.

For a more precise evaluation of bone piezoelectricity, Okino *et al* observed ultrasound using a 'bone' transducer, in which a bovine cortical bone disk from the mid shaft of the femur was used as a piezoelectric element [88]. The fabrication process of the unique transducer, including photos, is shown in figure 7.11. They fabricated two types of bone transducer: (Type A) a circular sample plate that was normal to the bone axis and (Type B) a circular sample plate that was normal to the radial direction of the bone axis. The bone transducers have a simple coaxial structure with an outer electric field shield, similar to conventional flat ultrasonic transducers. The output of the transducers resulting from ultrasound irradiation was approximately 1/1000 of that of a common poly(vinylidene fluoride) (PVDF) ultrasound transducer. The receiving sensitivity ranged from 10^{-2} to 10^{-3} μV Pa^{-1}. The electrical output from the transducer was small, which is consistent with the results of the low-frequency mechanical studies. Tsuneda *et al* evaluated the effects of water content in the bone on piezoelectricity by checking the electrical output as a function of the immersion time of dry bone transducers [89]. The output from the bone transducer was clearly observed from the initial dry state to the wet state, and there was minimal change, as shown in figure 7.12. The results show that the contribution of the streaming potential owing to the liquid in the pores seemed small, and the main mechanism of the electrical potentials might be piezoelectricity. Their results also showed a shift in the resonant frequency of the bone transducer resulting from the immersion time, indicating possible thickness and velocity changes due to swelling, as shown in figure 7.13.

As mentioned above, bone is not perfectly axisymmetric but is orthotropic and has nine independent elastic constants. Matsukawa *et al* investigated the anisotropic piezoelectric response of bone [90]. They fabricated three types of circular bone plate (thickness 3 mm) from the mid shaft of the bovine femur, which were cut normal to the radial direction of the bone axis (Type A), normal to the direction tangential to the

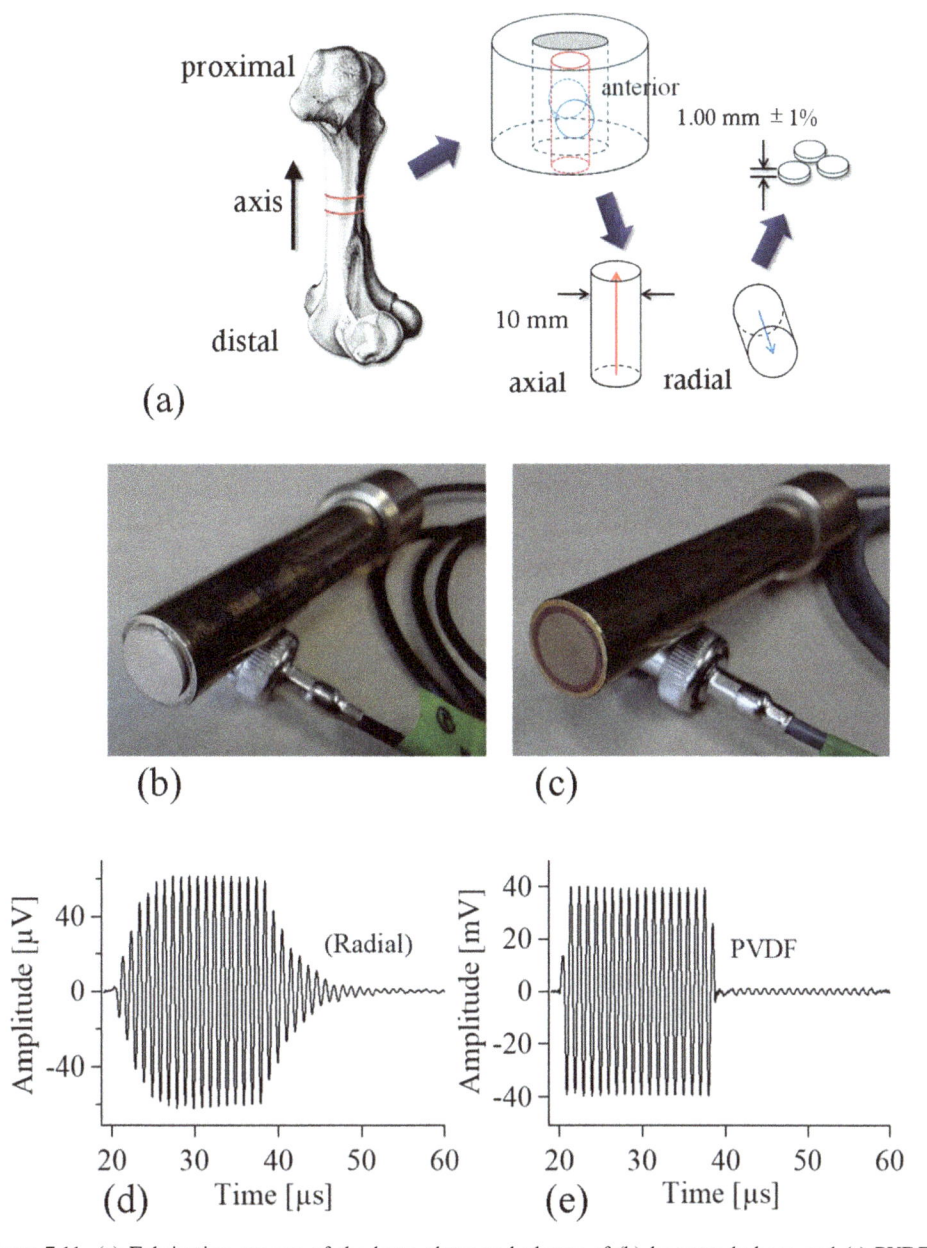

Figure 7.11. (a) Fabrication process of the bone plates and photos of (b) homemade bone and (c) PVDF transducers. Images (d) and (e) are observed ultrasonic waveforms. The wave amplitudes measured by the bone transducers were approximately 0.1% of those of the PVDF transducers. Reproduced from [88], with permission of AIP publishing.

bone axis (Type B), and normal to the bone axis (Type C). Bone transducers were fabricated using these plates. Here, the ultrasound transmitter and bone transducer were crossed at right angles in degassed water. As shown in figure 7.14, the maximum output values of the bone transducers were observed when the ultrasound propagation

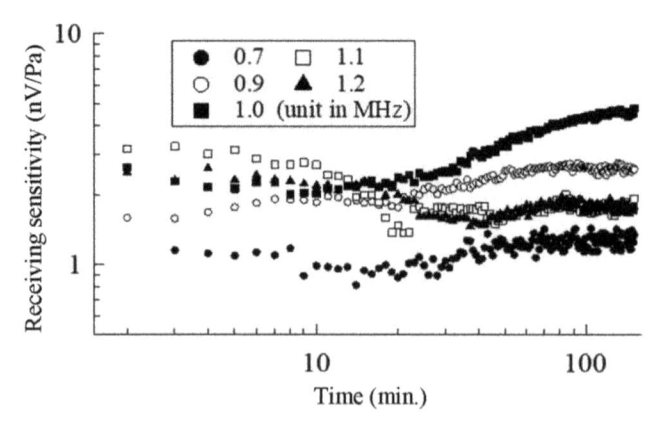

Figure 7.12. Typical receiving sensitivities of bone transducers as a function of immersion time. Reproduced from [89], with permission of AIP publishing.

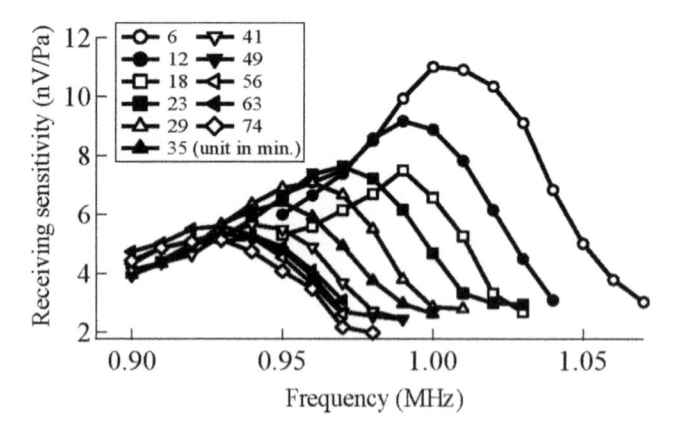

Figure 7.13. Shift of resonant frequency of a bone transducer (fabricated from a cortical bone that had a plexiform structure) as a function of immersion time. Reproduced from [89], with permission of AIP publishing.

direction was at an angle of approximately 45° to the three bone axes (the bone-axis, tangential, and radial directions). Interestingly, the minimum values were observed when ultrasound propagated in the three axial directions. Because the elastic properties in the radial and tangential directions were similar, the characteristic changes in the electrical output were not observed using the Type A transducer. These directivities of transducer output were not found in a transducer made from demineralized cortical bone plates [91]. Makino *et al* also confirmed the direct and converse piezoelectric effects of bone using bone transducers and showed that the maximum transmission sensitivity occurred when the bone plate was at an angle of approximately 45° from the axes [92]. A similar off-axis character of bone piezo-electricity was observed in low-frequency mechanical studies.

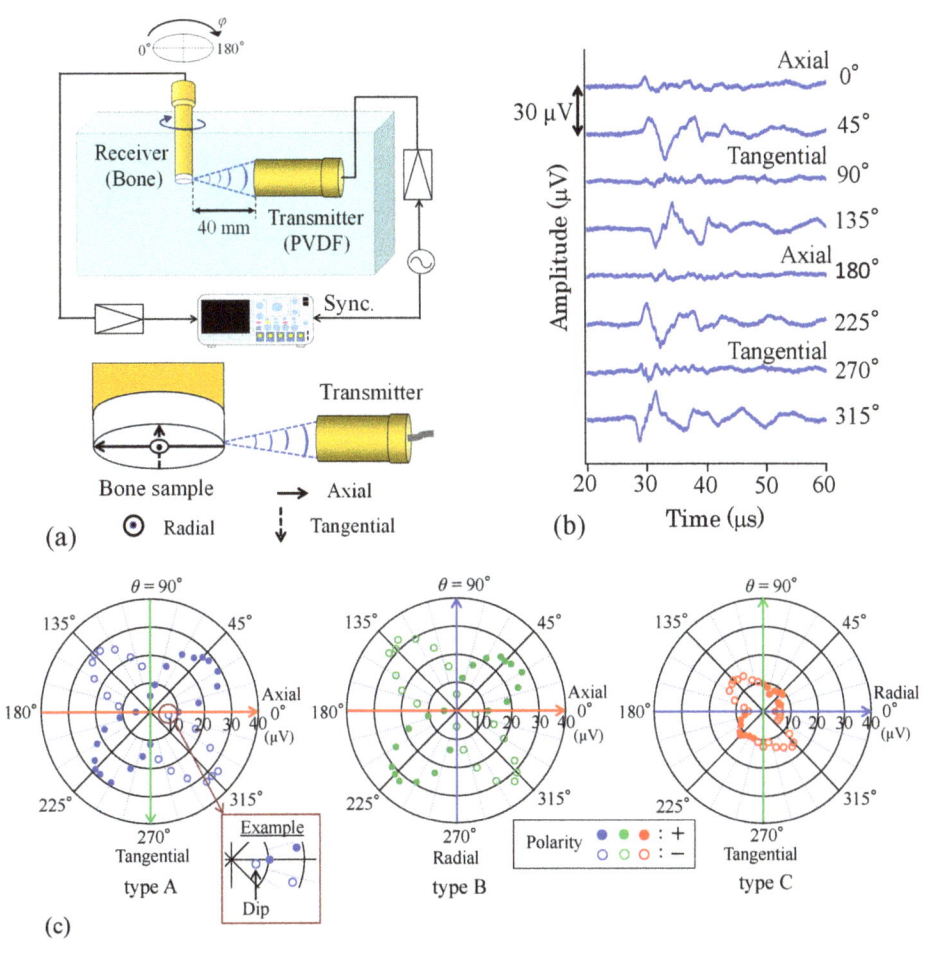

Figure 7.14. (a) Diagram of the experimental system. The transmitter and receiver were crossed at right angles in degassed water. The bone sample's side surface was located 40 mm from the transmitter (i.e. at the transmitter's focal length). Ultrasound measurements were taken at each rotation angle. (b) Waveforms observed for bone transducer Type A are shown. Image (c) shows the relationship between the polarity and peak-to-peak values of the stress-induced electric potentials and the ultrasound irradiation directions. Reproduced from [90], with permission of AIP publishing.

As Fukada and Yasuda reported, the crystallographic symmetry of the collagen in the bone is considered to be hexagonal [81]. However, the bone exhibits no apparent symmetry in its matrix of piezoelectric coefficients, due to its heterogeneity [84]. Because of the low ultrasound sensitivity of the bone transducers, the precise piezoelectric character is difficult to determine. Nakamura *et al* evaluated the site dependence of piezoelectricity in the megahertz range [93]. They fabricated bone plates from different bovine bones and showed that the largest output was produced by the radius bone transducer, followed by the tibia, femur, and humerus transducers, as shown in figure 7.15. Watanabe *et al* reported the success rates of human LIPUS therapy for delayed union and non-union fractures. These were approximately 90%, 87%, 82%,

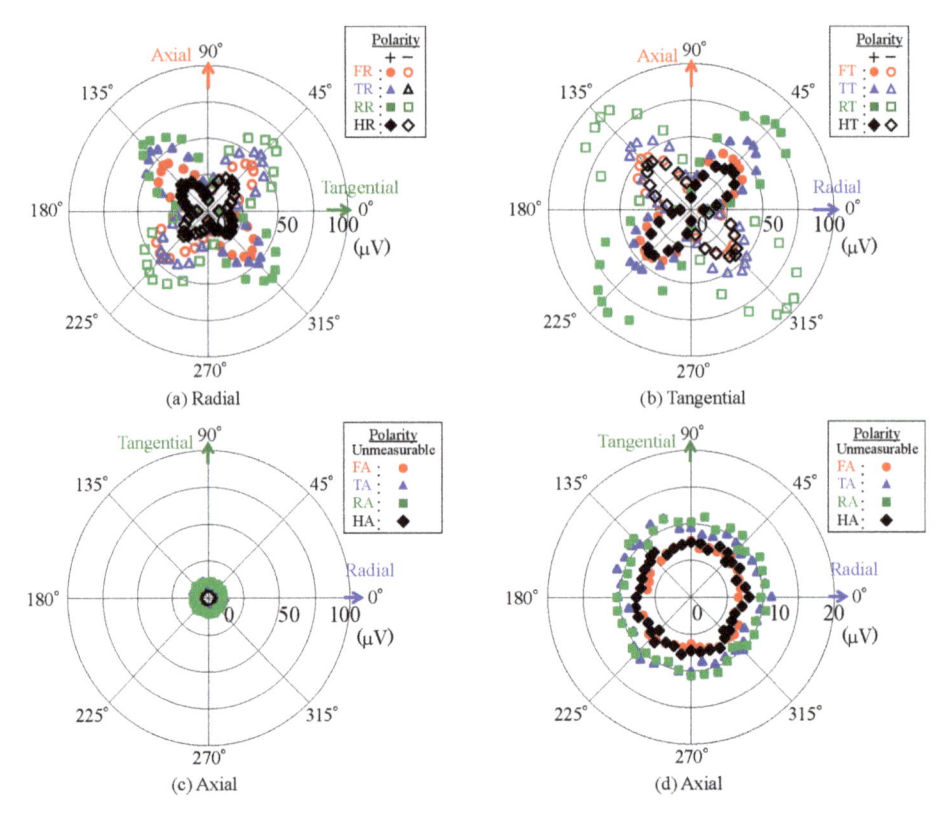

Figure 7.15. Relationships between the peak-to-peak values of the induced electrical potentials and the ultrasound irradiation directions. An ultrasonic pulse wave was radiated by the transducer (main frequency, 760 kHz; sound pressure, 7.4 kPa peak-to-peak). For bone ultrasound transducers, the femoral circular plates cut normal to the radial direction, normal to the tangential direction, and normal to the bone axis are referred to as FR, FT, and FA, respectively; similarly, the tibial samples cut in those three directions are referred to as TR, TT, and TA, respectively; the radial samples are referred to as RR, RT, and RA, respectively, and the humeral samples are referred to as HR, HT, and HA, respectively. Reproduced from [93], with permission of AIP publishing.

and 67% for the radius, tibia, femur, and humerus, respectively, which followed the same pattern as the electrical output of the Nakamura bone transducers [94]. Bovine cortical bone is different from human cortical bone, and interestingly, large electrical outputs were produced at sites where the success rate of human LIPUS therapy was high.

Electrical output was also observed in a cancellous bone transducer fabricated by Hosokawa *et al* [95]. He confirmed electrical output using water-filled cancellous bone transducers. Numerical simulations of the electromechanical responses in the bone were also performed using the piezoelectric finite-difference time-domain (PE-FDTD) method [96–98]. In addition, the application of bone piezoelectricity was considered. Ikushima *et al* created a bone evaluation system with micrometer-scale spatial resolution using acoustically stimulated electromagnetic (ASEM) responses. The system measured a small electromagnetic wave radiated by the bone as a result of ultrasonic stimulation. This response is based on piezoelectricity and is expected to be a new diagnostic system for collagen in bone [99, 100]. To date, osteoporotic bones have been evaluated.

7.3 Ultrasonic characterization of cancellous bone

7.3.1 Two-wave phenomenon and clinical application

Bone is an anisotropic and heterogeneous material with a complicated shape. In the process of bone evaluation, anisotropy and heterogeneity should also be recognized at the matrix and structural levels. In this section, we focus on the effects of bone structure and shape, which are greater than the effects of the material properties. In particular, an evaluation of cancellous bone, which is in the inner portion of the long bones, skull, and vertebrae [3], is discussed. Cancellous bone resembles a porous hard sponge with a 3D structure made of connected plates and/or rods. Cancellous bone is filled with viscous bone marrow [10], which results in temperature and frequency dispersion of ultrasonic wave velocity and attenuation during propagation [101]. In this complex structure, wave propagation mainly depends on the structure rather than the material properties of the bone and marrow, and it exhibits strong scattering and characteristic wave propagation phenomena. Because the main consequences of osteoporosis are dynamic structural changes, specifically a decrease in the bone volume fraction, structural changes in cancellous bones are expected to be a good indicator for the diagnosis of osteoporosis. However, *in vivo* ultrasonic evaluation of cancellous bone is difficult because its complex structure is filled with viscous marrow. The evaluation of wave propagation in cancellous bone seems difficult, as Kaufmann has stated. An analytical solution for wave propagation in cancellous bone is almost impossible because of its associated irregular geometry and inhomogeneous character [102].

The complicated structure of cancellous bone causes strong scattering, which has been widely investigated in through-transmission and pulse-echo measurements. There are well-known parameters of backscattered signals, such as the integrated reflection coefficient (IRC), broadband ultrasound backscatter (BUB), apparent integrated backscatter (AIB), time slope of apparent backscatter (TSAB), and frequency slope of apparent backscatter (FSAB). These parameters are expected to reflect the structure, density, composition, and elastic properties of cancellous bone [103–106]. They have been used for both *in vitro* and *in vivo* bone evaluations. One advantage of backscatter measurements is that it is possible to obtain such measurements using only one transducer. Therefore, this approach is applicable to skeletal sites, such as the hip and spine, where through-transmission measurements are difficult. One recent development of backscattering techniques for the calcaneus was described by Ta *et al* [107–109]. Their device has been applied clinically, and the measured backscattering coefficients show a good correlation with the BMD. Due to the simplicity of their system, the device can also be applied to neonatal bones to evaluate the small calcanei of babies. The recent application of linear arrays also enables the evaluation of pore diameter distribution in the cortical bone *ex vivo* [110]. Frequency analyses of signals reflected from the spine and femoral neck also provided good estimates of the BMD, which may also include scattering from the inside pores [19].

Hosokawa and Otani first experimentally observed two longitudinal wave propagations in bovine cancellous bone using a simple immersion pulse technique in the megahertz range [111, 112]. Several researchers have reported this phenomenon in human cancellous bone [113–117]. Longitudinal waves often separate into two waves (fast and slow waves) in cancellous bone, in which the trabecular thicknesses (Tv. Th.) and Tb. Sp. are on the same order as the ultrasound wavelength in the megahertz range. A precise analytical description of two-wave propagation in cancellous bone is difficult because of variations in the bone volume fraction and continuous changes in the trabecular orientation in cancellous bone.

A good approach to understanding this phenomenon is the use of computer simulations of ultrasound wave propagation, such as the finite-difference time-domain (FDTD) and finite element method (FEM) in which the actual 3D structure of cancellous bone is measured by high-resolution micro computed tomography (CT). Considering the anisotropic trabecular orientation in cancellous bone, a simulation clearly showed that wave separation occurred when ultrasound propagated parallel to the trabecular alignment [118–120]. Snapshots of the wave propagation simulation by Nagatani *et al* are shown in figure 7.16. These are the distributions of sound pressure in a cross section of a 3D simulation field using the cancellous bone from a bovine femur. As shown in this figure, the fast wave mainly propagates along the solid trabecular frame, and the wave properties reflect the state of the cancellous structure of the bone [121–123]. As a result of the propagation, the gradual formation of a fast wave front is observed in front of an intense slow wave, which propagates at approximately the speed of the liquid.

Fujita *et al* experimentally clarified the propagation mechanisms of fast and slow waves in the initial stage using a simple pulse immersion technique in an acoustic tube using degassed water [125]. As shown in figure 7.17, a rectangular cancellous bone sample, $22.4 \times 22.4 \times 8.7$ mm^3 in size, from the equine left radius was placed in the tube. Here, the wave propagation direction is parallel to the main bone axis. A single-cycle sinusoidal-wave electric pulse at 1 MHz was applied to a plane wideband PVDF transmitter (rectangular active area 15×15 mm in size, homemade). The ultrasonic waves that passed through the cancellous bone sample were observed by the same type of PVDF receiver or needle-type receiver (1.0 mm in diameter). The measurements were carried out using samples with different thicknesses ranging from 8.7 to 1.1 mm, obtained by precisely polishing the sample. Figure 7.18 shows the observed waveforms as a function of the thickness. Fast and slow waves were clearly observed in the thicker samples, whereas they overlapped in the thinner samples. Thus, a certain thickness of trabecular bone is required to observe a clear two-wave phenomenon. The wave front or first peak of the fast wave can still be identified in the thin samples, although most parts of the fast wave overlapped the slow wave. The wave front is not in phase during propagation in cancellous bone, as shown in the simulation studies in figure 7.16. An irregular wave front has been reported by several studies [119, 121, 126].

Since the aperture of the PVDF receiver used was larger than the wavelength, the spatial fluctuation of the phase at the wave front could be canceled at the receiver face. This phase cancellation is another mechanism that operates as a low-pass filter [127, 128].

(a) x-z plane   (b) y-z plane   5 mm   (c) x-y plane

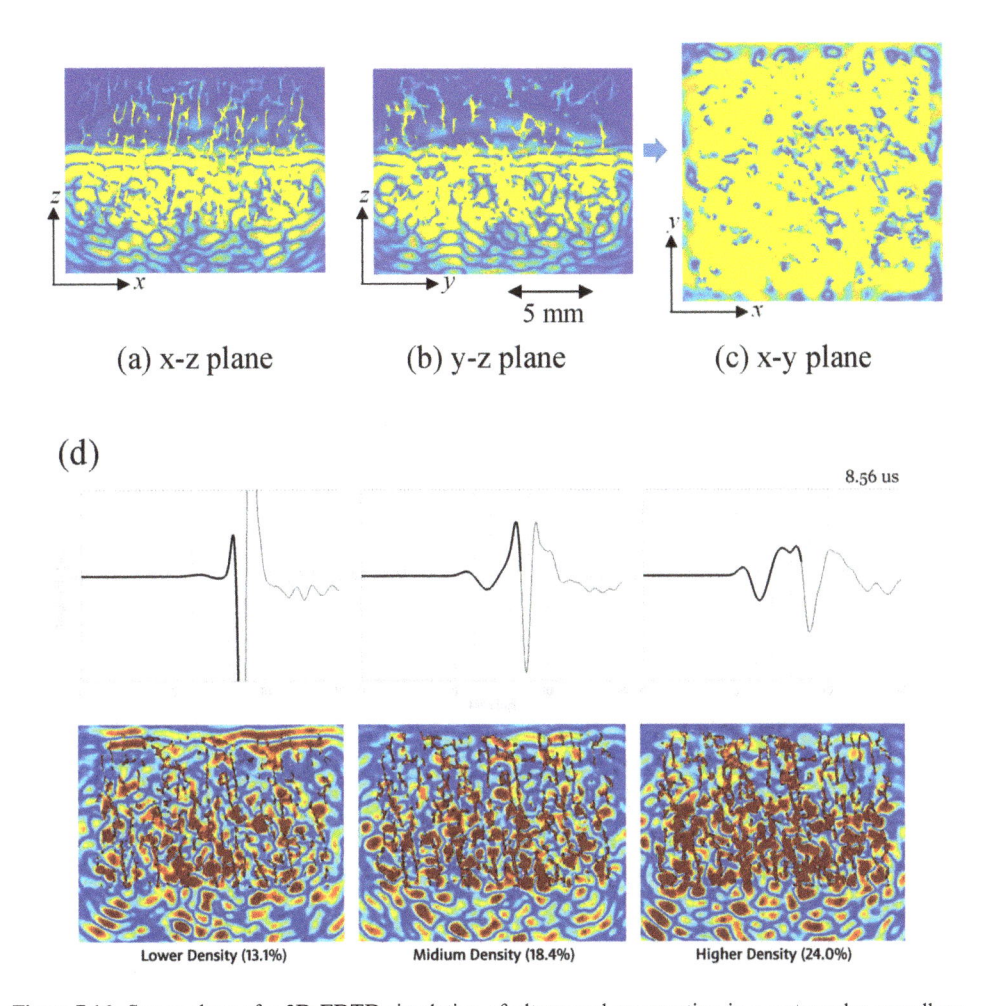

(d)

8.56 μs

Lower Density (13.1%)   Midium Density (18.4%)   Higher Density (24.0%)

Figure 7.16. Screen shots of a 3D FDTD simulation of ultrasound propagation in a rectangular cancellous bone specimen immersed in water. A digital bone model was created from x-ray computed tomography (CT) 3D reconstructed data of a bovine femur. One cycle of a sinusoidal wave at 1 MHz propagated from the bottom along the z-axis. Figure (d) shows simulated propagation images and waves observed by a large-aperture ultrasound receiver at the top of the cancellous bone (video available at https://doi.org/10.1088/978-0-7503-4936-9). Related discussions can be found in reference [124]. When the bone volume ratio of cancellous bone is high, the amplitude of the fast wave becomes high. (Courtesy of Dr Yoshiki Nagatani at Pixie Dust Technologies, Inc.)

Fujita *et al* observed spatial fluctuations of the wave front using a needle-type receiver. Figure 7.19 shows the waves observed after passing through a thin sample (thickness 1.1 mm). The fluctuations in the wave front are shown more clearly in the distribution of the wave arrival times in the measurement plane (figure 7.20). The standard deviation of the arrival time in one plane (441 measurement points) was 0.12 μs for the sample with a thickness of 1.1 mm. Figure 7.21 shows a comparison of the waves observed by the rectangular receiver and the summation of all the waves measured in one plane by the needle-type receiver. The waveform obtained by

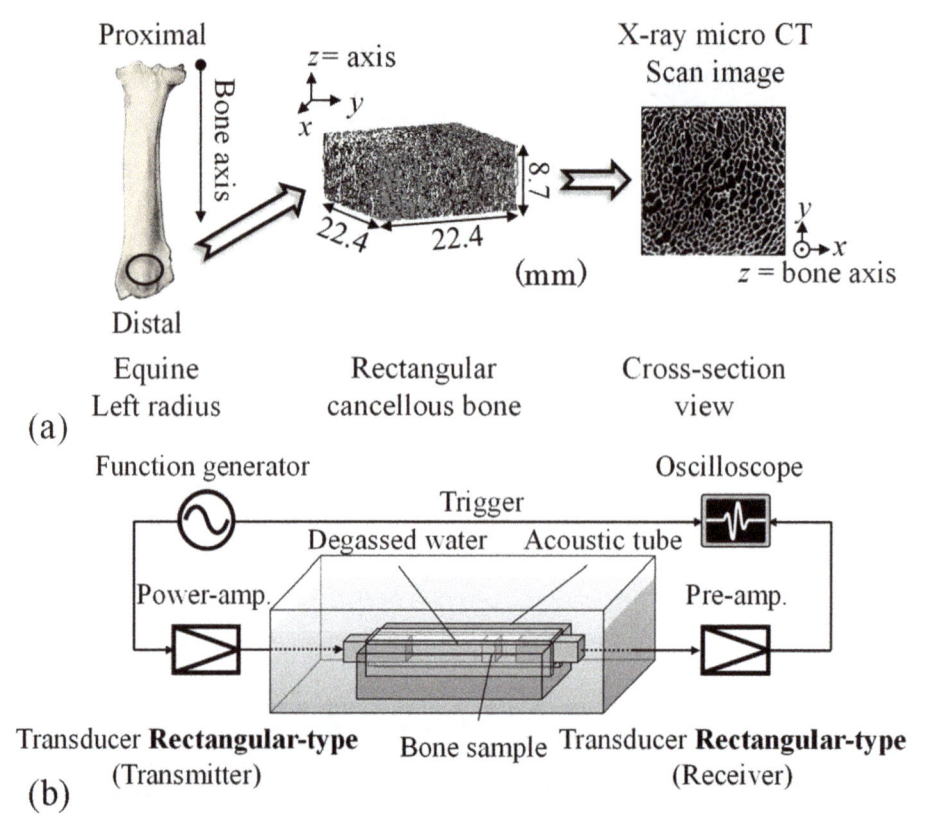

Figure 7.17. (a) Trabecular specimen preparation and an image of the sample scanned by x-ray micro CT. Image (b) shows the ultrasonic measurement configurations. The wall and bottom of the acoustic tube were covered by a foam polystyrene plate to avoid the invasion of the ultrasonic wave. The receiver was a rectangular PVDF transducer or a needle-type transducer. For the needle-type transducer, the receiver scanned in the plane normal to the wave propagation direction. Reproduced from [125], with permission of AIP publishing.

the rectangular transducer and the summation of the waveforms obtained by the needle sensor were similar. In comparison to the waves observed at each position by the needle-type receiver, the apparent nominal frequencies of the summation waves decreased because of the superposition of different waves at different positions in the plane. These data demonstrate the effect of the large aperture of the receiver on the measurement and show that the two observed wave properties also depend on the spatial averaging effect in the measurement system.

By focusing on ultrasonic transducers, Mizuno *et al* identified a relationship between the bone structure and a two-wave phenomenon using a spherical cancellous bone ball specimen obtained from the distal end of a bovine femur [124]. The wave propagation direction was changed by rotating the bone ball specimen (figure 7.22), and the propagated pulse wave was observed at 1 MHz. In strongly anisotropic specimens, fast and slow waves were clearly observed when the waves propagated in approximately the bone-axis (body weight) direction, which is

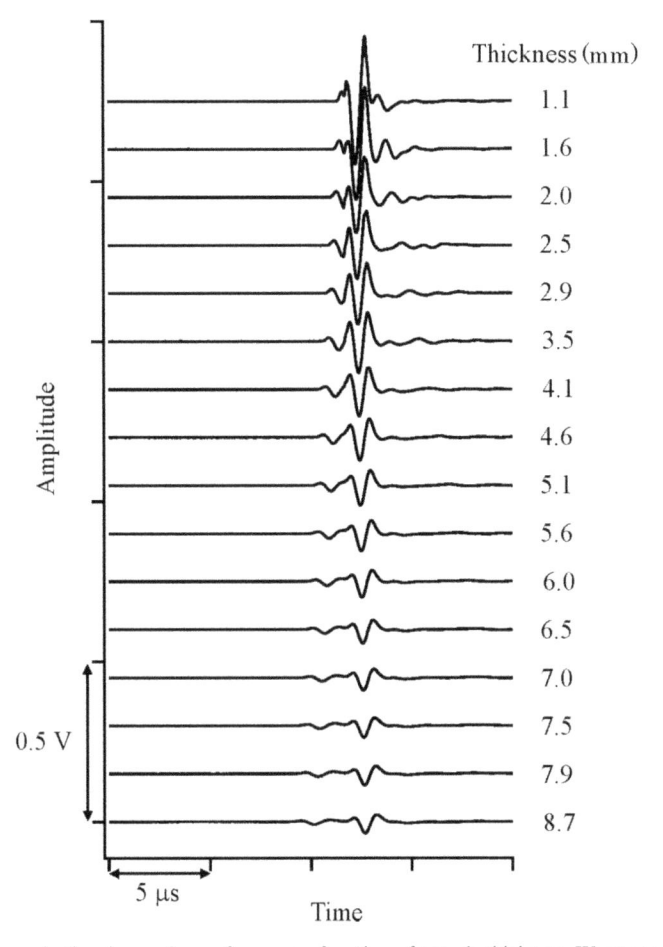

Figure 7.18. Changes in the observed waveforms as a function of sample thickness. Wave separation occurs in the thick cancellous bone specimen. Reproduced from [125], with permission of AIP publishing.

equal to the stress direction. In addition, they also observed separate waves in the direction orthogonal to the main trabecular direction (the A–P direction). In this directions, plate-like trabeculae exist, and strong trabecular alignments could be detected. Therefore, wave separation was observed when the waves propagated along the bone axis and the A–P cross section. This separation occurred because of the anisotropic structure of the cancellous bone. The velocities of the fast and slow waves were also dependent on the cancellous bone microstructure, especially the trabecular length and alignment. The maximum velocity was obtained when the wave propagated in the bone-axis direction. Figures 7.22 (b) and (c) show the characteristic behaviors of the observed waves as a function of the incident angle of the ultrasound. We observed two clear wave phenomena when the waves propagated along the trabeculae. In the M–L direction, the number of trabeculae was small, and the shape was rod-like. In this direction, wave separation was not observed; however, comparatively high-amplitude waves were detected.

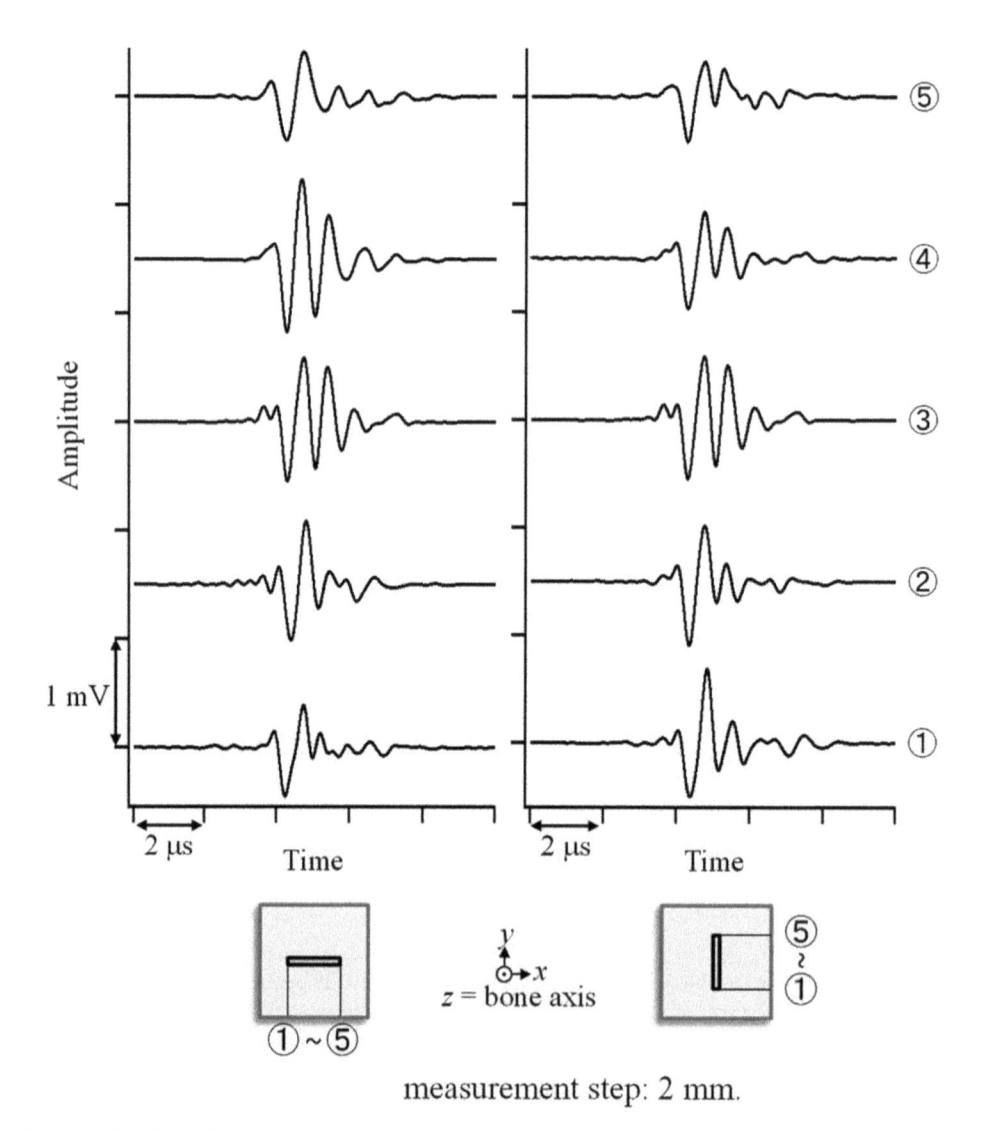

Figure 7.19. Ultrasonic waves observed at different positions in the plane perpendicular to the wave propagation direction after passing through the thin sample (thickness 1.1 mm). Reproduced from [125], with permission of AIP publishing.

The effects of the structure on the two-wave phenomenon were mainly observed in the fast wave propagation. Yamashita *et al* showed an apparent diffraction of fast waves owing to anisotropy by changing the angle between the incident angle of the wave and the main trabecular alignment direction [129]. The fast wave refracted to the main trabecular direction; however, the slow wave did not, because the fast wave propagated along the trabeculae, whereas the slow wave propagated in the liquid. These results indicate that the main trabecular alignment can be estimated based on directivity measurements of propagated ultrasound.

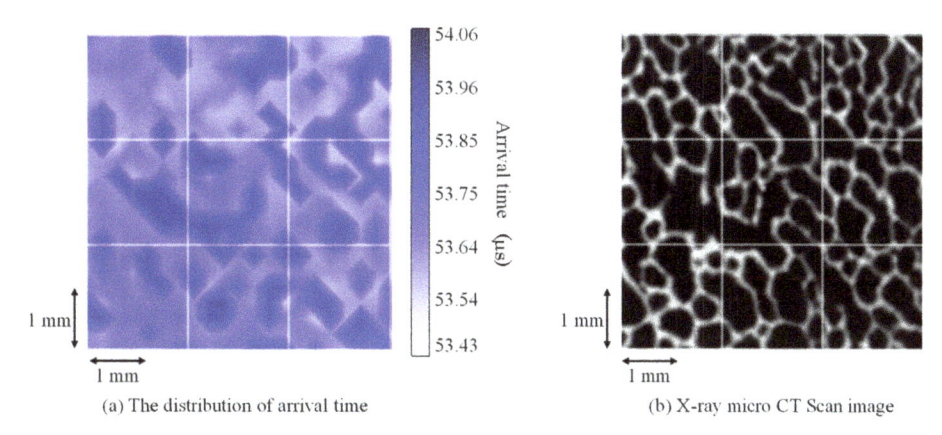

Figure 7.20. Distribution of the wave front in a plane after passing through the thin sample (thickness 1.1 mm) and micro CT data. Reproduced with permission from [125], with permission of AIP Publishing.

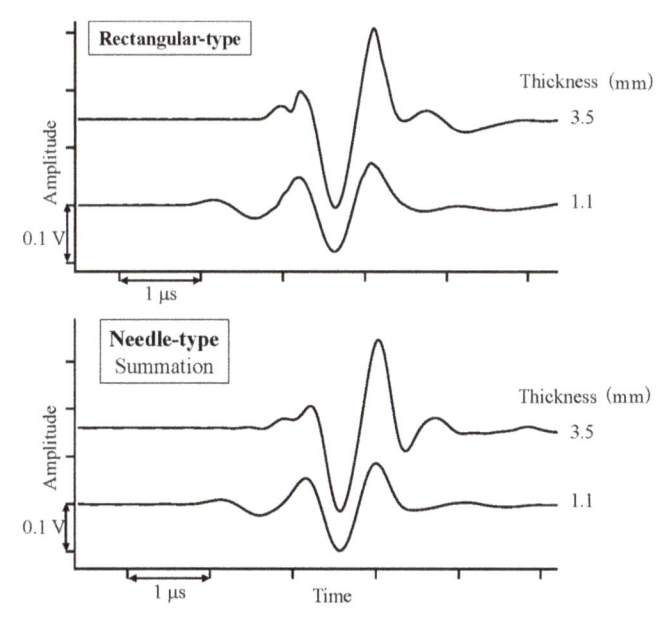

Figure 7.21. Comparison of the ultrasonic waves obtained by the different receivers: (a) waves measured by the rectangular large receiver, and (b) summation of all 441 waves in the plane measured by the needle-type receiver. Reproduced from [125], with permission of AIP publishing.

These data indicate that the characteristics of both fast and slow waves reflect the cancellous bone structure and bone volume fraction. This also indicates that they can provide bone structural information. Otani reported a negative relationship between the slow wave amplitude and bone volume fraction in cancellous bone, and this relationship was used as the basic idea for the development of a new bone

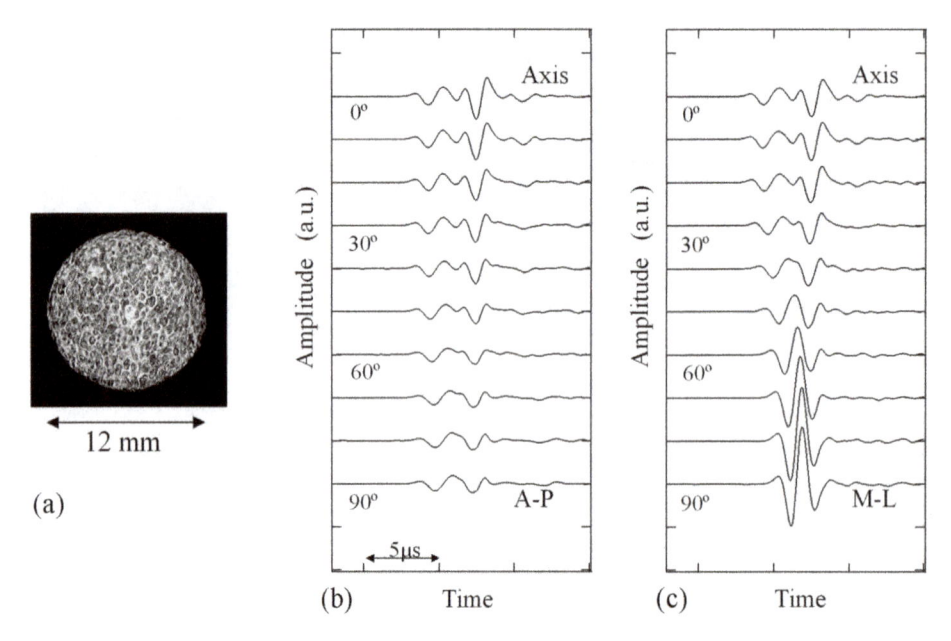

Figure 7.22. (a) Image of a cancellous bone ball. The measurements were performed by rotating the strongly anisotropic spherical specimen. Images (b) and (c) show typical waveforms observed at different angles. The waves were observed using the system shown in figure 7.4(b). Reproduced from [123], with permission of AIP publishing.

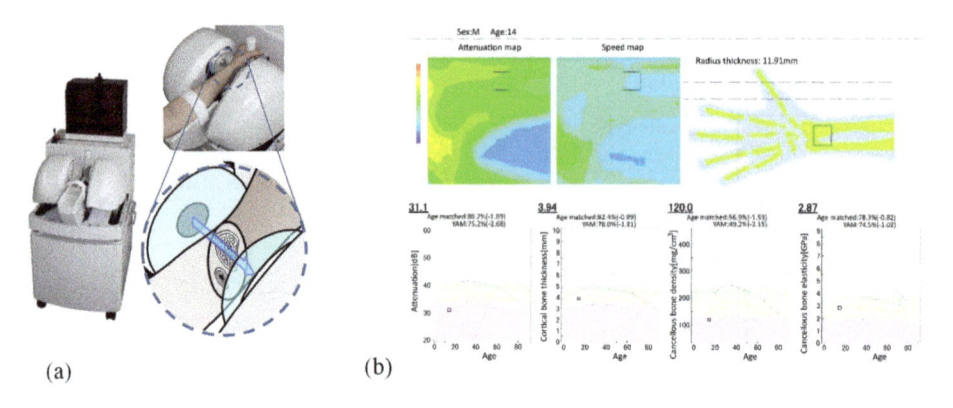

Figure 7.23. (a) *In vivo* two-wave apparatus for evaluation of the radius. (b) Measured results for a radius. Broadband ultrasonic attenuation (BUA) (left), cortical thickness, bone volume fraction of the trabecular part, and estimated elastic properties. The black line shows average values. The green and pink lines represent ±1 standard deviation (SD) and ±2 SD, respectively.

densitometry apparatus for the measurement of the radius [130–132]. The two-wave phenomenon is the basic concept of the original Japanese ultrasonic bone densitometry device for the radius, the LD-100 (Doshisha University, OYO Electric Co., Ltd, and Horiba, Ltd; see figure 7.23). In this system, ultrasonic pulsed waves in the megahertz range propagate from the back to the palm side or vice versa near the distal end of the radius, i.e. in the cancellous bone alignment direction. The system also measures the reflected wave at the surface of the bone, which is used to determine the total thickness of the radius and cortical. Using slow wave information, this system measures the density and elastic properties of the cancellous bone. The concept of this apparatus is totally different from that of conventional heel devices, because they only measure the average values of all tissues that the ultrasound passed through. The ultrasonically obtained density of the cancellous bone and cortical thickness show a strong correlation with the site-matched data obtained via peripheral quantitative CT (pQCT) [132]. The application of this apparatus has now grown beyond the diagnosis of osteoporosis. For evaluations of the effects of sport training, medicines, and teenage bone growth [133, 134], this safe ultrasonic device appears to be useful for people of various ages.

7.4 Conclusions

Bone is a complicated composite material that exhibits anisotropic, heterogeneous, and hierarchical structures, and also contains a viscous liquid (bone marrow). These acoustically difficult characteristics result in difficulties in the ultrasonic evaluation of bone. Using the definition provided by the World Health Organization, osteoporosis, which is one of the most common diseases of the bone, is considered to be 'a disease characterized by low bone mass and microarchitectural deterioration of bone tissue leading to enhanced bone fragility and a consequent increase in fracture risk'. X-ray techniques are considered to be most suitable for the evaluation of BMD and microarchitecture. Therefore, ultrasonic techniques cannot be used as the diagnostic criteria. However, ultrasonic techniques can provide information about bone quality, such as its elasticity, which cannot be measured by x-ray techniques.

Recently, bone studies have also begun investigating other diseases. Endocrine disorders, such as diabetes, are becoming a new topic of interest. These diseases also affect the bone structure; however, they affect the organic components, which cannot be evaluated using x-ray techniques. Ultrasonic techniques can provide information about a material's viscoelasticity, which is beyond the scope of x-ray techniques. Future studies of bone ultrasound may evaluate collagen, since it provides bone with flexibility and is also related to fracture risk.

References

[1] Laugier P and Haïat G (ed) 2011 *Bone Quantitative Ultrasound* (Dordrecht: Springer) ch 3
[2] Njeh C F, Hans D, Fuerst T, Glüer C-C and Genant H K (ed) 1999 *Quantitative Ultrasound* (London: Martin Dunitz) ch 4
[3] Currey J D 2002 *Bone* (Princeton, NJ: Princeton University Press) ch 1
[4] Wolff J 1892 *Das Gesetz der Transformation der Knochen* (Berlin, Hirschwald)
[5] Nair A K, Gautieri A, Chang S-W and Buehler M J 2013 *Nat. Commun.* **4** 1724
[6] Brown P W and Constantz B (ed) 1994 *Hydroxyapatite and Related Materials* (Boca Raton, FL: CRC Press)
[7] Giraud-Guille M M 1988 *Calcif. Tissue Int.* **42** 167–80

[8] Raum K 2008 *IEEE Trans. Ultrason. Ferroelect. Freq. Cont.* **55** 1417–31
[9] Raum K, Jenderka K V, Klemenz A and Brandt J 2003 *IEEE Trans. Ultrason. Ferroelect. Freq. Cont.* **50** 507–16
[10] Bain J B, Clark D M and Wilkins B S (ed) 2011 *Bone Marrow Pathology* 4th edn (Oxford: Wiley-Blackwell)
[11] Kubo T, Fujimori K, Cazier N, Saeki T and Matsukawa M 2011 *Ultrasound Med. Biol.* **37** 1923–29
[12] Lee K I 2012 *J. Acoust. Soc. Am.* **132** 296–302
[13] Recker R R, Kimmel D B, Parfitt A M, Davies K M, Keshawartz N and Hinders S 1988 *J. Bone Miner. Res.* **3** 133–44
[14] Laugier P and Haïat G (ed) 2011 *Bone Quantitative Ultrasound* (Dordrecht: Springer) chs 10 and 11
[15] Wear K 2020 *IEEE Trans. Ultrason. Ferroelect. Freq. Cont.* **67** 454–82
[16] Laugier P 2008 *IEEE Trans. Ultrason. Ferroelect. Freq. Cont.* **55** 1179–96
[17] Matsukawa M 2019 *Jpn. J. Appl. Phys.* **58** SG0802
[18] Ta D and Liu C 2017 *J. Acoust. Soc. Am.* **142** 2566
[19] Casciaro S *et al* 2016 *Ultrasound Med. Biol.* **42** 1337–56
[20] Otani T, Mano I, Tsujimoto T, Yamamot T, Teshima R and Naka H 2009 *Jpn. J. Appl. Phys.* **48** 07GK05
[21] Schwartz A V *et al* 2011 *J. Am. Med. Assoc.* **305** 2184–92
[22] Naylor K L *et al* 2014 *Kidney Int.* **86** 810–8
[23] Laugier P and Haïat G (ed) 2011 *Bone Quantitative Ultrasound* (Dordrecht: Springer) ch 2
[24] Cowin S (ed) 2001 *Bone Mechanics Handbook* (Boca Raton, FL: CRC Press)
[25] Laugier P and Haïat G (ed) 2011 *Bone Quantitative Ultrasound* (Dordrecht: Springer) ch 13
[26] Susan F L and Katz J L 1984 *J. Biomech.* **17** 241–9
[27] Yamato Y, Matsukawa M, Yanagitani T, Yamazaki K, Mizukawa H and Nagano A 2008 *Calcif. Tissue Int.* **82** 162–9
[28] Yamato Y, Matsukawa M, Mizukawa H, Yanagitani T, Yamazaki K and Nagano A 2008 *IEEE Trans. Ultrason. Ferroelect. Freq. Cont.* **55** 1298–303
[29] Laugier P and Haïat G (ed) 2011 *Bone Quantitative Ultrasound* (Dordrecht: Springer) ch 16
[30] Sasaki N and Sudoh Y 1997 X-ray pole figure analysis of apatite crystals and collagen molecules in bone *Calcif. Tissue Int.* **60** 361–7
[31] Nakano T, Kaibara K, Tabata Y, Nagata N, Enomoto S, Marukawa E and Umakoshi Y 2002 *Bone* **31** 479–87
[32] Ashman R B, Cowin S C, Van Buskirk W C and Rice J C 1984 *J. Biomech.* **17** 349–61
[33] Bensamoun S, Gherbezza J-M, de Belleval J-F and Ho Ba Tho M-C 2004 *Clin. Biomech.* **19** 639–47
[34] Lee S C, Coan B S and Bouxsien M L 1997 *Bone* **21** 119–25
[35] Yoon H S and Katz J L 1976 *J. Biomech.* **9** 459–62
[36] Lakes R S, Yoon H S and Katz J L 1986 *J. Biomed. Eng.* **8** 143
[37] Saulgozis J, Pontaga L, Lowet G and Van der Perre G 1986 *Physiol. Meas.* **17** 201
[38] Han S, Rho J, Medige J and Ziv I 1986 *Osteoporos. Int.* **6** 291
[39] Sasso M, Haïat G, Yamato Y, Naili S and Matsukawa M 2007 *Ultrasound Med. Biol.* **33** 1933
[40] Sasso M, Haïat G, Yamato Y, Naili S and Matsukawa M 2008 *J. Biomech.* **41** 347

[41] Nakatsuji T, Yamamoto K, Suga D, Yanagitani T, Matsukawa M, yamazaki K and Matsuyama Y 2011 *Jpn. J. Appl. Phys.* **50** 07HF18
[42] Xu K, Marrelec G, Bernard S and Grimal Q 2018 *IEEE Trans. Signal Process.* **67** 4–16
[43] Nightingale J P and Lewis D 1971 *Nature* **232** 334–5
[44] Chen H L and Gundjian A A 1974 *Med. Biol. Eng.* **14** 531–6
[45] Frantzl P, Groschner M and Vogl G 1992 *J. Bone Miner. Res.* **7** 329–34
[46] Frantzl P, Gupta H S and Paschalis E P *et al* 2004 *J. Mater. Chem.* **14** 2115–23
[47] Rinnerthaler S, Roschger P and Jakobs H F *et al* 1999 *Calcif. Tissue Int.* **64** 422–9
[48] Litniewski J 2005 *Ultrasound Med. Biol.* **31** 1361–6
[49] Raum K, Leguerney I, Chandelier F, Talmant M, Saied A, Peyrin F and Laugier P 2006 *Phys. Med. Biol.* **51** 733–46
[50] Raum K, Cleveland R O, Peyrin F and Laugier P 2006 *Phys. Med. Biol.* **51** 747–58
[51] Hofman T, Heyroth F, Meinhard H, Francel W and Raum K 2006 *J. Biomech.* **39** 2282–94
[52] Saied A, Raum K, Legurney I and Laugier P 2008 *Bone* **43** 187–94
[53] Laugier P and Haïat G (ed) 2011 *Bone Quantitative Ultrasound* (Dordrecht: Springer) ch 16
[54] Mandelstam L I 1926 *Zh Russ. Fiz-Khim. Ova.* **58** 381
[55] Brillouin L 1922 *Ann. Phys.* **9** 88–122
[56] Sandercock J R 1982 Light scattering in solids III ed M Cardona and G Guntherodt *Topics in Applled Physics* (Berlin: Springer) **51** 173–206
[57] Harley R, James D and Miller A *et al* 1977 *Nature* **267** 285–7
[58] Cusack S and Miller A 1979 *J. Mol. Biol.* **135** 39–51
[59] Scarcelli G and Yun S H 2008 *Nat. Photonics* **2** 39–43
[60] Scarcelli G and Yun S H 2012 *Opt. Express* **20** 9197–202
[61] Lees S, Tao N J and Lindsay S M 1989 *Acoust. Imag.* **17** 371–80
[62] Bassler H 1989 *Optical Techniques to Characterize Polymer Systems* (Amsterdam: Elsevier) ch 10
[63] Krüger J K, Embs J, Brierley J and Jiménez R 1998 *J. Phys. D* **31** 1913–7
[64] Sakamoto M, Kawabe M, Matsukawa M, Koizumi N and Ohtori N 2008 *Jpn. J. Appl. Phys.* **47** 4205–8
[65] Kawabe M, Matsukawa M and Ohtori N 2010 *Jpn. J. Appl. Phys.* **49** 07HB05
[66] Kawabe M, Fukui K, Matsukawa M, Granke M, Saied A, Grimal Q and Laugier P 2012 *JASA Exp. Lett.* **132** EL54–60
[67] Fukui K and Matsukawa M 2011 *Proc. Forum Acusticum* 2841–4
[68] Matsukawa M, Tsubota R, Kawabe M and Fukui K 2014 *Ultrasonics* **54** 1155–61
[69] Palombo F and Fioretto D 2019 *Chem. Rev.* **119** 7833–47
[70] Tsubota R, Fukui K and Matsukawa M 2014 *JASA Exp. Lett.* **135** EL109–14
[71] Akilbekova D, Ogay V, Yakupov T, Sarsenova M, Umbayev B, Nurakhmetov A, Tazhin K, Yakovlev V V and Utegulov Z N 2018 *J. Biomed. Opt.* **23** 097004
[72] Cardinali M A, Dallari D, Govini M, Stagni C, Marmi F, Tschon M, Brogini S, Fioretto D and Morresi A 2019 *Biomed. Opt. Express.* **10** 2606–11
[73] Mathieu V, Fukui K, Matsukawa M, Kawabe M, Vayron R, Soffer E, Anagnostou F and Haïat G 2011 *J. Biomech. Eng.* **133** 021006
[74] Vayron R, Matsukawa M, Tsubota R, Mathieu V, Barthel E and Haïat G 2014 *Phys. Med. Biol.* **59** 1389–406
[75] Fraulob M, Le Cann S, Voumard B, Yasui H, Yano K, Matsukawa M, Zysset P and Haïat G 2020 *J. Biomech. Eng.* **142** 121014

[76] Saito M and Marumo K 2010 *Osteoporosis Int.* **21** 195–214
[77] Wen C Y, Chen Y, Tang H L, Yan C H, Lu W W and Chiu K Y 2013 *Osteoarthr. Cartil.* **21** 1716–23
[78] Imoto Y, Tsubota R, Kawabe M, Saito M, Marumo K and Matsukawa M 2015 *Glycative Stress Res.* **2** 101–7
[79] Yasui H, Yano K, Kuzuhara Y, Ikegawa M and Matsukawa M 2020 *Calcif. Tissue Int.* **107** 381–8
[80] Yano K, Maekawa Y, Michimoto I and Matsukawa M 2021 *IEEE Trans. Ultrason. Ferroelect. Freq. Cont.* **68** 2727–32
[81] Fukada E and Yasuda I 1957 *J. Phys. Soc. Jpn.* **12** 1158–62
[82] Yasuda I 1977 *Clin. Orthop.* **124** 53–6
[83] Qin Y-X, Lin W and Rubin C 2002 *Ann. Biomed. Eng.* **30** 693–701
[84] Behari J 2009 *Biophysical Bone Behavior* (Singapore: Wiley) ch 2
[85] Leighton R, Watson J T, Giannouodis P, Papakostidis C, Harrison A and Steen R G 2017 *Injury* **48** 1339–47
[86] Padilla F, Puts R, Vico L and Raum K 2014 *Ultrasonics* **54** 1125–45
[87] Behari J and Singh S 1981 *Ultrasonics* **19** 87–90
[88] Okino M, Coutelou S, Mizuno K, Yanagitani T and Matsukawa M 2013 *Appl. Phys. Lett.* **103** 103701
[89] Tsuneda H, Matsukawa S, Takayanagi S, Mizuno K, Yanagitani T and Matsukawa M 2015 *Appl. Phys. Lett.* **106** 073704
[90] Matsukawa S, Makino T, Mori S, Koyama D, Takayanagi S, Mizuno K, Yanagitani T and Matsukawa M 2017 *Appl. Phys. Lett.* **110** 143701
[91] Mori S, Makino T, Koyama D, Takayanagi S, Yanagitani T and Matsukawa M 2018 *AIP Adv.* **8** 045007
[92] Makino T, Nakamura T, Bustamante L, Takayanagi S, Koyama D and Matsukawa M 2020 *IEEE Trans. Ultrason., Ferroelect., Freq. Contr.* **67** 1525–32
[93] Nakamura T, Takata M, Michimoto I, Koyama D and Matsukawa M 2021 *JASA Exp. Lett.* **1** 012002
[94] Watanabe Y, Matsushita M, Bhandari M, Zdero R and Schemitsch E H 2010 *J. Ortho. Trauma.* **24** S55–61
[95] Hosokawa A 2016 *JASA Exp. Lett.* **140** EL441–5
[96] Hosokawa A 2015 *Jpn. J. Appl. Phys.* **54** 07HF06
[97] Hosokawa A 2018 *Jpn. J. Appl. Phys.* **57** 07LF06
[98] Hosokawa A 2020 *Jpn. J. Appl. Phys.* **59** SKKE03
[99] Ikushima K, Watanuki S and Komiyama S 2006 *Appl. Phys. Lett.* **89** 194103
[100] Ikushima K, Kumamoto T, Ito K and Anzai Y 2019 *Phys. Rev. Lett.* **123** 238101
[101] Kawasaki S, Ueda R, Hasegawa A, Fujita A, Mihata T, Matsukawa M and Neo M 2015 *J. Acoust. Soc. Amer.* **138** EL83–7
[102] Kaufman J J, Luo G and Siffert R S 2008 *IEEE Trans. Ultrason. Ferroelect. Freq. Cont.* **55** 1205–18
[103] O'Donnell M and Miller J G 1981 *J. Appl. Phys.* **52** 1056–65
[104] Laugier P and Haïat G (ed) 2011 *Bone Quantitative Ultrasound* (Dordrecht: Springer) ch 6
[105] Wear K A 2008 *IEEE Trans. Ultrason. Ferroelectr. Freq. Control* **55** 1432–41
[106] Wear K A 2020 *IEEE Trans. Ultrason. Ferroelectr. Freq. Control* **67** 454–82

[107] Liu C, Xu F, Ta D, Tang T, Jiang Y, Dong J, Wang W-P, Liu X, Wang Y and Wang W-Q 2016 *J. Ultrasound Med.* **35** 2197–208
[108] Ta D and Liu C 2017 *J. Acoust. Soc. Am.* **142** 2566
[109] Ta D, Li Y, Li B, Zheng R and Le L H 2018 *J. Acoust. Soc. Am.* **144** 1822
[110] Lori G, Du Juan, Hackenbeck J, Kilappa V and Raum K 2021 *IEEE Trans. Ultrason. Ferroelectr. Freq. Control* **68** 1081–95
[111] Hosokawa A and Otani T 1997 *J. Acoust. Soc. Am.* **101** 558–62
[112] Hosokawa A and Otani T 1998 *J. Acoust. Soc. Am.* **103** 2713–22
[113] Cardoso L, Teboul F, Sedel L, Oddou C and Meunier A 2003 *J. Bone Miner. Res.* **18** 1803–12
[114] Nicholson P H F, Müller R, Lowet G, Cheng X G, Hildebrand T, Rüegsegger P, van de Perre G, Dequeker J and Boonen S 1998 *Bone* **23** 425–31
[115] Fellah Z E A, Chapelon J Y, Berger S, Lauriks W and Depollier C 2004 *J. Acoust. Soc. Am.* **116** 61–73
[116] Sebaa N, Fellah Z E A, Fellar M, Ogam E, Mitri F G, Depollier C and Lauriks W 2008 *IEEE Trans. Ultrason. Ferroelectr. Freq. Control* **55** 1516–23
[117] Mizuno K, Matsukawa M, Otani T, Laugier P and Padilla F 2009 *J. Acoust. Soc. Am.* **125** 3460–6
[118] Bossy E, Padilla F, Peyrin F and Laugier P 2005 *Phys. Med. Biol.* **50** 5545–56
[119] Nagatani Y, Imaizumi H, Fukuda T, Matsukawa M, Watanabe Y and Otani T 2006 *Jpn. J. Appl. Phys.* **45** 7186–90
[120] Haïat G, Padilla F, Peyrin F and Laugier P 2008 *J. Acoust. Soc. Am.* **123** 1694–705
[121] Hosokawa A, Otani T, Suzaki T, Kubo Y and Takai S 1997 *Jpn. J. Appl. Phys.* **36** 3233–7
[122] Mizuno K, Matsukawa M, Otani T, Takada M, Mano I and Tsujimoto T 2008 *IEEE Trans. Ultrason. Ferroelectr. Freq. Control* **55** 1480–7
[123] Mizuno K, Somiya H, Kubo T, Matsukawa M, Otani T and Tsujimoto T 2010 *J. Acoust. Soc. Am.* **128** 3181–9
[124] Nagatani Y and Tachibana R O 2014 *J. Acoust. Soc. Am.* **135** 1197–206
[125] Fujita F, Mizuno K and Matsukawa M 2013 *J. Acoust. Soc. Am.* **134** 4775–81
[126] Nagatani Y, Mizuno K, Saeki T, Matsukawa M, Sakaguchi T and Hosoi H 2008 *Ultrasonics* **48** 607–12
[127] Wear K A 2007 *IEEE Trans. Ultrason. Ferroelectr. Freq. Control* **54** 1352–9
[128] Nelson A M, Hoffman J J, Anderson C C, Holland M R, Nagatani Y, Mizuno K, Matsukawa M and Miller J G 2011 *J. Acoust. Soc. Am.* **130** 2233–40
[129] Yamashita K, Fujita F, Mizuno K, Mano I and Matsukawa M 2012 *IEEE Trans. Ultrason. Ferroelectr. Freq. Control* **59** 1160–6
[130] Otani T 2005 *Jpn. J. Appl. Phys.* **44** 4578–82
[131] Otani T, Mano I, Tsujimoto T, Yamamoto T, Teshima R and Naka H 2009 *Jpn. J. Appl. Phys.* **48** 1–5
[132] Sai H, Iguchi G, Tobimasu T, Takahashi K, Otani T, Horii K, Mano I, Nagai I, Iio H, Fujita T, Yoh K and Baba H 2010 *Osteoporos. Int.* **21** 1781–90
[133] Bréban S, Padilla F, Fujisawa Y, Mano I, Matsukawa M, Benhamou C L, Otani T, Laugier P and Chappard C 2010 *Bone* **46** 1620–5
[134] Ozaki E, Matsukawa M, Mano I, Matsui D, Yoneda Y, Masunuma M, Koyama T, Watanabe I, Maekawa M, Tomida S, Iwasa K, Umemura S, Kuriyama N and Uehara R 2020 *Bone* **141** 115669

IOP Publishing

Ultrasonics
Physics and applications
Mami Matsukawa, Pak-Kon Choi, Kentaro Nakamura, Hirotsugu Ogi and Hideyuki Hasegawa

Chapter 8

Acceleration and control of protein aggregation

Hirotsugu Ogi

Recent advances in ultrasound irradiation technology for solutions have made it possible to dramatically accelerate the aggregation reactions of various proteins, including amyloidogenic proteins. This not only contributes to the advancement of protein aggregation science, but also allows early definitive diagnosis of neurodegenerative diseases. In this chapter, recent studies of the control of protein aggregation reactions using ultrasound are introduced, and it is shown that the phenomenon of protein aggregation enhancement by ultrasound is a very promising method for the diagnosis of neurodegenerative diseases such as Alzheimer's disease (AD) and Parkinson's disease.

8.1 Introduction

Misfolded protein aggregates, such as amyloid fibrils, are deeply involved in the pathogenesis of various amyloidoses [1–4]. Each amyloidosis is caused by a specific protein, such as amyloid β (Aβ) for Alzheimer's diseases, α synuclein (αSyn) for Parkinson's disease, and $β_2$-microglobulin ($β_2$M) for dialysis-related amyloidosis. These amyloidogenic proteins commonly undergo a conformational change from a soluble monomeric state to highly ordered amyloid fibril, as shown in figure 8.1, which is referred to as the aggregation reaction. A general understanding of the aggregation reaction is as follows. In the early stage, oligomers (multimers such as hexamers and octamers as well as larger amorphous disordered aggregates) are produced, followed by the development of fibril nuclei after a long delay. The fibril elongation reaction subsequently proceeds to rapidly form amyloid fibrils with a needle-like morphology (~10 nm in diameter and several μm in length, as shown in figure 8.2). Amyloid fibrils are thermodynamically stable protein aggregates with a cross-β structure in which the β-strands are aligned perpendicular to the longitudinal direction of the fibril [5, 6]. The fibril formation process can be monitored during the aggregation reaction by a fluorometric analysis using thioflavin T (ThT), which specifically binds to the β-sheet structure of the amyloid fibrils and emits

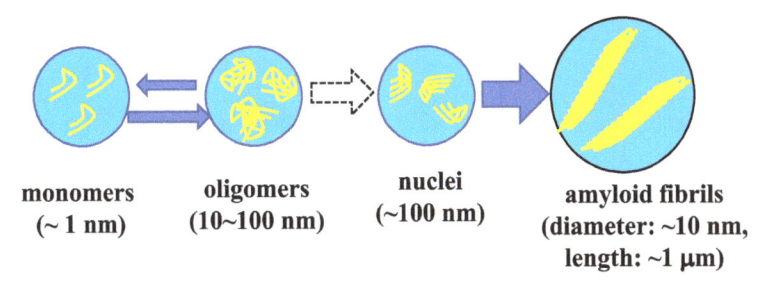

Figure 8.1. Aggregation reaction cascade from monomers toward amyloid fibrils.

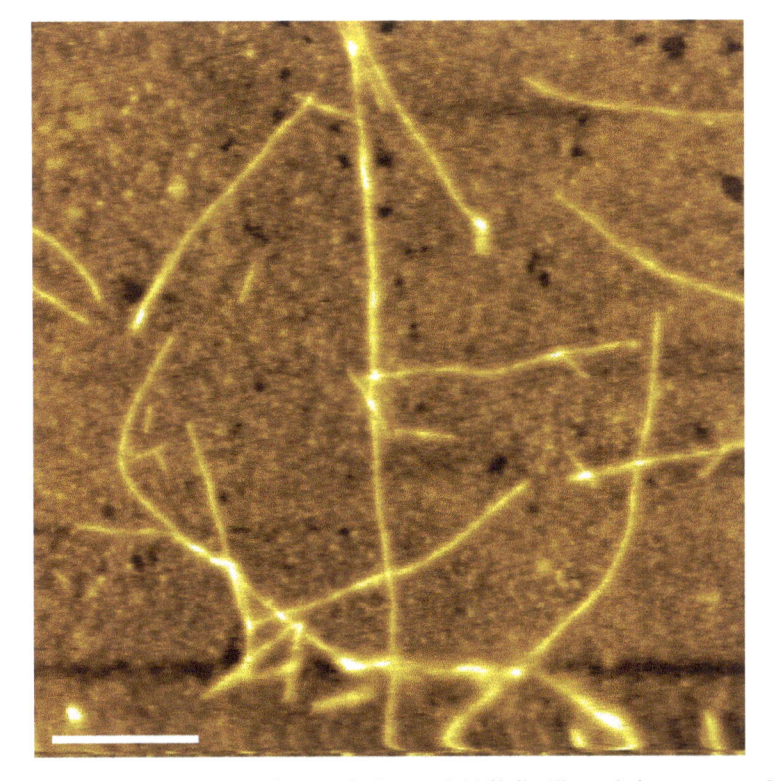

Figure 8.2. Atomic force microscopy image of αSyn amyloid fibrils. The scale bar represents 500 nm.

high-intensity fluorescence [7, 8]; an increase in ThT fluorescence intensity indicates an increase in the number of fibrils formed, as shown in figure 8.3. The aggregates produced in the aggregation reaction are deposited in tissues; they exhibit toxicity and cause tissue damage. Therefore, our understanding of the aggregation reaction remains a central issue in protein sciences and has a profound impact on related fields such as medicine, pharmacology, biology, and biotechnology. Although the fibril elongation reaction proceeds rapidly after nucleation, the energy barrier of the nucleation reaction is very high, and this reaction becomes the rate-limiting step of the aggregation reaction [9, 10], making the aggregation reaction very slow.

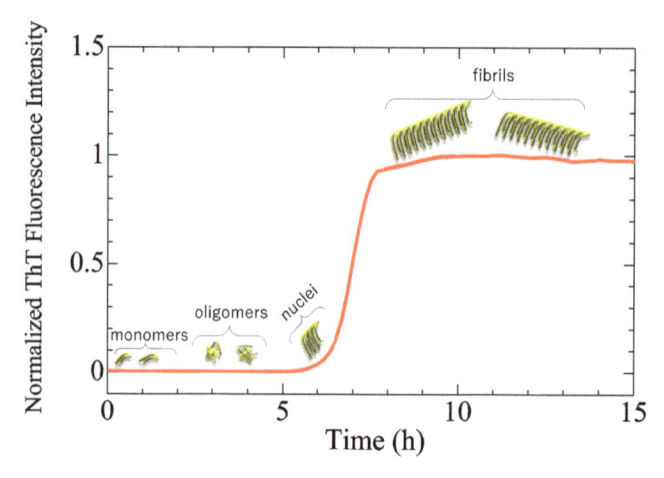

Figure 8.3. Example of change in thioflavin T fluorescent intensity during an aggregation reaction observed in a β_2M solution.

This slowness has hindered the elucidation of the fibrillation reaction and thus the pathogenic mechanism of each amyloidosis; therefore, there is a need to establish an effective acceleration method.

It has been found that the aggregation reaction for fibrillation can be dramatically accelerated using ultrasonic irradiation. This phenomenon was first suggested by Stathopulos *et al* [11], who showed that ultrasonication (at 20 kHz and 30 W) produced fibril-like aggregates in protein solutions and also found that the addition of some preformed aggregates accelerated their aggregation reactions. The latter is now recognized as the seeding effect. Today, the enhancement of the protein aggregation reaction by ultrasound has been confirmed for a variety of amyloidogenic proteins, including β_2M [12], αSyn [13], prion protein [14], and Aβ [15]. Goto *et al* investigated this phenomenon in more detail [12, 13, 16] as described in review papers [17, 18] and developed a high-throughput ultrasound amyloid-assay system called HANABI (*HAN*dai *a*myloid *b*urst *i*nducer) [19–22]. They further proposed a new concept, which was that the protein aggregation reaction can be explained by precipitation from a supersaturated state [16, 22–25]. The acceleration mechanism has been intensively studied by Nakajima and co-researchers [26–28], who have shown that local protein enrichment and local heating due to the collapse of ultrasonic cavitation bubbles accelerate the nucleation reaction. Recently, it has been suggested that ultrasound irradiation with optimized frequency and power can promote not only the nucleation reaction but also the seeding reaction, and it is expected that early diagnosis of amyloidosis can be achieved using this principle [20, 22].

In this chapter, the mechanism of ultrasonically accelerated aggregation reaction is first discussed, and then the usefulness of the nonlinear components of the ultrasonic field inside the solution is demonstrated for a quantitative evaluation of the effect of ultrasound on the aggregation reaction. A new concept for understanding protein aggregation, 'precipitation from supersaturation,' and the development of a high-throughput ultrasound assay system are then described.

8.2 Mechanism of acceleration of protein aggregation

It is known that ultrasound irradiation has a profound effect on a variety of chemical reactions. For example, it can trigger reactions that would not normally proceed or accelerate certain reaction steps. Most of these behaviors are due to ultrasonic cavitation, and such reactions are called sonochemical reactions [29–31]. Ultrasonic cavitation usually promotes decomposition reactions in organic materials [32–35]. Cavitation bubbles repeatedly grow and collapse, causing a significant temperature increase at bubble collapse, which accelerates the thermal decomposition of soluble chemicals inside and near the bubbles. The extreme temperature rise also generates radical species from the water, which oxidize the dissolved organic substances [36–38]. Such sonochemical reactions have also been used to generate seeds for fibril growth. Okumura and Itoh [39] performed a molecular dynamics simulation and found that bubbles are selectively formed at the hydrophobic residues under negative pressure, and they collapse when the pressure becomes positive, causing water molecules to collide with the hydrophilic residues and fragmentate the fibrils. Because monomers dissolved in the solution attach to the ends of the fibrils and cause the fibrils to grow, the total amount of fibril aggregates increases with fibril fragmentation [40, 41].

The promotion of the aggregation reaction by ultrasound, however, results in the polymerization of the monomer, which is the opposite of the decomposition reaction. This mechanism was clarified by Nakajiama *et al* [26] using $A\beta_{1-40}$ peptides, as shown below. It has been recognized that the structural change from monomer to fibril proceeds through two principal reaction processes: a nucleation reaction and a subsequent fibril growth reaction [42, 43], although various modified models have been proposed, including the transient presence of a secondary nucleus [44, 45]. Since the energy barrier of the nucleation reaction is much higher than that for fibril growth [9, 10], the acceleration of the aggregation reaction by ultrasound was attributed to acceleration of the nucleation reaction.

Cavitation bubbles are generated in the negative-pressure process of ultrasound. At low ultrasonic-pressure amplitudes, nearly sinusoidal bubble-radius oscillation occurs, but at high pressure amplitudes, bubble growth and rapid contraction processes are repeated with the ultrasound period, and at the time of collapse, when the bubble diameter is at its minimum, the temperature and pressure in the bubble undergo a strong transient increase. The temperature at the time of bubble collapse exceeds 10 000 K when the liquid is sufficiently degassed to generate only a single bubble [46] and remains as high as 5000 K, even when many bubbles are generated by normal plane-wave ultrasound irradiation [47]; it is greatly influenced by the frequency and pressure of the driving ultrasound waves [48]. Therefore, ultrasonically accelerated aggregational behavior was systematically investigated at various frequencies and pressures for $A\beta_{1-40}$ peptides. Figure 8.4 shows the experimental system developed by Nakajima *et al* [26]. A Langevin-type ultrasonic transducer was attached to the bottom of a stainless-steel container. Five sample tubes containing the $A\beta$ solution were placed near the water surface of the reaction container and irradiated with ultrasonic waves from below. The water in the reaction container was degassed using a degassing device to prevent the ultrasound pressure from being reduced by scattering from cavitation bubbles in the

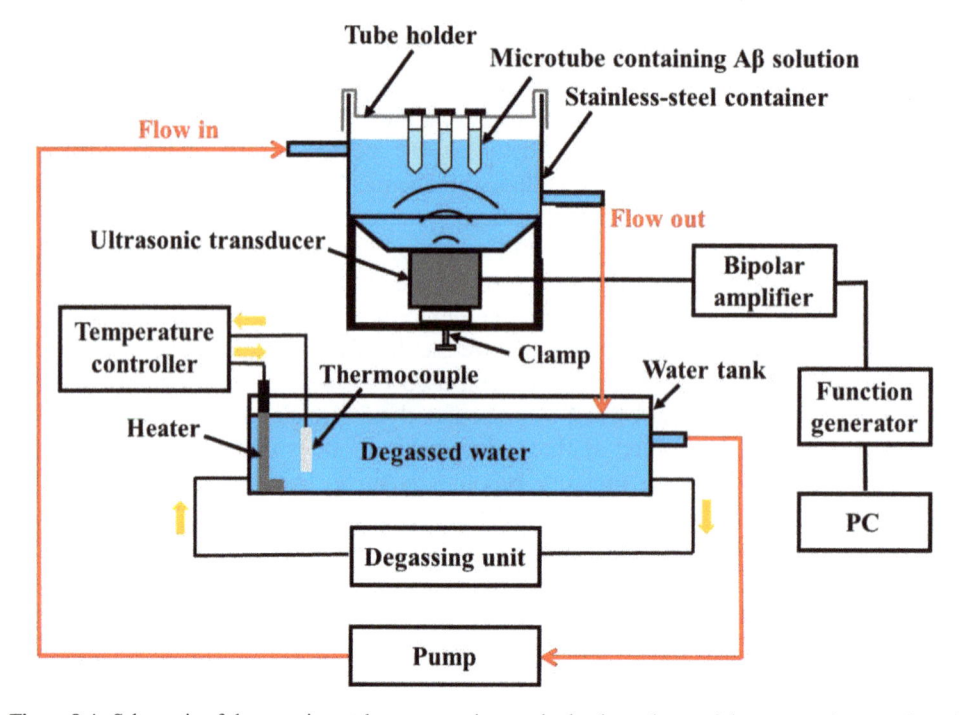

Figure 8.4. Schematic of the experimental system used to study the dependence of the aggregation reaction of Aβ$_{1-40}$ peptide on the frequency and pressure of the ultrasonic waves. A Langevin-type ultrasonic transducer was attached to the bottom surface of the container. The water was degassed by the degassing unit, and its temperature was kept at 37 °C by the temperature control system. The maximum power applied to the solution was about 50 W. Reproduced from [26]. Copyright 2016, The author(s). With permission of Springer.

container. The temperature of the solution in the sample tubes was kept at 37 °C by adjusting the temperature of the degassed water in the buffer tank using a temperature controller. In this experimental system, the five sample tubes were arranged in a circular pattern, and the ultrasonic irradiation experiments were conducted simultaneously on the five samples. A sequence of 1 min of irradiation followed by 9 min of incubation was repeated for approximately 10 h. Every 30 min, 5 μL of the Aβ sample was taken from each sample tube, mixed with 50 μL of the ThT solution, and placed in a quartz cell. The cell was placed in a spectrophotometer to measure the fluorescent intensity of the ThT.

Figure 8.5 shows the accelerated behavior of the aggregation reaction subjected to ultrasonic irradiation, as measured by the experimental system shown in figure 8.4. In the absence of ultrasound irradiation, no aggregation reaction was observed even after 10 h, and the circularly polarized dichroism (CD) spectrum was almost the same as before the experiment, indicating that the secondary structure remained a random coil in the absence of ultrasound irradiation. However, ultrasound irradiation markedly accelerated the aggregation reaction, and the CD spectrum showed a minimum value at 220 nm, indicating the formation of amyloid fibrils with a β-sheet-rich structure. (The CD spectrum provides information related to the secondary structure of protein aggregates, and the negative peak at around 220 nm indicates the presence of β structures [49].)

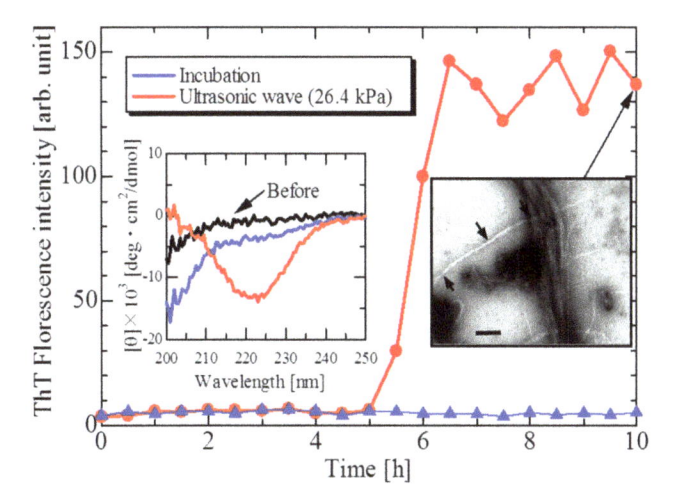

Figure 8.5. Aggregation reaction of 10 μM Aβ$_{1-40}$ peptide caused by ultrasonic irradiation. The left-hand inset shows the CD spectra of the initial monomer solution (black), a solution incubated for 10 h (blue), and a solution after ultrasonic irradiation (red). The right-hand inset shows a TEM image of aggregates formed by ultrasonic-wave irradiation for 10 h. The scale bar denotes 100 nm. The arrows in the TEM image indicate the minimum diameters of the twisted fibrils. Reproduced from [26]. Copyright 2016, The author(s). With permission of Springer.

In fact, transmission electron microscopy (TEM) images of the aggregates formed under ultrasound irradiation showed fibrils that had a morphology similar to that formed without ultrasound irradiation: amyloid fibrils with ~7 nm diameters have been found in brain tissue from AD patients [50], and periodic twisted fibril structures with a period of 80–250 nm have been observed without ultrasound irradiation [50–52]. In the TEM image in figure 8.5, fibrils with diameters of 6–10 nm and periodic twisted fibrils with periods of about 150 nm were observed, confirming that the fibrils formed under ultrasound irradiation show identical morphology to those in AD patients.

In order to study the frequency dependence of the aggregation reaction, ultrasonic irradiation experiments were performed at different frequencies between 19 and 240 kHz. The acoustic pressure in each sample tube was measured by a needle-type hydrophone, and the pressure of the second-harmonic component was set to the same value at all frequencies to precisely evaluate the frequency dependence. (Ultrasonic amplitude in the fundamental mode cannot be used as a measure of ultrasonic energy because it saturates or decreases with increasing sound power due to generation of cavitation bubbles.) Since cavitation bubbles exhibit highly nonlinear dynamics and produce strong harmonic components, the amplitude of the harmonic-component wave is more suitable for evaluating the sound power in the sample tube. In fact, previous reports have experimentally shown that the amplitude of the second-harmonic component is positively correlated with the input sound power [53, 54]. The pressure at each frequency was thus controlled so as to achieve nearly the same pressure value of the second-harmonic component of ~15 kPa, as shown in figure 8.6(a). The evolution of the ThT fluorescence intensity over time is shown for each frequency in figure 8.6(b).

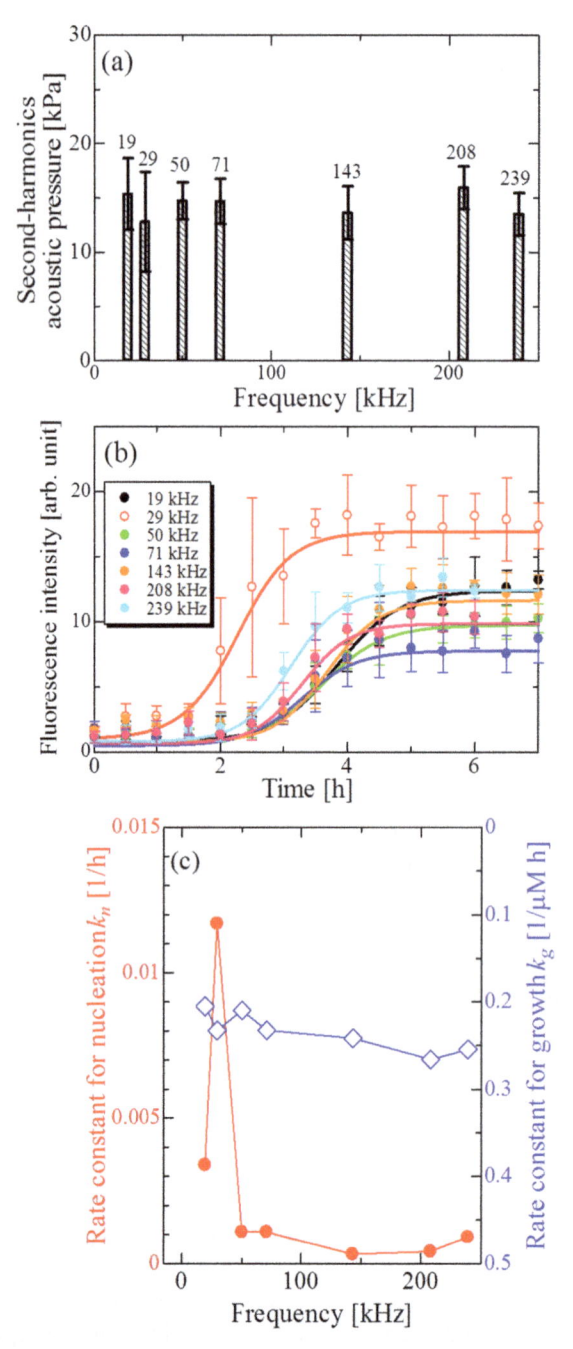

Figure 8.6. Frequency dependence of the aggregation reaction of 10 μM Aβ$_{1-40}$ peptide. (a) Averaged acoustic pressure of the second-harmonic component of the ultrasonic wave at each frequency. The numbers denote the fundamental frequencies in kHz. (b) Evolution of ThT fluorescence intensity over time caused by ultrasonic-wave irradiation at various frequencies. The solid lines denote curves fitted by the two-step model. (c) Frequency dependence of the rate constants for nucleation (solid circles), k_n, and for growth (open diamonds), k_g. Reproduced from [26]. Copyright 2016, The author(s). With permission of Springer.

The ThT fluorescence intensity change was analyzed using the two-step (Finke–Watzky) model, which assumes that the aggregation reaction proceeds through nucleation and growth processes [42, 43]. The concentration of fibrils $[F]$ at time t can be written as

$$[F] = [M]_0 \left\{ 1 - \frac{k_n + k_g[M]_0}{k_n e^{(k_n + k_g[M]_0)t} + k_g[M]_0} \right\}. \tag{8.1}$$

Here, $[M]_0$ denotes the initial concentration of the monomer. By fitting this two-step model to the experimental data, the reaction-velocity constant for nucleation (k_n) and that for fibril growth (k_g) were obtained. The solid lines in figure 8.6(b) denote the curves fitted by the two-step model, and figure 8.6(c) shows the frequency dependences of the reaction-velocity constants. The k_n value strongly depends on the frequency and has a maximum value at 29 kHz, which is 35 times higher than the minimum value at 143 kHz. On the other hand, the k_g value is found to be almost independent of frequency. The optimum frequency is thus 29 kHz for the ultrasound-induced nucleation reaction of Aβ peptide. The higher the ultrasound frequency, the more the maximum size of the cavitation bubble is limited and the lower the temperature rise at the time of bubble collapse. However, the numbers of collapse events per unit time and per unit volume increase as the frequency increases. Therefore, the rate for the aggregation reaction is determined by a trade-off between the temperature rise at the time of bubble collapse and the number of collapse events, which results in the optimum frequency.

The dependence of the acceleration behavior on the acoustic pressure was further investigated at the optimum frequency of 29 kHz. Figure 8.7(a) shows the evolution of the ThT fluorescence intensity at each acoustic pressure, including incubation data without ultrasonic irradiation, and figure 8.7(b) shows the pressure dependences of the rate constants. To avoid excessive temperature rises in the sample tube due to ultrasonic irradiation, which would have affected the aggregation reaction, the acoustic pressure range was selected so that the temperature change was less than 0.2 °C, as shown in figure 8.7(c). The aggregation reaction is accelerated by higher acoustic pressures. Surprisingly, the k_n value increases by a factor of ~1000 under the optimum ultrasonic irradiation condition, compared to the quiescent condition, while the k_g value is less affected and remains within the same order of magnitude. As the acoustic pressure increases below 53 kPa, k_n increases, but it decreases at 75 kPa (see the inset in figure 8.7(b)). The latter indicates a decomposition reaction due to very high acoustic pressure, which is a typical sonochemical reaction.

The following theoretical calculations were performed to reproduce these observations [26]. First, the bubble-radius change caused by an ultrasonic plane wave was calculated based on the Keller–Miksis equation [46] given below:

$$\left(1 - \frac{\dot{R}}{c}\right)\rho \ddot{R} R + \frac{3}{2}\left(1 - \frac{\dot{R}}{3c}\right)\rho \dot{R}^2 = \left(1 + \frac{\dot{R}}{c}\right)\{p_g - P_0 - P\} + \frac{R\dot{p}_g}{c} - 4\eta\frac{\dot{R}}{R} - 2\sigma\frac{1}{R}, \tag{8.2}$$

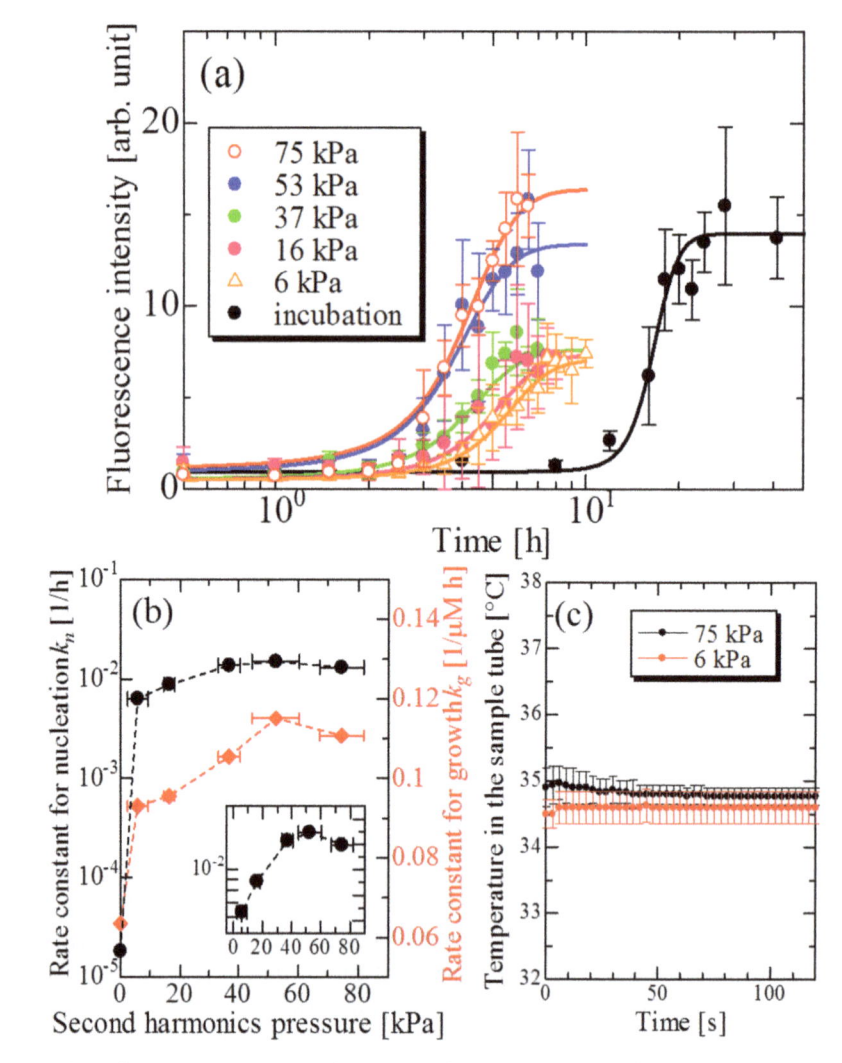

Figure 8.7. Acoustic pressure dependence of the aggregation reaction of Aβ peptide. (a) Evolutions of the ThT fluorescence intensity under ultrasonication for various second-harmonic-component acoustic pressures. The solid lines denote curves fitted by the two-step model. (b) Relationship between the second-harmonic-component pressure of the ultrasonic wave and the rate constants for nucleation k_n (circles) and for growth k_g (diamonds). (c) Temperature change in the sample tube measured just after 1 min of ultrasonic-wave irradiation at 75 and 6 kPa. Reproduced from [26]. Copyright 2016, The author(s). With permission of Springer.

$$p_g = \left(P_0 + \frac{2\sigma}{R_0}\right)\left(\frac{R_0}{R}\right)^{3\gamma}, \tag{8.3}$$

$$P = P_a \sin\left\{\omega\left(t + \frac{R}{c}\right)\right\}. \tag{8.4}$$

Here, R denotes the bubble radius, R_0 the equilibrium bubble radius, and c the sound velocity. ρ, η, and σ are density, viscosity, and the surface tension of water, respectively. p_g and P denote the gas pressure inside the bubble and the acoustic pressure of the ultrasonic wave which has a pressure amplitude of P_a and an angular frequency of ω, respectively. Because the bubble collapse occurs instantaneously (<~10 ns), the process can nearly be regarded as an adiabatic compression process, and the relationship between the bubble radius and the gas temperature inside the bubble is approximately given by $T = T_0(R_0/R)^{3(\gamma-1)}$ using the ratio of specific heat γ. Figure 8.8 shows the simulated results of the variation of the bubble radius and the gas temperature inside the bubble for three different pressure amplitudes at the optimum frequency of 29 kHz. The maximum bubble radius and the gas temperature at the time of the bubble collapse significantly increase with increasing acoustic pressure.

Second, the temperature distribution after the bubble collapse was evaluated by solving the thermal-diffusion equation in the spherical coordinate system. The temperature distribution in the solution at the time of the bubble collapse was assumed to be stepwise, in which the temperature in the region corresponding to the bubble region at the collapse was considered to be that of the heated water region and the temperature outside that region was considered to be at room temperature. With this initial condition, the subsequent change in the temperature distribution was calculated (figure 8.9). The bubble radius continues to change after collapse, which affects the temperature distribution. However, since the high-temperature region disappears rapidly (within ~1 μs), the temperature distribution was assumed to be independent of the bubble dynamics after the collapse for simplicity.

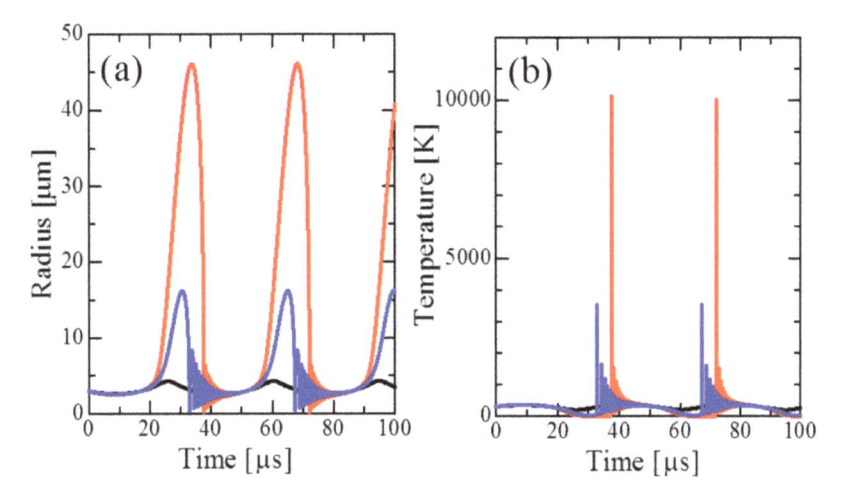

Figure 8.8. Changes in (a) bubble radius and (b) temperature of the gas inside the bubbles calculated by the Keller–Miksis equation for three acoustic pressures of P_a = 100 kPa (black line), 125 kPa (blue line), and 150 kPa (red line) at a frequency of 29 kHz. R_0 was assumed to be 2 μm. Reproduced from [26]. Copyright 2016, The author(s). With permission of Springer.

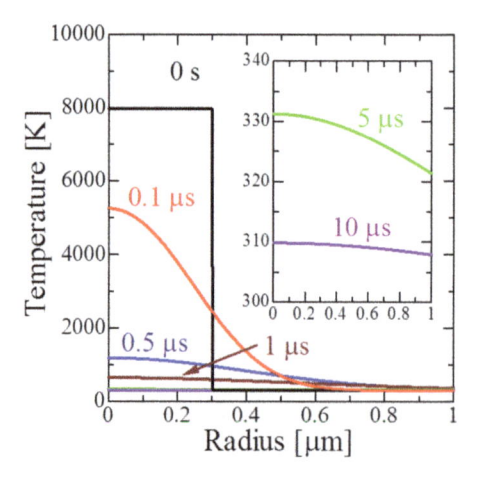

Figure 8.9. Change in the temperature distribution in the solution after bubble collapse (0 s). The horizontal axis indicates the distance from the center of the bubble. Reproduced from [26]. Copyright 2016, The author(s). With permission of Springer.

Third, the rate constant for nucleation was calculated using the following assumptions. Since Aβ monomers contain highly hydrophobic amino acid residues [55, 56], they are adsorbed on the bubble surface (liquid–gas interface) by hydrophobic interactions and are attracted to the center of the bubble during the process of bubble contraction, causing monomer condensation and then accelerating the nucleation reaction. In addition, since this contraction process occurs in a very short time, it causes an almost adiabatic compression process, which significantly increases the temperature of the solution around the bubble and contributes to further acceleration of the nucleation reaction. Thus, the nucleation reaction is promoted by local condensation and local heating, as illustrated in figure 8.10. In the theoretical calculation, it was assumed that the number of peptides adsorbed on the bubble surface was equal to the number of peptides that would have been present in the volume of the maximum-sized bubble, and that, at the bubble collapse, these peptides remained at a distance of the minimum radius $R_{\min}$ from the center, where they were exposed to the temperature change $T(R_{\min}, t)$. Also, the volume fraction φ of the bubble at its maximum was assumed to have a constant value of 10^{-4} [57], which was independent of frequency and acoustic power. The number of peptides excited into forming a nucleus was estimated using the factor $N\exp\left(-\frac{E_a}{k_B T}\right)$, where N, E_a, and k_B denote the total peptide number, the activation energy required for nucleation, and the Boltzmann constant, respectively. The time-averaged rate constant for nucleation k_n is then obtained as follows:

(a) (b) (c)

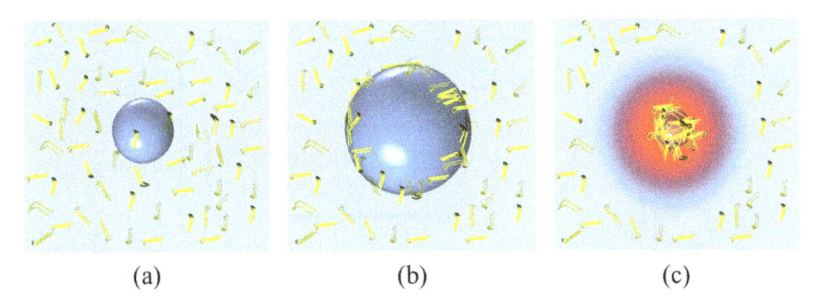

Figure 8.10. Schematic of a model of an accelerated protein aggregation reaction, focusing on the dynamics of cavitation bubbles. (a) Bubbles are generated in the solution by the negative pressure of ultrasound. (b) They grow under the negative pressure of ultrasound, and Aβ monomers (yellow hairpin-shaped rods) are adsorbed on the bubble surface by a hydrophobic interaction. (c) When the acoustic pressure becomes positive, the bubbles contract and collapse. The Aβ monomers are then condensed near the center of the bubbles, where the temperature significantly increases, accelerating the nucleation reaction. Reproduced from [26]. Copyright © 2016, The author(s). With permission of Springer.

$$k_n = \frac{A\varphi}{T_{ac}} \int_0^{T_{ac}} \exp\left(-\frac{E_a}{k_B T(R_{min}, t)}\right) dt + A\left\{(1-\varphi)\exp\left(-\frac{E_a}{k_B T_\infty}\right)\right\}. \quad (8.5)$$

Here, A, T_{ac}, and T_∞ are the prefactor, the period of the ultrasonic wave, and the temperature in the far region that is not affected by bubble dynamics. The first term refers to the nucleation probability of peptides in the heat-affected region, while the second term represents the nucleation probability of peptides in the non-heat-affected region, which corresponds to spontaneous nucleation. Note that the temperature rise in the solution after bubble collapse is more pronounced at lower ultrasonic frequencies, but the number of collapse events per unit time is higher at higher frequencies, indicating that there is an optimum frequency. Figure 8.11 compares the calculated results for the frequency dependence and the acoustic pressure dependence of k_n with the experimental results. As shown in figure 8.11(a), there is a sharp peak in the frequency dependence, which has an optimum frequency near 30 kHz, and the rate constant increases significantly by many orders of magnitude as the acoustic pressure increases (figure 8.11(b)), reproducing important trends of the aggregation reaction under ultrasonic-wave irradiation. The quantitative discrepancy between the calculated and experimental values may be caused by the uncertainty of the parameters used in the calculation, such as the volume fraction of the bubble, the heat transport loss from gas to water during collapse, and the driving sound pressure. Furthermore, some peptides are not able to follow the fast movement of the bubble wall during the contraction process, and they become detached from the bubble surface and left behind in the low-temperature region. Therefore, the k_n value obtained from the calculation is overestimated. Regardless of the uncertainty of these parameters, however, the important reaction properties are maintained, indicating the validity of the proposed model.

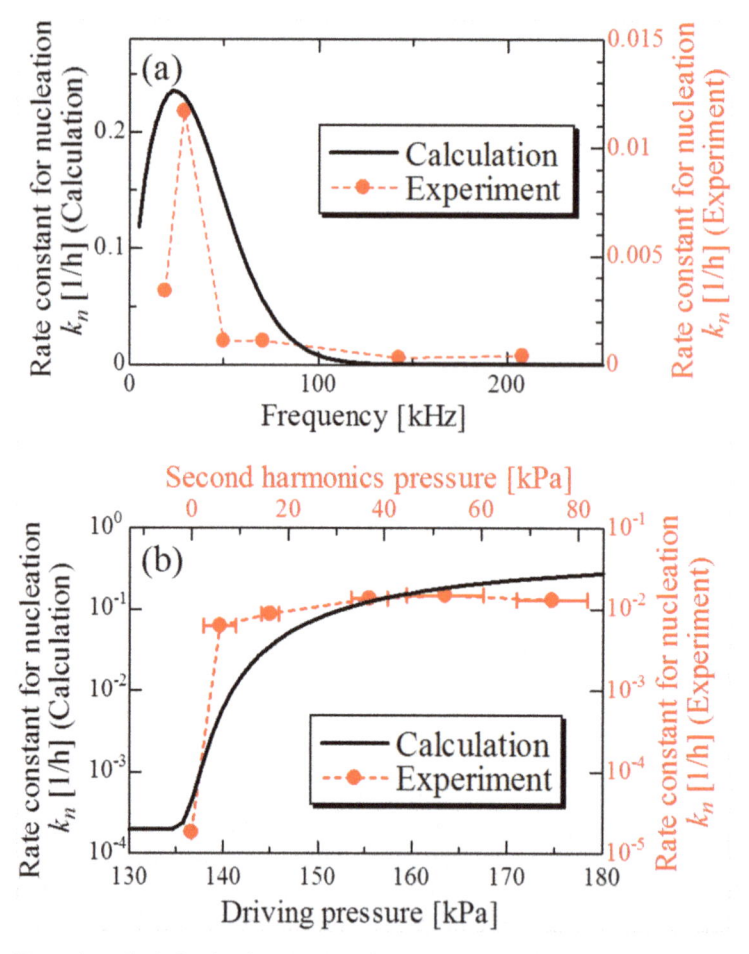

Figure 8.11. Comparison of calculated and measured (a) frequency and (b) acoustic pressure dependences of the rate constant for nucleation, k_n. Reproduced from [26]. Copyright 2016, The author(s). With permission of Springer.

8.3 Nonlinear components as indicators for the aggregation reaction

As mentioned in the previous section, it is not appropriate to use the acoustic pressure of the fundamental frequency component of the ultrasonic wave to evaluate the actual acoustic energy supplied to the solution, because cavitation bubbles are created in the solution and their nonlinear motion generates nonlinear components, such as harmonic and subharmonic components, into which the energy of the fundamental wave is converted. Since cavitation bubbles behave as catalysts for the nucleation reaction as demonstrated in the previous section, the nonlinear components of the ultrasonic wave have been adopted as measures for the aggregation reaction.

Uesugi et al [15] investigated the relationship between the acoustic pressure of the harmonic components and the degree of acceleration of the aggregation reaction of $A\beta_{1-40}$ peptide. They simultaneously irradiated 10 microtubes containing 500 μL $A\beta_{1-40}$ solution with ultrasonic waves using a 26 kHz transducer set in a water bath whose

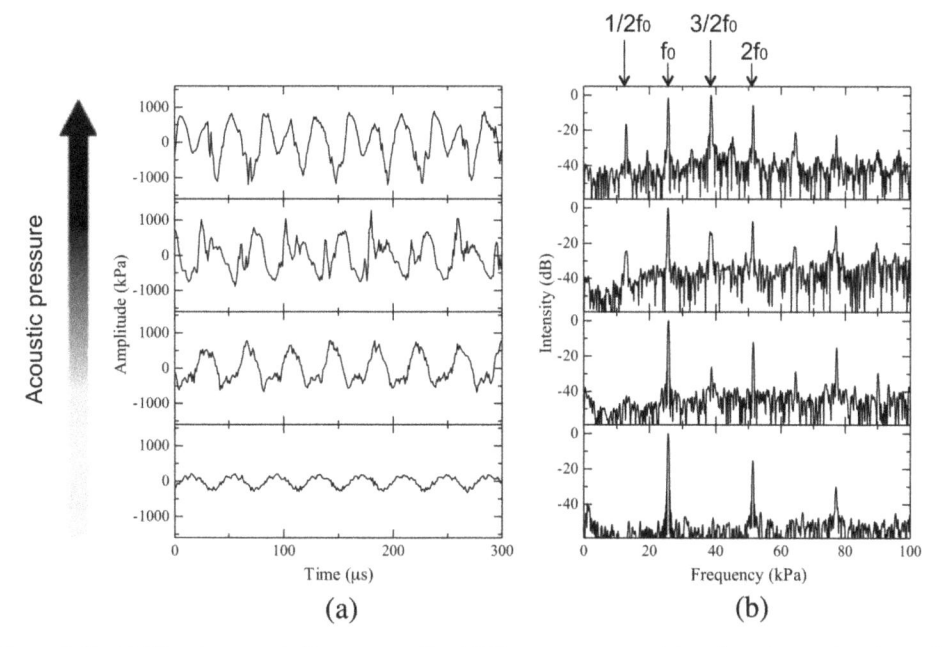

Figure 8.12. (a) Waveforms and (b) corresponding FFT spectra measured in microtubes under ultrasonic irradiation at 26 kHz. Here, f_0 denotes the fundamental frequency. Reproduced with permission from [15]. Copyright 2013 The Japan Society of Applied Physics.

temperature was maintained at 15 °C. The ultrasonic waveforms in the microtubes were acquired using a lead–zirconium–titanium (PZT) probe with a diameter of 1 mm, and the amplitudes of the fundamental and higher harmonics were extracted by fast Fourier transform (FFT) (figure 8.12) and converted to pressure values through calibration performed using a needle-type hydrophone. In their experiments, because the maximum ThT fluorescence appeared at around 5 h, the influence of the acoustic pressure on the acceleration degree was investigated using the ThT value at 5 h. The results are shown in figure 8.13. The correlation of the ThT level with the acoustic pressure of the fundamental component is poorer than those with the pressures of the second and third harmonics, indicating that monitoring the acoustic pressure of a harmonic component is more suitable for optimizing the acoustic field in the solution for the aggregation reaction. They also investigated the effect of argon gas on the aggregation reaction, because it is known that the temperature at the bubble collapse becomes higher if the dissolved gas is replaced by argon, due to its larger specific-heat ratio. The ultrasonic-wave irradiation for argon-gas-saturated $A\beta_{1-40}$ solution enhances the ThT level (inverted triangles in figure 8.13), indicating that the high-temperature region around the bubbles contributes to the nucleation reaction. The solubility of proteins often decreases as the temperature increases, which is dependent on the characteristics of the hydrophobic residues [58]. This effect enhances the supersaturation degree. In addition, the reaction rate for nucleation is increased at elevated temperatures. Furthermore, they investigated the effect of protein charging on the aggregation reaction by varying the pH value. It is known that cavitation bubbles are negatively charged [59, 60], and

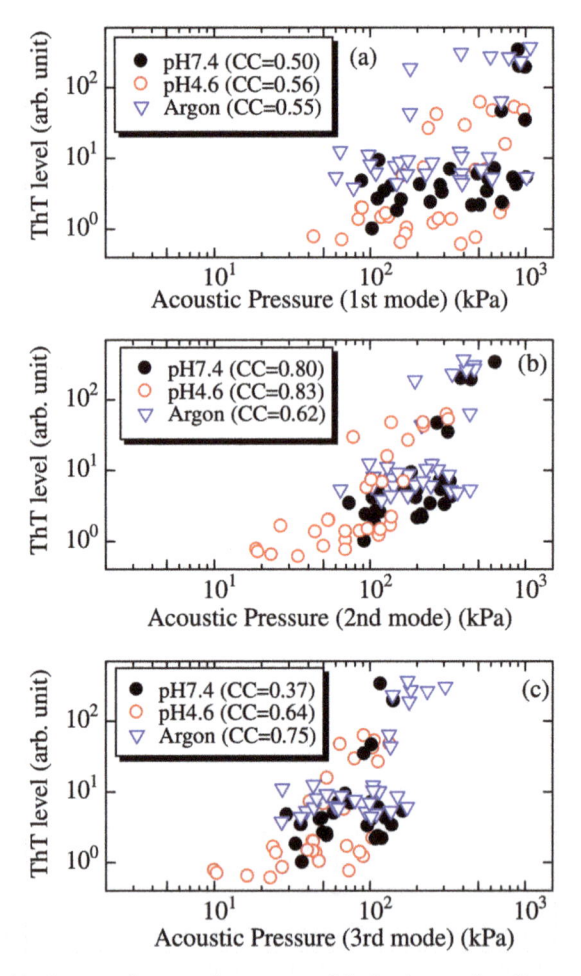

Figure 8.13. Relationships between the acoustic pressures of the fundamental and harmonic waves for the ThT fluorescence increment at 5 h caused by the ultrasonic irradiation. (a), (b), (c) show the relationships between the fundamental, second-harmonic-component, and third-harmonic-component pressures, respectively. The black and red circles denote the results for solutions at pH 7.4 and 4.6, respectively, and blue inverted triangles represent the results for the Ar-gas-saturated solution at pH 7.4. The linear correlation coefficients (CC) are shown. Reproduced with permission from [15]. Copyright 2013 The Japan Society of Applied Physics.

positively charged proteins may be collected by electrostatic interactions near the surface of the bubbles. The isoelectric point of the Aβ peptide is pH 5.2, and it should be positively and negatively charged at pH 4.6 and 7.4, respectively. If the electrical interaction were dominant, the increase in the ThT level would be expected to be trivial at pH 7.4 because of the repulsive interaction between the peptide and the bubbles. However, as shown in figure 8.13, the ThT level at pH 7.4 is comparable to or higher than that at pH 4.6, indicating that this electrical interaction is not the dominant factor.

Nakajima *et al* [28] investigated the relationship between the subharmonic component and the acceleration behavior for an aggregation reaction using insulin, which has been widely used as a model protein in amyloid fibril research [61–63]. Insulin has a native folded structure at neutral pH near room temperature and is extremely stable, making it difficult for the aggregation reaction to proceed with standard agitation, including a high-speed stirring agitation. However, it has been found that the fibrillation reaction of insulin proceeds hundreds of times faster with optimal ultrasound irradiation than with high-speed stirring agitation at a rotational speed of 1200 rpm when the subharmonic intensity exceeds a threshold.

The experimental system they developed is shown in figure 8.14(a). An ultrasonic transducer with a fundamental frequency of 26 kHz was placed in a water bath filled with degassed water treated with a deaerator to avoid the scattering loss of ultrasonic waves due to cavitation bubbles. Microtubes containing the sample solution were placed near the water surface of the water bath and irradiated with ultrasonic waves through the degassed water. The temperature of the degassed water was controlled by a temperature controller. Figure 8.14(b) shows the change in the normalized subharmonic-component intensity when the output level of the ultrasonic generator was increased to the maximum. The sample solutions were irradiated with the ultrasonic wave for 1 min and incubated for 4 min. This 5 min sequence was repeated for ~7 h. Every 0.5 h, 5 µL sample solution was taken and mixed with a 5 µM ThT solution, and its fluorescent intensity was measured. The temperature change in the microtube during the ultrasonic irradiation was measured by a non-contact radiation thermometer. The acoustic pressure was measured by inserting a PZT needle probe into a microtube containing only buffer solution without insulin.

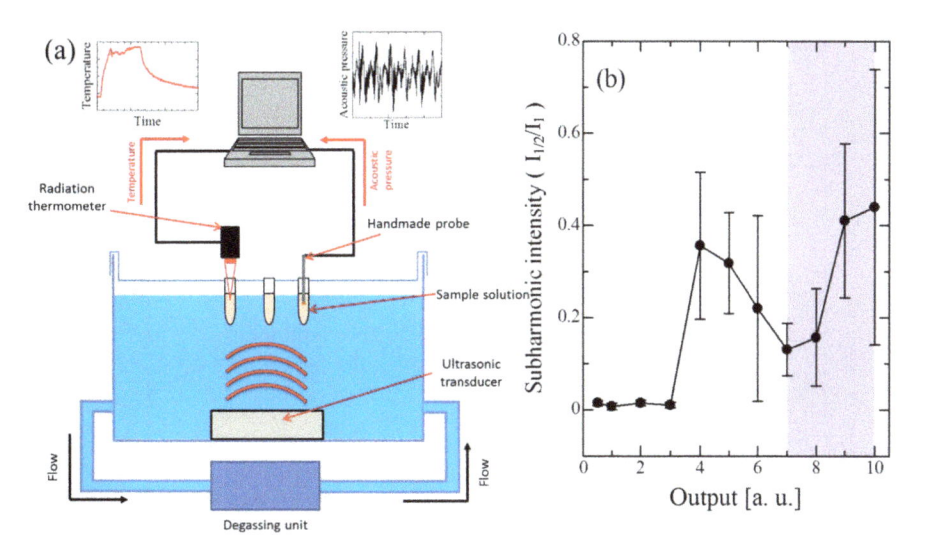

Figure 8.14. (a) Experimental system used for the ultrasonic irradiation experiment for insulin. Microtubes filled with insulin sample solution were placed near the water surface and irradiated with 26 kHz ultrasound from below. The temperature and sound field in the microtubes were measured by a non-contact radiation thermometer and a needle-shaped PZT probe, respectively. (b) Variation of the normalized subharmonic-component intensity with increasing power levels of the ultrasound generator. The shaded area indicates the output level used for the aggregation reaction of insulin. The maximum power (level 10) is about 200 W. Reproduced from [28]. Copyright (2017), with permission from Elsevier.

The subharmonic-component intensity increases significantly when the output level of the ultrasound generator exceeded level three, decreased temporarily between levels four and seven, and increased again when the level exceeded seven. This two-threshold behavior of the subharmonic component was reported by Neppiras [64] and interpreted as follows. The first increase in subharmonic intensity is due to nonlinear oscillations of stable bubbles, and the second increase above level seven indicates the appearance of collapsing bubbles, which repeat the growth–collapse–rebound sequence, as shown in figure 8.8(a). This behavior was also theoretically confirmed by Eller and Flynn [65]. It was found that insulin cannot be fibrillated at the first subharmonic peak, and a power level between seven and ten was employed to fibrillate insulin.

Figure 8.15(a) shows four examples of changes in the ThT fluorescence intensity during ultrasonication: two of the examples show an increase in fluorescence intensity

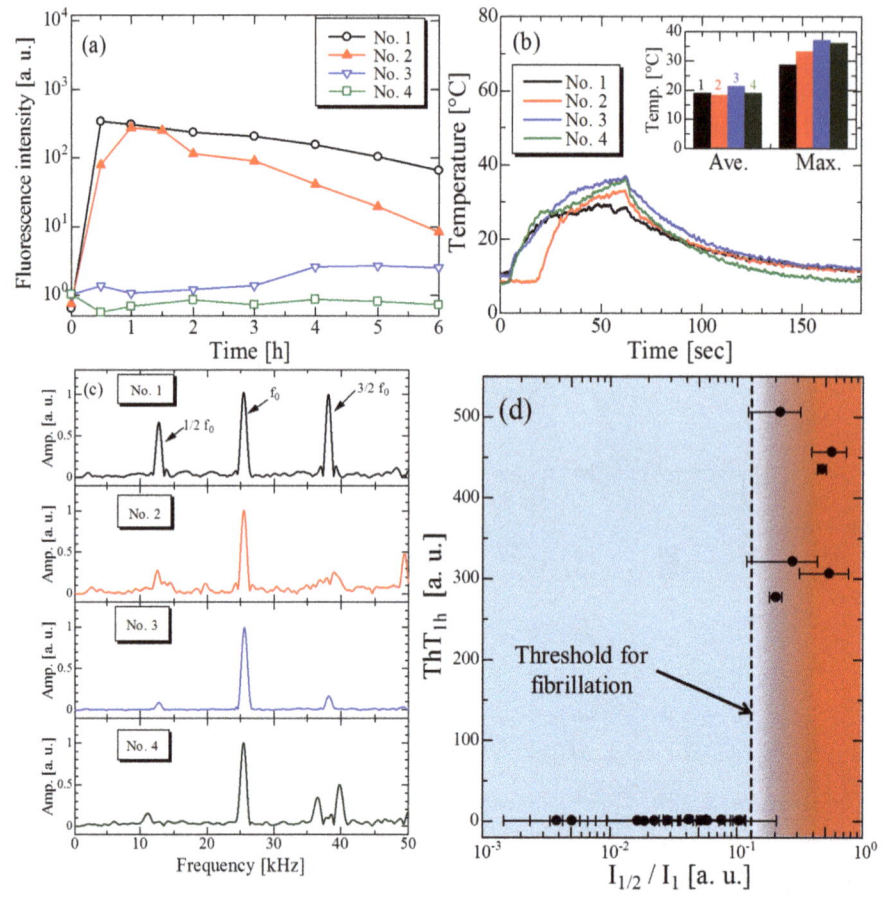

Figure 8.15. (a) Examples of changes in the ThT fluorescence of four samples. (b) Temperature change of each sample in (a). The inset shows the average and maximum temperatures of the four measurements (the same color is used for each corresponding measurement). (c) FFT spectra of the acquired waveforms of the measurements shown in (a) and (b). (d) Relationship between normalized subharmonic-component intensity and ThT fluorescence intensity. The vertical axis shows the ThT fluorescence intensity 1 h after the start of the experiment. Reproduced from [28]. Copyright (2017), with permission from Elsevier.

within 30 min, and in two, it failed to increase even after 6 h. Figure 8.15(b) shows the corresponding temperature changes in the sample solutions. It is important to note that there is no obvious difference in the temperature profiles. The temperature of the sample solution reaches a maximum value of 35 °C during ultrasonication and then cools down to the base temperature in the subsequent incubation period. This result indicates that the temperature of the solution is not a major factor in promoting the fibrillation of insulin. Figure 8.15(c) shows FFT spectra for measurements corresponding to figures 8.15(a) and (b). The subharmonic intensity was higher in the measurements with increased ThT fluorescence intensity (No. 1 and No. 2) and lower in the measurements without increased ThT fluorescence intensity (No. 3 and No. 4). Figure 8.15(d) shows the relationship between the subharmonic intensity normalized by the fundamental component ($I_{1/2}/I_1$) and the ThT fluorescence intensity at 1 h. Since the subharmonic intensity must exceed a threshold ($I_{1/2}/I_1 > 0.1$) for the fibrillation reaction to occur, and this threshold is approximately equal to the occurrence of the collapsing bubbles (figure 8.14(b)), it is clear that the acceleration of the fibrillation is caused by the collapsing bubbles. The drastic acceleration of the aggregation reaction is thus explained by the mechanism described in the previous section.

8.4 Supersaturation: a new concept for protein aggregation phenomenon

Recently, a new concept has been proposed, which is that the phenomenon of protein aggregation can be interpreted as precipitation from a supersaturated state, similar to that of solid crystals [16, 23]. Figure 8.16 is a schematic representation of this concept. Proteins in solution never form aggregates below their solubility (soluble region). Even when a solution is supersaturated above the solubility, the protein is still soluble because the supersaturated state remains relatively stable (metastable region). As the supersaturation degree is further enhanced, the

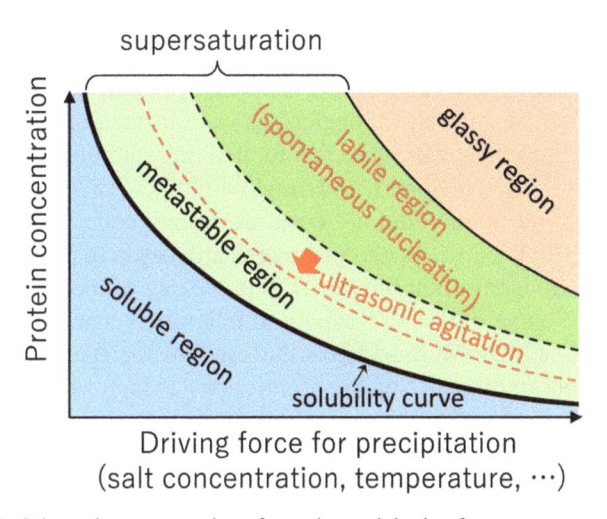

Figure 8.16. Schematic representation of protein precipitation from a supersaturated state.

solution state becomes unstable, and after a long delay, spontaneous nucleation is expected to occur, leading to the formation of amyloid fibrils (labile region). When the protein concentration or driving force (salt concentration, temperature, etc.) is excessively high, amorphous aggregates precipitate (glassy region).

The important point is that amyloidogenic proteins are usually in the metastable region at *in vivo* concentrations [23], and amyloid fibrils should not be formed since they are sufficiently stable under supersaturated conditions. However, the fact that their aggregates have been observed in patients indicates that some stimulus can move the boundary between the labile and metastable regions toward the metastable region. Therefore, it is important to maintain a metastable region in order to inhibit the development of amyloidosis, and this can be achieved by controlling the agitation factor. Furthermore, finding an important agitation factor corresponds to a new biomarker for the amyloidosis. In fact, many contaminants are present in the body, and some of them increase the driving force or move the labile–metastable boundary downward in figure 8.16. However, it takes a very long time to investigate their effects independently, because the spontaneous nucleation happens after a long delay due to the high stability of supersaturated proteins. Ultrasound can be a powerful agitation tool for moving the labile region downward to break the supersaturation and greatly contributes to the screening process used to find factors that inhibit or promote aggregation reactions.

Nakajima *et al* [22] systematically studied the effect of ultrasonication and shaking agitation on the phase diagram as shown in figure 8.16 by introducing a half-time heat map. The half-time is defined as the time at which the fluorescence intensity of ThT reaches half of its maximum value, and it represents the instability of the state or the strength of the driving force in the phase diagram. Using NaCl as a driving force factor, they investigated the half-time of the aggregation reaction of β_2M. Figure 8.17 shows the results. At quiescence (without any agitation) (figure 8.17(a)), the monomer in the solution containing 30 mM NaCl remained soluble for 100 h. As the salt concentration was increased, the curve of the ThT evolution followed a typical sigmoidal function, and fibril-like aggregates were observed in the solution. However, at NaCl concentrations above 240 mM, the ThT evolution deviated from the sigmoid curve; it continued to increase after the initial sharp increase. As a result, spherical aggregates rather than fibrils were observed, indicating that amorphous aggregates were formed at excess NaCl concentrations. When the solution was subjected to shaking agitation (figure 8.17(b)), the aggregation reaction was accelerated, and amyloid fibrils were formed even at 30 mM NaCl. Note that fibril formation did not occur at this salt concentration at quiescence. However, above 240 mM NaCl, amorphous aggregates began to form, as was the case at quiescence. Under ultrasonication (figure 8.17(c)), the aggregation reaction was further accelerated, and the curve of the ThT evolution followed a sigmoidal function up to a NaCl concentration of 240 mM. In addition, the resultant aggregates were amyloid fibrils in the solutions. Importantly, at NaCl concentrations as high as 240 mM, amorphous aggregates were obtained under quiescence and shaking conditions, but amyloid fibrils were formed by ultrasound irradiation.

Figures 8.17(d)–(f) show the relationships between the half-time values in the aggregation reaction and the monomer concentrations under the three conditions at

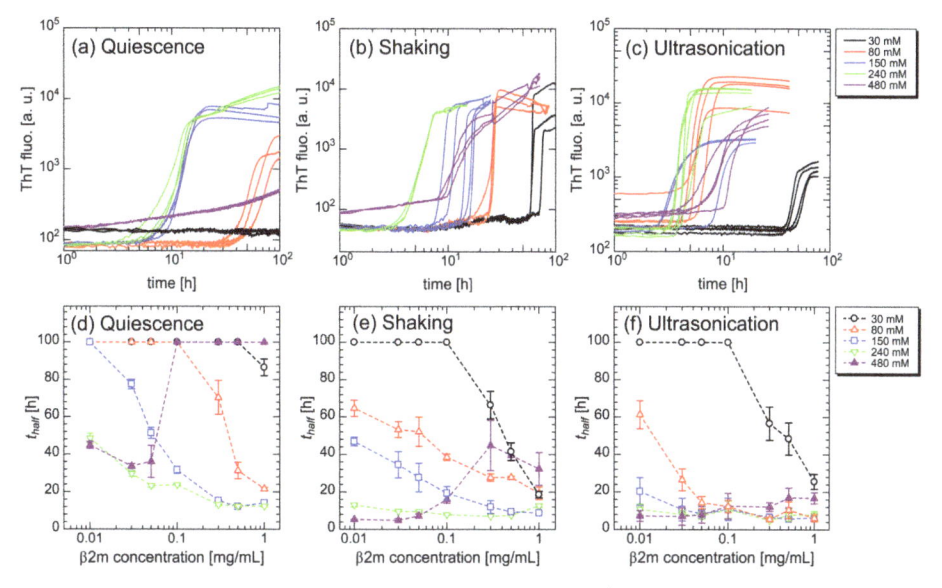

Figure 8.17. Changes in the ThT fluorescence intensity of 0.3 mg mL^{-1} β$_2$M monomer solution at various salt concentrations subjected to (a) quiescence, (b) shaking, and (c) ultrasonication ($n > 3$). Relationships between the half-time value (t_{half}) and monomer concentration in the aggregation reaction under conditions of (d) quiescence, (e) shaking, and (f) ultrasonication at various salt concentrations. Reproduced with permission from [22]. Copyright 2021 American Chemical Society.

various salt concentrations. The plots on the 100 h line indicate measurements for solutions that remained soluble without an increase in the ThT level within 100 h. At low NaCl concentrations (30, 80, and 150 mM), the monomer concentration and the half-time are inversely correlated, as expected, for quiescence and shaking (figures 8.17(d) and (e)). At higher NaCl concentrations (240 and 480 mM), samples with higher monomer concentrations exhibited longer half-time values than those with lower concentrations. Under these conditions, amorphous aggregates were formed. It has been reported that the slower rate of the aggregation reaction at higher protein concentrations is due to the formation of amorphous species [66]. Therefore, the longer half-time values in the region of higher monomer and higher salt concentrations indicate the formation of amorphous aggregates. A possible mechanism for this phenomenon is that the partial formation of amorphous aggregates reduces the concentration of active free monomer in the solution, resulting in a lower apparent monomer concentration and a slower reaction rate. Another reason for this slow rate is that the rapidly formed amorphous aggregates are slowly converted to fibrils [67].

Under ultrasound irradiation (figure 8.17(f)), only the sample containing 30 mM NaCl shows an inverse correlation between the monomer concentration and the half-time. For samples with NaCl concentrations of 240 mM or less, the half-time decreases in the region of low monomer concentration, but reaches almost the same value (~10 h) in the region of high monomer concentration, regardless of monomer concentration. In the 480 mM NaCl sample, the half-time increases with increasing

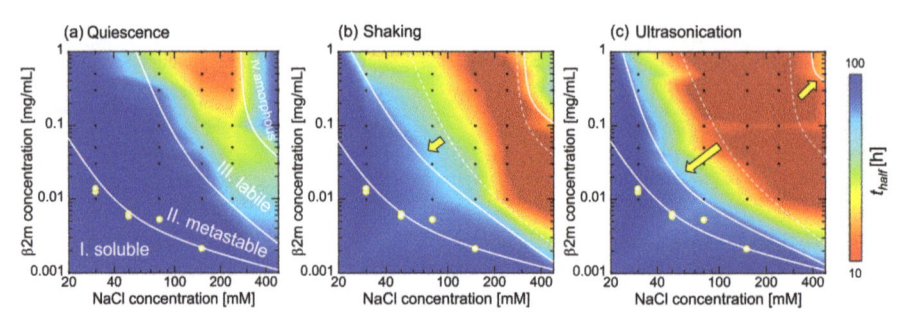

Figure 8.18. Half-time (t_{half} value) heat maps of aggregation reactions under conditions of (a) quiescence, (b) shaking, and (c) ultrasonication. The yellow dots denote the solubility of $β_2$M monomer at each salt concentration measured by ultracentrifugation and ELISA assay. The dotted lines in (b) and (c) indicate the phase boundaries under quiescence, which are varied by agitation. Reproduced with permission from [22]. Copyright 2021 American Chemical Society.

monomer concentration because of the formation of amorphous aggregates. This trend is similar to that for shaking, but the half-times of these samples are significantly smaller than those of the samples exposed to shaking, suggesting that ultrasonication promotes the conversion from amorphous aggregates to fibrils.

Figure 8.18 is a visual summary of these observations using phase diagrams. The boundary between the soluble and metastable regions was defined as the condition in which no fibrils were formed within 100 h. When samples are exposed to shaking (figure 8.16(b)), the metastable–labile boundary shifts downward and the metastable region becomes narrower than that at quiescence (figure 8.18(a)), whereas the labile–amorphous boundary remains nearly unchanged. On the other hand, ultrasonication not only shifts the metastable–labile boundary downward significantly, but also shifts the labile–amorphous boundary upward (figure 8.18(c)). Shaking fails to accelerate the aggregation reaction for solutions with low monomer concentrations (<0.1 mg mL^{-1}). This is the case because the reaction acceleration due to shaking is based on the mechanism of decreasing the apparent mean-free path between monomers and increasing the probability of intermolecular interaction, which is effective for highly concentrated solutions with small intermolecular distances, but not for dilute solutions.

On the other hand, ultrasound maintains a high acceleration ability even for dilute monomer solutions. As described in section 8.2, cavitation bubbles act as catalysts for the nucleation reaction. The cavitation bubbles generated by the negative pressure of ultrasound attract monomers to their surfaces during the bubble expansion phase because the hydrophobic amino acid residues prefer the air–water interface. The subsequent bubble collapse causes the monomers attached to the bubble surface to condense at the collapse center, which heats the solution locally and temporarily, promoting the nucleation reaction. The bubble expands to a radius of several tens of micrometers and then shrinks to less than 1 μm at the time of collapse, resulting in an instantaneous shrinkage of volume by a factor of 1000. This rapid volume change causes a localized increase in the monomer concentration near the bubble-collapse point, and with the addition of an instantaneous increase in temperature, the nucleation reaction is accelerated even in a dilute monomer solution. On the other hand, when the surface of the bubble is completely covered with monomers, the effect of local condensation becomes saturated. This explains why the half-time of a sample with a high monomer concentration does not fall below the lower limit of ~10 h under ultrasonication (figure 8.17(f)).

8.5 Multichannel ultrasonication system for amyloid assay: HANABI

Goto *et al* developed a high-throughput and high-speed amyloid-assay system by integrating a multichannel fluorescence spectrophotometer with an ultrasonic irradiation system, and named it HANABI (*Han*dai *a*myloid *b*urst *i*nducer; 'Handai' is the abbreviation for 'Osaka University' in Japanese) [18, 68]. In the HANABI system, a 96-well microplate containing sample solutions was placed in a large water bath (14 L) and was irradiated with ultrasonic waves generated simultaneously in three areas below the bath (directly below and diagonally below it), and the fluorescence intensity of each well was measured from the top. The frequency and power of the ultrasonic wave were about 20 kHz and 350 W, respectively. The HANABI system has successfully promoted the aggregation reaction of various proteins including hen egg-white lysozyme, β_2M, and Aβ peptide [68]. However, it was difficult to achieve a reproducible measurement, because the acoustic field produced in each sample solution could not be controlled.

A modified HANABI system was then developed and named HANABI-2000, as shown in figure 8.19 [21]. In this system, the water bath is removed and rod-shaped ultrasonic transducers (figures 8.20(a) and (b)) are placed on individual wells. The resonant frequency of each transducer is set to about 30 kHz, which is the optimum

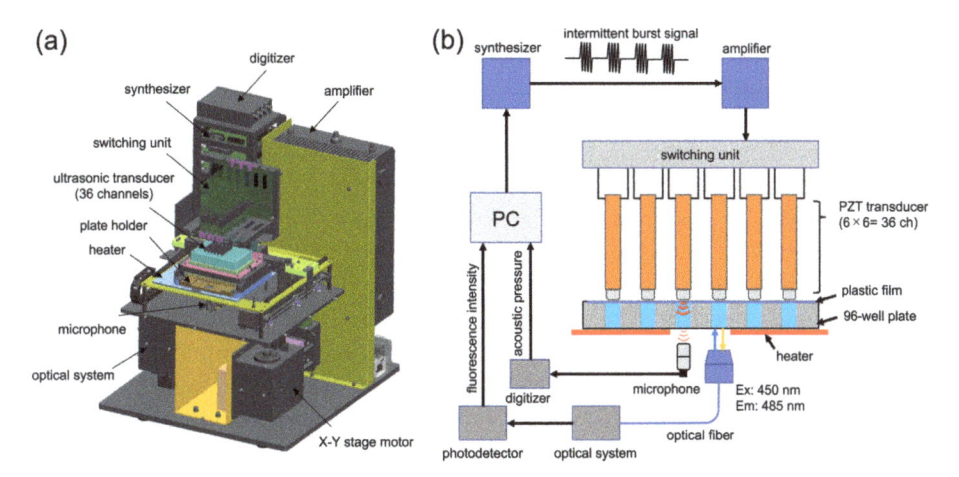

Figure 8.19. (a) Schematic illustration of the multichannel high-speed amyloid-assay instrument, the HANABI-2000. (b) Block chart of the control units of the HANABI-2000. Reproduced with permission from [21]. Copyright 2021 Elsevier.

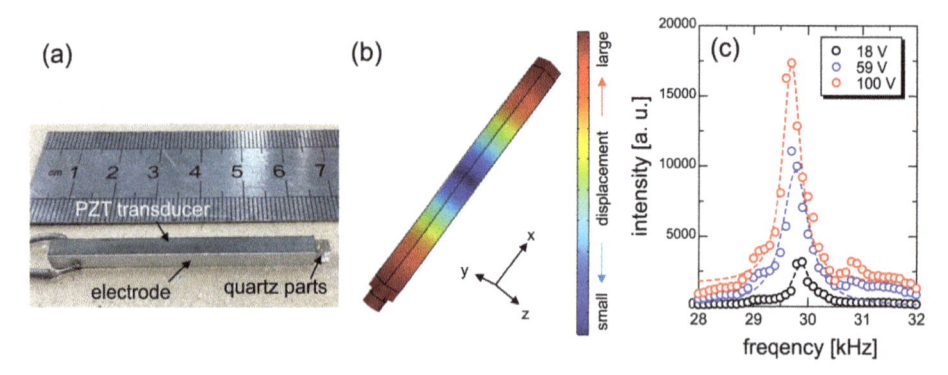

Figure 8.20. (a) A PZT transducer used in the HANABI-2000. (b) Modal analysis for the transducer, which was used to estimate the resonant frequency by the finite element method (FEM). (c) The resonant spectra of the PZT transducer at different applied voltages. Reproduced with permission from [21]. Copyright 2021 Elsevier.

frequency given in section 8.2. A microphone is placed below the microplate so that the ultrasound field in the solution in each well can be monitored, and the amplitude and frequency of the driving voltage of each transducer can be adjusted individually with reference to the output of the microphone. A photodetector is also installed below the microplate to measure the fluorescence signal and monitor the progress of the aggregation reaction in each well. A 0.1 mm thick plastic film is used to seal the solution in the microplate. The transducers contact this plastic film, from which optimized ultrasound waves are emitted towards the solutions. All transducers are connected to a signal switching unit and are driven sequentially by a tone-burst signal. The frequency and amplitude of the burst signal can be set individually. The generated burst signal is amplified by an amplifier and sent to each transducer in turn via the switching unit. A typical burst length is 300 ms, with a switching time of 500 ms. Before an assay takes place, the resonant frequency of each individual transducer in contact with the film is individually determined by sweeping the excitation frequency and measuring the acoustic intensity with a microphone to obtain the resonance spectrum (figure 8.20(c)). The transducers are thus driven at their resonant frequencies.

The HANABI-2000 system was first used to study the acceleration of amyloid fibril formation by ultrasound irradiation in the presence of amyloid seeds. Figure 8.21 shows such results for $\beta_2 M$ and is an example of many experiments performed simultaneously in one microplate, with and without sonication, and for solutions at various seed concentrations. The seeding reaction principally consists of three reactions: first, spontaneous nucleation by soluble monomers (primary nucleation); second, the fibril elongation reaction, in which monomers are adsorbed on the ends of the seed or fibrils to grow fibrils; and third, the fragmentation reaction, in which fibrils are fragmented by some kind of agitation. Based on these three reactions, a theoretical model was proposed, in which the mass concentration of fibrils at time t, $M(t)$, is given by [69]

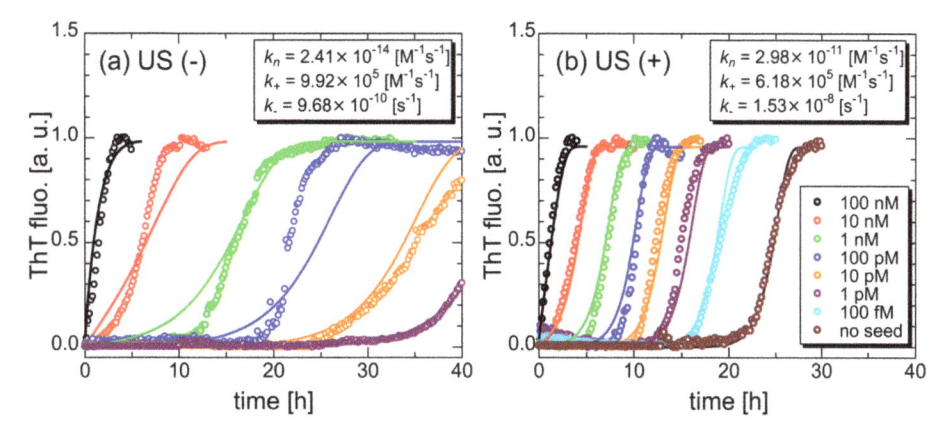

Figure 8.21. Changes of ThT fluorescence intensity in the presence of amyloid seeds at concentrations from 0 and 100 nM for β$_2$M (a) without (US(−)) and (b) with (US(+)) ultrasonic irradiation, obtained simultaneously in one microplate using the HANABI-2000 system. Solid lines indicate fitted theoretical curves. Reproduced with permission from [21]. Copyright 2021 Elsevier.

$$M(t) = m_0 \left\{ 1 - \exp\left(-C_+ e^{\kappa t} + C_- e^{-\kappa t} + \frac{m_0^{n_C-1} k_n}{k_-} \right) \right\}. \quad (8.6)$$

where k_n and k_- denote the rate constants for primary nucleation and fragmentation, respectively. m_0 is the initial monomer concentration, and n_C is the minimum number of monomers required in order to stabilize the aggregate, which was set to two [21]. $\kappa = \sqrt{2 m_0 k_+ k_-}$ and $C_\pm = (k_+ P_0/\kappa) \pm (M_0/2 m_0) \pm (k_n m_0^{n_C-1}/2 k_-)$, where P_0 and M_0 denote the number and mass concentrations of the initial seeds, respectively, and k_+ is the rate constant for fibril growth. The three rate constants k_n, k_+, and k_- were inversely determined by fitting the theory (equation (8.6)) to the experimental results in figure 8.21. Ultrasonic irradiation changed k_n, k_+, and k_- by 1240, 0.623, and 15.8 times, respectively, indicating that ultrasonication accelerates the fibril-forming reaction by promoting the primary nucleation and fragmentation reactions, but affects the fibril growth reaction less.

The HANABI-2000 system was then applied to the detection of amyloid seeds [22]. Figure 8.22 shows the results of observing the seeding reaction under three conditions; quiescence, shaking, and ultrasonication. In the absence of seeds, the half-time t_{half} of the fibril formation reaction was about 44 h at quiescence (figure 8.22(a)), but it was reduced to about 4 h in the presence 10 nM seeds, indicating that the seeds added at the beginning of the experiment acted as points of origin for fibril growth. With the addition of 10 pM seeds, the seeding effect was clearly observed. However, at a seed concentration of 100 fM, the seeding effect was not evident, indicating that the detection limit of the seed was about 1 pM at quiescence. Regardless of the seed concentration, the shaking agitation accelerated the seed reaction compared to the reaction at quiescence (figure 8.22(b)), resulting in rapid seed detection. However, the ThT change curves of the samples with seed concentrations of 10 fM and 100 fM overlapped with those of the unseeded samples,

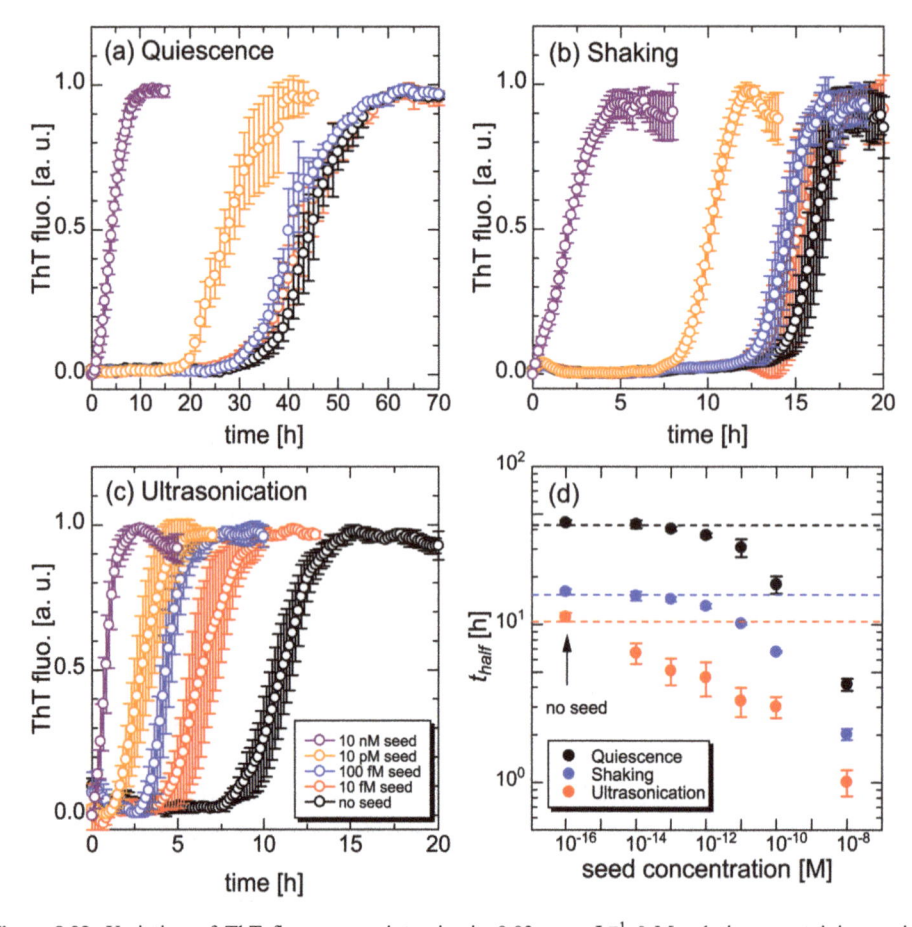

Figure 8.22. Variation of ThT fluorescence intensity in 0.03-mg mL^{-1} β$_2$M solutions containing various concentrations of seeds (a) at quiescence, (b) exposed to shaking, and (c) ultrasonic irradiation. (d) The relationship between seed concentration and half-time (t_{half}) for the three different types of agitation. Reproduced with permission from [22]. Copyright 2021 American Chemical Society.

as in the assay at quiescence. Therefore, the detection limit of the seed is also about 1 pM for samples exposed to shaking, indicating that shaking promotes the formation of fibrils but fails to improve the detection limit. Ultrasonication results in further acceleration of the seeding reaction (figure 8.22(c)). It is noteworthy that the ThT curve of the sample with 10 fM seeds is clearly separate from that without seeds, demonstrating a seed detection limit of less than 10 fM under ultrasonication. This fact indicates that the seeding assay under ultrasonication is less time-consuming and more sensitive than shaking, and this is a very important advantage for clinical applications.

8.6 Summary and future prospects

It is a scientifically and practically interesting fact that ultrasound irradiation, which has been conventionally adopted for the decomposition reaction of organic compounds in liquids, can dramatically accelerate the polymerization reaction of proteins by optimizing the conditions. Importantly, ultrasound irradiation can not only accelerate the formation of amyloid fibrils from monomer solutions, but also accelerate the seeding reaction. The latter can be applied to the diagnosis of neurodegenerative diseases: in the early stages of the onset of Alzheimer's disease and Parkinson's disease, it is suggested that the seeds of causative proteins are formed. Therefore, it is possible to evaluate the presence of the seeds by adding body fluids, such as cerebrospinal fluid, to a monomer solution of the causative protein and monitoring the aggregation reaction. However, the completion of such a seeding reaction takes a very long time (>10 days) [3], and its acceleration is required. Optimized ultrasonic irradiation systems such as HANABI-2000 are, therefore, expected to contribute greatly to the early diagnosis of these diseases.

References

[1] Chiti F and Dobson C M 2017 *Annu. Rev. Biochem.* **86** 27–68
[2] Nakamura A *et al* 2018 *Nature* **554** 249–54
[3] Shahnawaz M *et al* 2020 *Nature* **578** 273–7
[4] Kakuda K *et al* 2019 *Sci. Rep.* **9** 6001
[5] Cohen F E and Kelly J W 2003 *Nature* **426** 905–9
[6] Chiti F and Dobson C M 2006 *Annu. Rev. Biochem.* **75** 333–66
[7] Naiki H, Higuchi K, Hosokawa M and Takeda T 1989 *Anal. Biochem.* **177** 244–9
[8] Naiki H, Hashimoto S, Suzuki H, Kimura K, Nakakuki K and Gejyo F 1997 *Amyloid* **4** 223–32
[9] Jerrett J T and Lansbury P T Jr. 1993 *Cell* **73** 1055–8
[10] Chatani E, Lee Y-H, Yagi H, Yoshimura Y, Naiki H and Goto Y 2009 *Proc. Natl Acad. Sci.* **106** 11119–24
[11] Stathopulos P B, Scholz G A, Hwang Y M, Rumfeldt J A, Lepock J R and Meiering E M 2004 *Protein Sci.* **13** 3017–27
[12] Ohhashi Y, Kihara M, Naiki H and Goto Y 2005 *J. Biol. Chem.* **280** 32843–8
[13] Kim H J, Chatani E, Goto Y and Paik S R 2007 *J. Microbiol. Biotechnol.* **17** 2027–32
[14] Yamaguchi K, Matsumoto T and Kuwata K 2012 *Protein Sci.* **21** 38–49
[15] Uesugi K, Ogi H, Fukushima M, So M, Yagi H, Goto Y and Hirao M 2013 *Jpn. J. Appl. Phys.* **52** 07HE10
[16] Yoshimura Y, Lin Y, Yagi H, Lee Y-H, Kitayama H, Sakurai K, So M, Ogi H, Naiki H and Goto Y 2012 *Proc. Natl Acad. Sci.* **109** 14446–51
[17] Yoshimura Y, So M, Yagi H and Goto Y 2013 *Jpn. J. Appl. Phys.* **52** 07HA01
[18] Goto Y, Nakajima K, Yamaguchi K, So M, Ikenaka K, Mochizuki H and Ogi H 2022 *Neurochem. Int.* **153** 105270
[19] So M, Yagi H, Sakura K, Ogi H, Naiki H and Goto Y 2011 *J. Mol. Biol.* **412** 568–77
[20] Kakuda K *et al* 2019 *Sci. Rep.* **9** 6001
[21] Nakajima K, Noi K, Yamaguchi K, So M, Ikenaka K, Mochizuki H, Ogi H and Goto Y 2021 *Ultrason. Sonochem.* **73** 105508
[22] Nakajima K, Toda H, Yamaguchi K, So M, Ikenaka K, Mochizuki H, Goto Y and Ogi H 2021 *ACS Chem. Neurosci.* **12** 3456–66
[23] Noji M, Sasahara K, Yamaguchi K, So M, Sakurai K, Kardos J, Naiki H and Goto Y 2019 *J. Biol. Chem.* **294** 15826–35

[24] Furukawa K *et al* 2020 *Curr. Res. Struct. Biol.* **2** 35–44
[25] Noji M *et al* 2021 *Commun. Biol.* **4** 120
[26] Nakajima K, Ogi H, Adachi K, Noi K, Hirao M, Yagi H and Goto Y 2016 *Sci. Rep.* **6** 22015
[27] Nakajima K, So M, Takahashi K, Tagawa Y, Hirao M, Goto Y and Ogi H 2017 *J. Phys. Chem.* B **121** 2603–13
[28] Nakajima K, Nishioka D, Hirao M, So M, Goto Y and Ogi H 2017 *Ultrason. Sonochem.* **36** 206–11
[29] Suslick K S 1990 *Science* **247** 1439–45
[30] Brenner M P, Hilgenfeldt S and Lohse D 2002 *Rev. Mod. Phys.* **74** 425–84
[31] Koda S, Kimura T, Kondo T and Mitome H 2003 *Ultrason. Sonochem.* **10** 149–56
[32] Thomas J R 1959 *J. Phys. Chem.* **63** 1725–29
[33] Shestakova M, Vinatoru M, Mason T J and Sillanpää M 2015 *Ultrason. Sonochem.* **23** 135–41
[34] Choi P-K 2017 *Jpn. J. Appl. Phys.* **56** 07JA01
[35] Shimakage K, Kobayashi D, Naya M, Matsumoto H, Shimada Y, Otake K and Shono A 2016 *Jpn. J. Appl. Phys.* **55** 07KE01
[36] Merouani S, Hamadaoui O, Saoudi F and Chiha M 2010 *J. Hazard. Mater.* **178** 1007–14
[37] Neuenschwander U, Neuenschwander J and Hermans I 2012 *Ultrason. Sonochem.* **19** 1011–4
[38] Stricker L and Lohse D 2014 *Ultrason. Sonochem.* **21** 336–45
[39] Okumura H and Itoh S G 2014 *J. Am. Chem. Soc.* **136** 10549–52
[40] Saborio G P, Permanne B and Soto C 2001 *Nature* **411** 810–3
[41] Saa P, Castilla J and Soto C 2006 *J. Biol. Chem.* **281** 35245–52
[42] Watzky M A and Finke R G 1997 *J. Am. Chem. Soc.* **119** 10382–400
[43] Watzky M A, Morris A M, Ross E D and Finke R G 2008 *Biochemistry* **47** 10790–800
[44] Cohen S I A, Linse S, Luheshi L M, Hellstrand E, White D A, Rajah L, Otzen D E, Vendruscolo M, Dobson C M and Knowles T P J 2013 *Proc. Natl. Acad. Sci.* **110** 9758–63
[45] Yagi H, Abe Y, Takayanagi N and Goto Y 2014 *Biochim. Biophys. Acta* **1844** 1881–8
[46] McNamara W B III, Didenko Y T and Suslick K S 1999 *Nature* **401** 772–5
[47] Lohse D 2005 *Nature* **434** 33–4
[48] Keller J B and Miksis M 1980 *J. Acoust. Soc. Am.* **68** 628–33
[49] Woody R W 1995 *Methods Enzymol.* **246** 34–71
[50] Lu J-X, Qiang W, Yau W-M, Schwieters C D, Meredith S C and Tycko R 2013 *Cell* **12** 1257–68
[51] Nybo M, Svehag S-E and Nielsen E H 1999 *Scand. J. Immunol.* **49** 219–23
[52] Goldsbury C, Frey P, Olivieri V, Aebi U and Müller S A 2005 *J. Mol. Biol.* **352** 282–98
[53] Neppiras E 1980 *Phys. Rep.* **61** 159–251
[54] Frohly J, Labouret S, Bruneel C, Looten-Baquet I and Torguet R 2000 *J. Acoust. Soc. Am.* **108** 2012–20
[55] Vassar R *et al* 1999 *Science* **286** 735–41
[56] Jean L, Lee C F and Vaux D J 2012 *Biophys. J.* **102** 1154–62
[57] Burdin F, Tsochatzidis N A, Guiraud P, Wilhelm A M and Delmas H 1999 *Ultrason. Sonochem.* **6** 43–51
[58] Rosenberger F, Howard S B, Sowers J Q and Nyce T A 1993 *J. Cryst. Growth* **129** 1–12
[59] Watmough D J, Shiran M B, Quan K M, Sarvazyan A P, Khizhnyak E P and Pashovkin T N 1992 *Ultrasonics* **30** 325–31
[60] Takahashi M 2005 *J. Phys. Chem.* B **109** 21858–64

[61] Bryant C, Spencer D B, Miller A, Bakaysa D L, McCune K S, Maple S R, Pekar A H and Brems D N 1993 *Biochemistry* **32** 8075–82
[62] Ivanova M I, Sievers S A, Sawaya M R, Wall J S and Eisenberg D 2009 *Proc. Natl. Acad. Sci.* **99** 18990–5
[63] Noormägi A, Valmsen K, Tõugu V and Palumaa P 2015 *Protein J.* **34** 398–403
[64] Neppiras E A 1969 *J. Acoust. Soc. Am.* **46** 587–601
[65] Eller A and Flynn E G 1969 *J. Acoust. Soc. Am.* **46** 722–7
[66] Hasecke F *et al* 2018 *Chem. Sci.* **9** 5937–48
[67] Adachi M, So M, Sakurai K, Kardos J and Goto Y 2015 *J. Biol. Chem.* **290** 18134–45
[68] Umemoto A, Yagi H, So M and Goto Y 2014 *J. Biol. Chem.* **289** 27290–9
[69] Knowles T P J, Waudby C A, Devlin G L, Cohen S I A, Aguzzi A, Vendruscolo M, Terentjev E M, Welland M E and Dobson C M 2009 *Science* **326** 1533–7

IOP Publishing

Ultrasonics
Physics and applications
Mami Matsukawa, Pak-Kon Choi, Kentaro Nakamura, Hirotsugu Ogi and Hideyuki Hasegawa

Chapter 9

High-frame-rate medical ultrasonic imaging

Hideyuki Hasegawa

Ultrasound is a highly beneficial modality for the noninvasive imaging of living bodies. Since an imaging frame rate of up to 100 Hz is available even in clinical ultrasonic equipment, ultrasound is often used for functional imaging, such as blood flow imaging and cardiac motion imaging. Recently, the benefits of ultrasound have been significantly enhanced by the introduction of high-frame-rate ultrasonic imaging, which achieves an extremely high frame rate of over 10 000 Hz. This chapter describes the principle of high-frame-rate medical ultrasonic imaging. The extremely high temporal resolution is highly beneficial for the measurement of dynamic tissue properties. This chapter also describes the applications of high-frame-rate ultrasonic imaging.

9.1 Introduction

In early medical ultrasound imaging, an ultrasonic image was obtained by mechanically translating or rotating a single-element transducer [1]. Such imaging methods were strongly influenced by underwater sonar imaging [2]. Subsequently, array transducers were developed to translate the transmit–receive aperture and control the ultrasonic field [3, 4] to obtain ultrasound images in real time. Owing to this historical background, current clinical ultrasound systems generate focused beams in both transmission and reception, and the transmit–receive event is repeated after translating the aperture position using an array transducer. In such a sequence, a number of transmit–receive events are required to obtain the received lines which are required to compose an ultrasound image, and thus, the imaging frame rate is limited to less than 100 Hz (this sequence is referred to as 'line-by-line acquisition' in this chapter). Nevertheless, this temporal resolution (frame rate) is much better than those of other modalities, such as computed tomography (CT) and magnetic resonance imaging (MRI). The concept of high-frame-rate imaging based on illuminating a target with a wide ultrasonic beam and creating received lines in parallel from backscattered echoes was introduced in medical ultrasonic imaging to further increase the frame rate [5, 6]. High-frame-rate ultrasonic imaging enables the measurement of the transient propagation of shear waves produced in tissue due to its extremely high temporal resolution [7] and is also used in various applications for functional imaging [8].

9.2 High-frame-rate ultrasonic imaging

In line-by-line acquisition, which is commonly used in clinical ultrasound systems, one or a few received beams are created for each emission of a focused transmitted beam. Using this approach, a number of emissions are required to obtain the received beams (referred to as scan lines or received lines in this chapter) required to construct an ultrasonic image. In contrast to the approach used in line-by-line acquisition, in high-frame-rate ultrasonic imaging, a plane wave illuminates a wide region, as illustrated in figure 9.1(a). During reception, multiple received beams are created in parallel, as illustrated in figure 9.1(b). In the extreme case, an imaging field of view can be illuminated by just a single shot of a plane wave, and then all the received beams required to construct an ultrasound image can be created at once. In this case, the imaging frame rate is the same as the pulse repetition frequency (PRF). The speed of sound in biological soft tissue is approximately 1500 m s^{-1}; thus, the PRF is 10 000 Hz when the maximum imaging depth is 75 mm. This imaging frame rate is significantly higher than that in a line-by-line acquisition at less than 100 Hz.

As described above, ultrasound imaging that uses single emission of a plane wave realizes an extremely high frame rate. On the other hand, the lateral resolution and contrast are significantly degraded because of the loss of focus in transmission. Image quality in high-frame-rate ultrasonic imaging can be improved by sending plane waves to each imaging point from multiple directions. This is called the coherent plane-wave compounding (CPWC) technique. It has theoretically been shown that CPWC produces a similar effect to the use of a focused transmitted beam [9]. The maximum available steering angle θ_{max} of a plane wave is determined by the

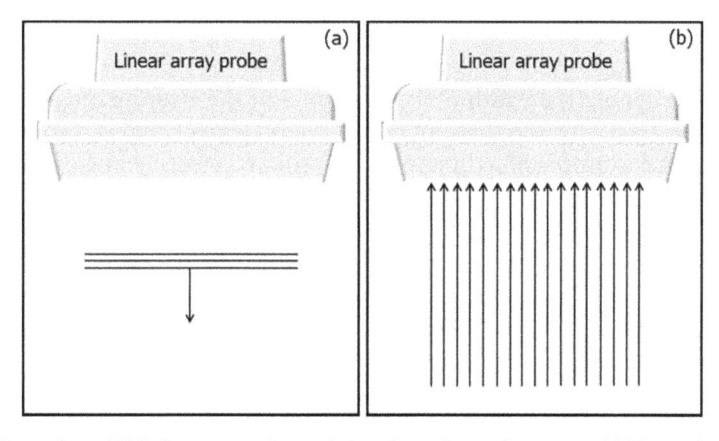

Figure 9.1. Illustration of high-frame-rate ultrasonic imaging using a plane wave. (a) Transmission of a plane wave. (b) Parallel receive beamforming.

element pitch d of an array. The wave number k_x of a plane wave with a steering angle of θ_{max} is given by $k_0 \sin\theta_{max}$, where k_0 is the wave number in the direction of ultrasonic propagation. The spatial frequency $k_x/2\pi$ of the plane wave in the lateral direction should be less than half the spatial sampling frequency $1/d$ in the lateral direction. This condition yields a relationship expressed as

$$\frac{k_0 \sin\theta_{max}}{2\pi} = \frac{1}{2d} \implies \sin\theta_{max} = \frac{\lambda}{2d}, \tag{9.1}$$

where λ is the ultrasonic wavelength in the direction of propagation. A typical value of λ/d ranges between one and two for medical ultrasound probes. Therefore, θ_{max} theoretically ranges from 30° to 90°. When the array is composed of N elements, all the information available from this array is retained by N components at spatial frequencies of i/Nd ($i = -N/2, \ldots, N/2 - 1$).

Compounding multiple plane waves at different steering angles corresponds to synthetic transmit focusing, and the correspondence between CPWC and conventional cylindrical focusing has been proven theoretically [9]. CPWC achieves a lateral resolution which is the same as that of conventional cylindrical focusing, using n of the N elements, where n is expressed as

$$n = \frac{Nd}{\lambda F}. \tag{9.2}$$

The f-number in receive beamforming is denoted by F. The value of n is 96 when $d = \lambda$, $N = 192$, and $F = 2$. Under these conditions, the plane wave should be steered within ±15°. It is to be expected that the resolution can be improved further by increasing the steering angle. However, one should be wary of grating-lobe artifacts, particularly when the receiving beams are also steered, as in vector Doppler flow imaging [10]. Under a far-field approximation, the directivity $D(\theta)$ in the direction of observation θ is expressed as

$$D(\theta) = \left| \frac{\sin\left(\pi\frac{a}{\lambda}\sin\theta\right)}{\pi\frac{a}{\lambda}\sin\theta} \right| \left| \frac{\sin\left(\pi N \frac{d}{\lambda}(\sin\theta - \sin\theta_0)\right)}{\sin\left(\pi \frac{d}{\lambda}(\sin\theta - \sin\theta_0)\right)} \right| \equiv D_e(\theta) D_a(\theta), \tag{9.3}$$

where a and θ_0 denote the width of an element and the steering angle, respectively, and $D_e(\theta)$ and $D_a(\theta)$ are the directivities of each element and an array with ideal point sources. An example of a directivity pattern at a steering angle of 20° is shown in figure 9.2(a). The parameters N, a, d, and λ are set to 192, 0.18, 0.2, and 0.2 mm, respectively. Additionally, the corresponding ratio of the main-lobe level to the grating-lobe level (main-lobe/grating-lobe ratio) was calculated, as shown in figure 9.2(b). As shown in figure 9.2(b), the grating-lobe level increases significantly with increasing steering angles. Therefore, beam steering in receive beamforming is typically limited to a maximum steering angle of 10° for motion estimation when the element pitch d is comparable to the ultrasonic wavelength λ [10–12].

Additionally, increasing the plane-wave steering angle reduces the fully compounded region, as illustrated in figure 9.3. When the steering angles of the received

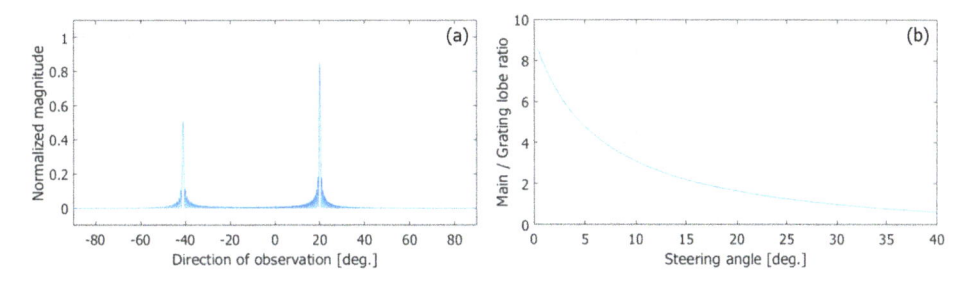

Figure 9.2. (a) Far-field directivity pattern at a steering angle of 20°. (b) Main-lobe to grating-lobe ratio.

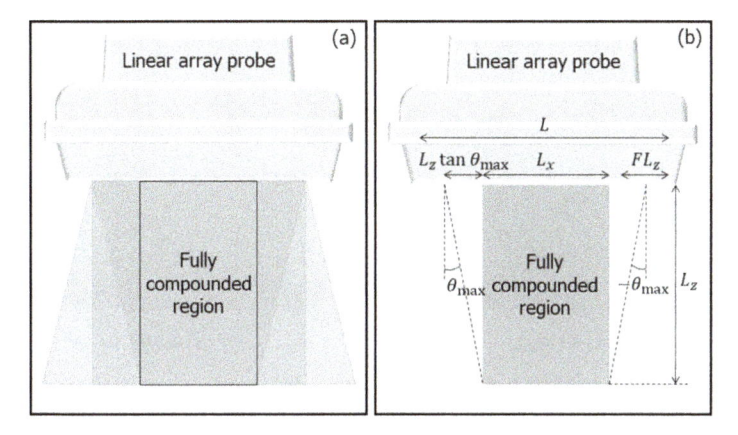

Figure 9.3. (a) Illustration of the fully compounded region. (b) Relationship between the lateral size of the fully compounded region and parameters in the beamforming process.

beams are zero, as in [9], the relationship between the lateral size L_x of the fully compounded region and the physical aperture size L is expressed as

$$L = L_x + 2L_z \tan\theta_{max}$$

$$\Longrightarrow L_x = L - 2L_z \tan\theta_{max}, \tag{9.4}$$

where L_z is the vertical size of the fully compounded region. In this case, the aperture for receive beamforming can be omitted except in the case in which the maximum steering angle θ_{max} is very small.

On the other hand, when the steering angle of the receiving beams is the same as that of the transmitted plane wave [10, 12], the relationship between the lateral size L_x of the fully compounded region and the physical aperture size L is expressed as

$$L = L_x + 2L_z \tan\theta_{max} + \frac{L_z}{F}$$

$$\Longrightarrow L_x = L - 2L_z \tan\theta_{max} - \frac{L_z}{F}, \tag{9.5}$$

where F is the f-number in receive beamforming, and L_z/F corresponds to the largest aperture size in receive beamforming.

Figure 9.4 shows the ratio of the lateral size of the fully compounded region to the physical aperture size obtained using equation (9.4) at an f-number of two in receive beamforming. As shown in figure 9.4, the lateral size of the fully compounded region is significantly increased by increasing the maximum steering angle. As described above, the imaging parameters, including the maximum steering angles, should be optimized depending on the application. Basically, an ultrasonic probe with a fine element pitch (low d/λ) can suppress grating lobes, and large steering angles are feasible using such a probe. On the other hand, a greater number of elements are also required to maintain a sufficient imaging field of view.

Figures 9.5 and 9.6 show examples of line-by-line and CPWC imaging obtained by simulations using the Field II software [13, 14]. Figures 9.5(a)–(c) show B-mode

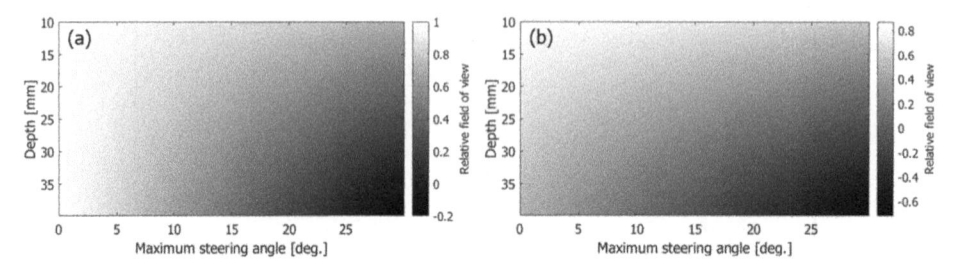

Figure 9.4. Ratio of the lateral field of view to physical aperture size at an f-number of two in receive beamforming. (a) No steering in reception. (b) Same steering angle in reception as in the emission of plane waves.

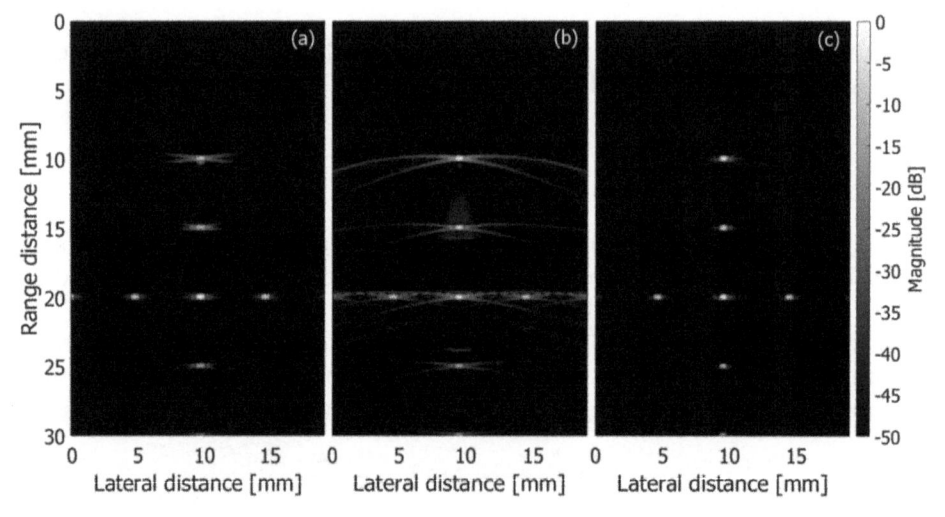

Figure 9.5. B-mode images of point targets obtained by Field II simulations. (a) Line-by-line acquisition with a transmitted beam focused at 20 mm. (b) Plane-wave imaging (single emission, no steering). (c) Plane-wave imaging (97 emissions, steering angles: ±15°).

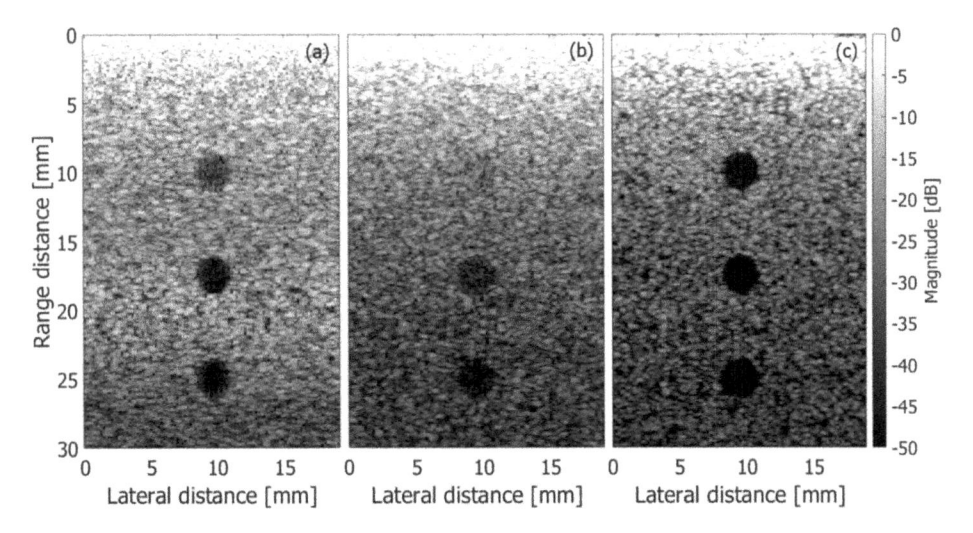

Figure 9.6. B-mode images of anechoic cyst targets obtained by Field II simulations. (a) Line-by-line acquisition with a transmitted beam focused at 20 mm. (b) Plane-wave imaging (single emission, no steering). (c) Plane-wave imaging (97 emissions, steering angles: ±15°).

images of point targets obtained using line-by-line acquisition with a transmitted beam focused at 20 mm, a single emission of a nonsteered plane wave, and CPWC imaging with 97 emissions at steering angles within ±15°, respectively. Similar results for anechoic cyst phantoms are shown in figure 9.6.

Imaging with a single emission of a plane wave achieves an extremely high frame rate that corresponds to the PRF (a typical PRF used to image superficial tissues, such as a carotid artery, is 10 kHz). On the other hand, the side-lobe level is high, as shown in figure 9.5(b). CPWC imaging reduces the side-lobe level, as shown in figure 9.5(c), which is similar to that of line-by-line acquisition in figure 9.5(a) around the transmission's focal position of 20 mm. Since coherent compounding is performed over the entire imaging field of view, CPWC imaging achieves similar side-lobe levels at different depths, as shown in figure 9.5(c).

The high side-lobe level in single-emission plane-wave imaging also affects the imaging of anechoic cyst targets. The contrast between the anechoic cyst region and the speckle background is significantly degraded, as shown in figure 9.6(b), compared with the B-mode image obtained by line-by-line acquisition in figure 9.6(a). Reduction of the side-lobe level by CPWC imaging improves the contrast of the cyst targets at different depths, as shown in figure 9.6(c).

As demonstrated by the results shown in figures 9.5 and 9.6, CPWC imaging offers great flexibility to control the trade-off between temporal and spatial resolutions. Imaging that uses fewer emissions realizes an extremely high frame rate. On the other hand, image quality can be improved by increasing the number of emissions at different steering angles, while the imaging frame rate is reduced. One of the major issues in compound high-frame-rate imaging is the artifacts induced by target motion between emissions, because target motion decreases the coherence between images obtained using plane waves at different steering angles. Methods for motion correction have been developed to improve image quality in compound imaging [15].

In CPWC imaging, a beamformed radio-frequency (RF) signal is obtained for each transmit–receive event. The beamformed RF signal obtained per plane-wave emission in high-frame-rate imaging corresponds to a low-resolution image in synthetic aperture imaging [16], in which spherical waves are sequentially emitted by individual transducer elements. Therefore, a spherical wave is also used in high-frame-rate ultrasound imaging. This is particularly beneficial in cardiac imaging, because a wide field of view should be realized using a small-footprint probe (aperture size). To increase the penetration depth, a spherical wave is often emitted using multiple transducer elements to emulate a spherical wave produced by a virtual point source behind an array. In high-frame-rate imaging with spherical transmitted beams and a small footprint, it is more difficult to perform a compounding process than in plane-wave imaging with a relatively large footprint. In such cases, compounding is performed by linearly translating the virtual point source within a limited footprint [17] or by steering the spherically diverging wave [18].

9.3 Motion estimators

For functional ultrasonic imaging, such as blood flow imaging and the measurement of tissue mechanical properties, motion estimators are indispensable. This section describes representative motion estimators used in medical ultrasonic imaging.

9.3.1 Autocorrelation method

It was initially demonstrated that cardiac blood flow could be detected by the ultrasonic Doppler method [19]. Using the Doppler method, velocity components along an ultrasonic beam, i.e. axial velocity, can be estimated. Later, the autocorrelation method was developed to image the spatial distribution of axial flow velocities in real time [20]. Let us consider an ultrasonic signal received from a target to be a regionally sinusoidal wave at frequency f_0. In such a case, the complex analytic signal of the received signal $\tilde{s}_1(t)$ resulting from the first emission can be modeled as follows:

$$\tilde{s}_1(t) = e^{j\omega_0 t}, \tag{9.6}$$

where $\omega_0 = 2\pi f_0$ and the amplitude of the received signal is omitted. When the target moves in the direction of ultrasonic propagation at velocity v, the complex received signal $\tilde{s}_2(t)$ resulting from the second emission can be expressed as follows:

$$\tilde{s}_2(t) = \exp\left\{j\omega_0\left(t - \frac{vT}{c_0}\right)\right\}, \tag{9.7}$$

where T and c_0 are the time intervals between emissions and the speed of sound, respectively. The correlation function $\gamma(\tau, \delta n)$ of $\tilde{s}_i(t)$ at temporal lag τ and emission lag δn is expressed as

$$\gamma(\tau, \delta n) = \frac{1}{2T_w} \int_{-T_w}^{T_w} s_1^*(t) \cdot s_{1+\delta n}(t + \tau) dt, \quad (9.8)$$

where T_w determines the length of a correlation kernel size, and * denotes the complex conjugate. From the relationships of equations (9.6)–(9.8), the target velocity v can be estimated to be

$$\hat{v} = -\frac{\omega_0 c_0}{T} \angle \gamma(0, 1), \quad (9.9)$$

where $\hat{}$ and $\angle$ denote an estimate and the phase angle of a complex value, respectively. The angular frequency ω_0 of the received signal can also be estimated using

$$\hat{\omega}_0 = \frac{\angle \gamma(T_s, 0)}{T_s}, \quad (9.10)$$

where T_s denotes the sampling interval of the received signal.

9.3.2 Vector Doppler method

The autocorrelation method described in section 9.3.1 estimates the velocity component in the direction of ultrasonic propagation, i.e. the axial velocity. Therefore, the true magnitude and direction of the target motion velocity cannot be estimated by the autocorrelation method. To overcome this limitation, the multiangle Doppler method was developed. Although 3D estimation is required to obtain the true motion velocity, 2D estimation is considered in this chapter.

As illustrated in figure 9.7, let us define the beam-steering angles θ_i and φ_j used for the ith transmission and the jth received beam, respectively, with respect to a target

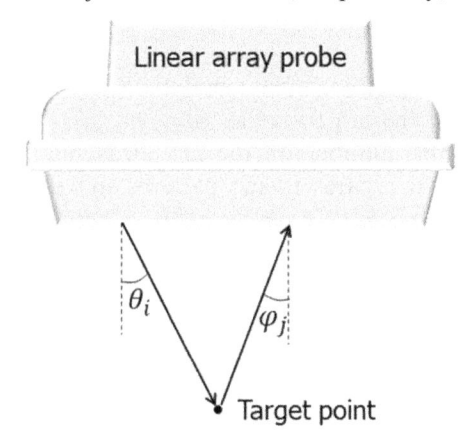

Figure 9.7. Illustration of beam-steering angles in transmission and reception.

point. The axial velocity $v_{\text{ax}}(i, j)$ measured using transmitted and received beams at steering angles of θ_i and φ_j, respectively, can be expressed using the lateral and vertical components of the target velocity, v_x and v_z, respectively, as follows [21]:

$$v_x(\cos\theta_i + \cos\varphi_j) + v_z(\sin\theta_i + \sin\varphi_j) = 2v_{\text{ax}}(i, j). \quad (9.11)$$

By measuring the axial velocities $v_{\text{ax}}(i, j)$ from multiple directions of transmission and reception, the relationships obtained can be formulated in matrix form:

$$\begin{bmatrix} \cos\theta_1 + \cos\varphi_1 & \sin\theta_1 + \sin\varphi_1 \\ \vdots & \vdots \\ \cos\theta_{B_t} + \cos\varphi_{B_r} & \sin\theta_{B_t} + \sin\varphi_{B_r} \end{bmatrix} \begin{bmatrix} v_x \\ v_z \end{bmatrix} = \begin{bmatrix} v_{\text{ax}}(1, 1) \\ \vdots \\ v_{\text{ax}}(B_t, B_r) \end{bmatrix}$$

$$\Longrightarrow \mathbf{A}\mathbf{v} = \mathbf{v}_{\text{ax}}, \quad (9.12)$$

where B_t and B_r are the numbers of transmitted and received beams, respectively. The solution of equation (9.12) is given by [10]:

$$\hat{\mathbf{v}} = (\mathbf{A}^T\mathbf{A})^{-1}\mathbf{A}^T\mathbf{v}_{\text{ax}}, \quad (9.13)$$

where ^{T} denotes the transpose operation, and the entity $(\mathbf{A}^T\mathbf{A})^{-1}\mathbf{A}^T$ is the pseudoinverse of A.

9.3.3 Block-matching method

To realize good accuracy in the estimation of lateral velocities using the multiangle Doppler method, the beam-steering angle used should be as large as possible. However, the available maximum steering angle depends on the relationship between the size of the probe footprint and the maximum observation depth. Therefore, it is difficult to apply the multiangle Doppler method to a scenario in which the probe footprint is small relative to the maximum observation depth, such as cardiac imaging. In such a situation, the block-matching method, which is often called the speckle-tracking method, is used for 2D or 3D motion estimation in echocardiography.

Let us define the sampled complex analytic signal of the 2D beamformed ultrasonic echo signal in the nth frame as $\tilde{s}(m_x, m_z, n)$, where m_x and m_z are the lateral and vertical sample numbers of the 2D ultrasonic signal, respectively. The block-matching method compares image patterns in kernels (regions of interest (ROIs)) assigned in two images (2D signals here). A kernel is assigned in the earlier image frame, and its position is fixed. Another kernel is assigned in the later image frame, and its position is movable. The block-matching method evaluates the similarity between the patterns in the two kernels assigned in the two images by shifting the position of the kernel in the later image. By evaluating the similarity between the signals at each position of the kernel in the later frame, the similarity function reaches a maximum at the lateral and vertical shifts (lags) that correspond to the displacement of the target between the two image frames. To evaluate the similarity between the patterns in the two kernels, the normalized cross-correlation function is commonly used, which is expressed as

$$\gamma(m_x, m_z, n; \delta m_x, \delta m_z) = \frac{\sum_{i=-M_x}^{M_x} \sum_{j=-M_z}^{M_z} \tilde{s}^*(m_x + i, m_z + j, n) \cdot \tilde{s}(m_x + i + \delta m_x, m_z + j + \delta m_z, n + 1)}{\sqrt{\sum_{i=-M_x}^{M_x} \sum_{j=-M_z}^{M_z} |\tilde{s}^*(m_x + i, m_z + j, n)|^2} \sqrt{\sum_{i=-M_x}^{M_x} \sum_{j=-M_z}^{M_z} |m_x + i + \delta m_x, m_z + j + \delta m_z, n + 1|^2}}, \quad (9.14)$$

where M_x and M_z determine the kernel sizes in the lateral and vertical directions, respectively, and δm_x and δm_z are lateral and vertical lags, respectively. The lateral and vertical displacements u_x and u_z between the two frames are estimated as follows:

$$(u_x, u_z) = (\delta \hat{m}_x \cdot \delta x, \delta \hat{m}_z \cdot \delta z), \quad (9.15)$$

$$(\delta \hat{m}_x, \delta \hat{m}_z) = \arg \max_{\delta m_x, \delta m_z} \gamma(m_x, m_z, n; \delta m_x, \delta m_z). \quad (9.16)$$

Other functions, such as the sum of the absolute difference and the sum of the squared difference, are also used to evaluate the similarity between image patterns [22]. The correlation function defined by equation (9.14) is obtained for the lateral and vertical intervals δx and δz, respectively, which correspond to those of the sampled ultrasonic signal. Consequently, the resolution of the estimated displacements is limited by the sampling interval. To estimate a subsample small displacement, interpolation of the similarity function, such as reconstructive interpolation [23], is necessary.

The block-matching method is used for various purposes, such as the measurement of myocardial contraction and relaxation [22, 24], tissue elastography [23], vascular elastography [25, 26], and blood flow imaging [27, 28]. Although it is preferable to use RF signals to achieve good accuracy in the estimation of axial displacement, envelope signals provide more accurate estimates of lateral displacements than RF signals [29]. It should be noted that the axial direction is generally closer to the vertical direction than the lateral direction, because the beam-steering angle is limited by the limited physical size of an ultrasonic probe and the increased grating-lobe level, as described in section 9.2.

9.3.4 Spectrum-based motion estimator

The block-matching method described in section 9.3.3 can be applied to any type of image and is thus very useful for motion estimation. However, its high computational cost is a challenging issue. As described in section 9.3.3, the block-matching method with a normalized cross-correlation function requires interpolation of the correlation function for the estimation of subsample small displacements. For accurate interpolation of the correlation function, the correlation function should be calculated for a wide range of lags δm_x and δm_z. In high-frame-rate ultrasonic imaging, the time intervals between frames are small, and thus, the displacement of a target between frames tends to decrease more than the sampling interval of the correlation function (which is the same as that of the ultrasonic echo signal). Additionally, a large number of frames (up to 10 000 frames per second in the measurement of carotid arteries) need to be processed. Therefore, computational efficiency is important in motion estimation based on high-frame-rate ultrasonic imaging.

For the efficient estimation of 2D motion, a phase-sensitive motion estimator based on a frequency analysis of ultrasonic echo signals was developed [30]. Phase-sensitive motion estimators do not require any interpolation process to estimate subsample displacements, although they suffer from the aliasing effect. Phase-sensitive motion estimators are beneficial for the efficient estimation of target motion in high-frame-rate ultrasonic imaging, because target displacements between two consecutive frames tend to be smaller than the sampling intervals and do not cause the aliasing effect.

Let us define the 2D spatial frequency spectrum of a 2D beamformed ultrasonic RF signal $s(m_x, m_z, n)$ in the nth frame as $S(m_x, m_z, n; k_x, k_z)$, where k_x and k_z are wave numbers in the lateral and axial directions, respectively. The spatial frequency spectrum $S(m_x, m_z, n; k_x, k_z)$ is obtained by applying a Fourier transform to the beamformed RF signal $s(m_x, m_z, n)$ around a spatial position $(m_x \delta x, m_z \delta z)$. The spatial frequency spectrum $S(m_x, m_z, n; k_x, k_z)$ can be expressed as

$$S(m_x, m_z, n; k_x, k_z) = |S(m_x, m_z, n; k_x, k_z)| \exp\{j(k_x x + k_z z)\}, \tag{9.17}$$

where the initial phase of the ultrasonic signal is omitted. Under target displacements u_x and u_z in the lateral and vertical directions, respectively, the spatial frequency spectrum $S(m_x, m_z, n+1; k_x, k_z)$ in the $(n+1)$th frame can be expressed as

$$\begin{aligned} &S(m_x, m_z, n+1; k_x, k_z) \\ &= |S(m_x, m_z, n+1; k_x, k_z)| \times \exp[j\{k_x(x - u_x) + k_z(z - u_z)\}]. \end{aligned} \tag{9.18}$$

The cross spectrum $C(m_x, m_z, n; k_x, k_z; \delta k_x, \delta k_z, \delta n)$ is defined as

$$\begin{aligned} &C(m_x, m_z, n; k_x, k_z; \delta m_x, \delta m_z, \delta n) \\ &= S^*(m_x, m_z, n; k_x, k_z) \cdot S(m_x + \delta m_x, m_z + \delta m_z, n + \delta n; k_x, k_z), \end{aligned} \tag{9.19}$$

where δk_x, δk_z, and δn are lags in the directions of the lateral wave number, the vertical wave number, and the frame, respectively. Based on the models described in equations (9.17) and (9.18), the relationship described by equation (9.20) can be derived:

$$\angle C(m_x, m_z, n; k_x, k_z; 0, 0, 1) = -k_x u_x - k_z u_z. \tag{9.20}$$

Let us define the mean squared difference α between the phase of the cross spectrum and the model described in equation (9.20) as follows:

$$\alpha = \frac{1}{K} \sum_{k_x, k_z \in \Omega} w(k_x, k_z) \{\angle C(m_x, m_z, n; k_x, k_z; 0, 0, 1) + k_x u_x + k_z u_z\}^2, \tag{9.21}$$

where Ω is the range of the wave numbers used for the calculation of α and K is the number of wave number components in Ω. To determine the lateral and vertical displacements $\hat{u}_x$ and $\hat{u}_z$, which minimize the mean squared difference α, the partial derivatives of equation (9.21) with respect to u_x and u_z are set to zeros, as follows:

$$u_x \sum_{k_x,k_z \ni \Omega} w(k_x, k_z)k_x^2 + u_z \sum_{k_x,k_z \ni \Omega} w(k_x, k_z)k_x k_z$$

$$= - \sum_{k_x,k_z \ni \Omega} w(k_x, k_z) \angle C(m_x, m_z, n; k_x, k_z; 0, 0, 1)k_x$$

$$u_x \sum_{k_x,k_z \ni \Omega} w(k_x, k_z)k_x k_z + u_z \sum_{k_x,k_z \ni \Omega} w(k_x, k_z)k_z^2$$

$$= - \sum_{k_x,k_z \ni \Omega} w(k_x, k_z) \angle C(m_x, m_z, n; k_x, k_z; 0, 0, 1)k_z$$

$$\Rightarrow \mathbf{Ku} = -\mathbf{C}, \tag{9.22}$$

where

$$\mathbf{u} = (u_x u_z)^{\mathrm{T}}, \tag{9.23}$$

$$\mathbf{K} = \begin{pmatrix} w(k_x, k_z) \sum_{k_x,k_z \ni \Omega} k_x^2 & w(k_x, k_z) \sum_{k_x,k_z \ni \Omega} k_x k_z \\ w(k_x, k_z) \sum_{k_x,k_z \ni \Omega} k_x k_z & w(k_x, k_z) \sum_{k_x,k_z \ni \Omega} k_z^2 \end{pmatrix}, \tag{9.24}$$

$$\mathbf{C} = \begin{pmatrix} \sum_{k_x,k_z \ni \Omega} w(k_x, k_z) \angle C(m_x, m_z, n; k_x, k_z; 0, 0, 1)k_x \\ \sum_{k_x,k_z \ni \Omega} w(k_x, k_z) \angle C(m_x, m_z, n; k_x, k_z; 0, 0, 1)k_z \end{pmatrix}, \tag{9.25}$$

and $w(k_x, k_z)$ is a weighting function. The magnitude of the cross spectrum could be used as the weighting function $w(k_x, k_z)$. The least-squares solution to equation (9.22) is obtained using

$$\hat{\mathbf{u}} = -\mathbf{K}^{-1}\mathbf{C}, \tag{9.26}$$

where $^{-1}$ denotes an inverse matrix. The wave numbers k_x and k_z in the lateral and axial directions are also estimated using

$$\hat{k}_x = \frac{\angle C(m_x, m_z, n; k_x, k_z; 1, 0, 0)}{\delta x} \tag{9.27}$$

$$\hat{k}_z = \frac{\angle C(m_x, m_z, n; k_x, k_z; 0, 1, 0)}{\delta z}. \tag{9.28}$$

This method can be extended to a 3D phase-sensitive motion estimator [31].

9.4 Applications of high-frame-rate ultrasonic imaging

High-frame-rate ultrasonic imaging is now used for various purposes, from tissue elasticity imaging [7] to monitoring the generation of cavitation bubbles in high-intensity focused ultrasound (HIFU) therapy [32]. However, this article focuses on applications for cardiovascular dynamic measurements.

9.4.1 Strain or strain-rate imaging

The intima–media thickness (IMT) of the carotid artery is widely used for the ultrasonic diagnosis of atherosclerosis, because the IMT becomes larger during the progression of atherosclerosis, leading to the formation of atherosclerotic plaque [33]. Atherosclerotic plaque itself carries a risk of occluding the arterial lumen at its own sites when its size becomes very large. On the other hand, atherosclerotic plaques can possibly cause serious cardiovascular events, such as myocardial and cerebral infarction, even when their sizes are not extremely large. Atherosclerotic plaques often accumulate lipids in the intima–media region, and lipid-rich plaques, which are referred to as 'vulnerable atherosclerotic plaques,' are prone to rupture due to hemodynamic forces caused by cardiac pulsation [34]. Since the amount of lipids should affect the deformability of plaques, a method that can measure the elasticity of the arterial wall has the potential to evaluate the threat of atherosclerotic plaques.

Elastography was first developed for the evaluation of tissue elasticity by measuring strains by pressing tissues (applying external force) using an ultrasonic probe [23]. In arteries, cardiac pulsation changes the internal pressure of the artery almost once per second. This change in internal pressure during a cardiac cycle spontaneously produces deformation of the arterial wall, which corresponds to radial strain, and its magnitude is less than 0.1 mm within the intima–media complex, which has a typical thickness of 0.5 mm. In initial investigations, a 1D phase-sensitive estimator [35] and block-matching method [36] were used for the measurement of these minute deformations. The measurement of strain or strain rate requires high accuracy in estimating the displacement or motion velocity, because spatial differentiation is necessary to obtain the strain or strain rate. The least-squares strain estimator was developed for the stable estimation of strain or strain rate [37].

To estimate each strain component using the least-squares method, the spatial distributions of the lateral and vertical displacements u_x and u_z are assumed to be linear functions of the lateral and axial positions x and z. In the 2D case, the relationships are described by

$$u_x = a_x x + b_x z + c_x, \quad (9.29)$$

$$u_z = a_z x + b_z z + c_z, \quad (9.30)$$

where a_x, b_x, c_x, a_z, b_z, and c_z are coefficients describing the linear functions in equations (9.29) and (9.30). In this case, each component of strain is described using coefficients a_x, b_x, a_z, and b_z as follows:

$$\varepsilon_{xx} = \frac{\partial u_x}{\partial x} = a_x, \qquad (9.31)$$

$$\varepsilon_{zz} = \frac{\partial u_z}{\partial z} = b_z, \qquad (9.32)$$

$$\varepsilon_{zx} = \frac{1}{2}\left(\frac{\partial u_z}{\partial x} + \frac{\partial u_x}{\partial z}\right) = \frac{1}{2}(a_z + b_x), \qquad (9.33)$$

where ε_{xx} and ε_{zz} are normal strains in the lateral and axial directions, respectively, and ε_{zx} is the shear strain. From the relationships given in equations (9.32) and (9.33), one can see that each component of strain can be estimated by fitting the linear relationships in equations (9.29) and (9.30) to the measured lateral and vertical displacements in a region of interest (strain kernel) using the least-squares method. Similarly, the strain rates are estimated by replacing the lateral and vertical displacements u_x and u_z with the lateral and vertical velocities v_x and v_z, respectively. One-dimensional estimation of the radial strain of an arterial wall makes it possible to image the artery in the longitudinal axis view [35] or place an intravascular ultrasonic probe at the center of an artery [36], because the direction of an ultrasonic beam almost corresponds to the radial direction of the artery in such situations. On the other hand, more accurate strain estimates can be obtained using 2D or 3D measurements [38–40].

It is possible to evaluate the accuracy of motion and deformation estimates using simulation. A numerical model is typically constructed by distributing point scatterers. Figure 9.8(a) shows an example of a horizontally aligned cylindrical simulation phantom [40]. In the cylindrical phantom, point scatterers are randomly distributed in a cylindrical shape. The scattering coefficients of the scatterers are also assigned randomly. The displacement of a cylindrical shell during an increase in its internal pressure is analytically obtained, as it is inversely proportional to the distance from the central axis of the cylinder. To simulate this motion of the phantom, the distributed scatterers are moved according to

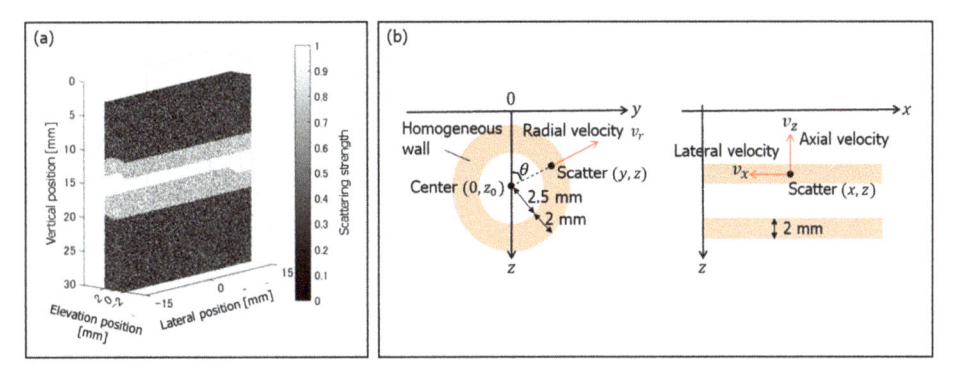

Figure 9.8. Illustration of a numerical cylindrical phantom. Adapted from [40]. Copyright 2019 The Japan Society of Applied Physics. All rights reserved. (a) Distributed point scatterers. (b) Scatterer's motion velocity.

$$v_x = V_l, \quad (9.34)$$

$$v_y = v_r \sin\phi, \quad (9.35)$$

$$v_z = v_r \cos\phi, \quad (9.36)$$

$$v_r = \frac{V_r}{\sqrt{y^2 + (z-z_0)^2}}, \quad (9.37)$$

$$\phi = \tan^{-1}\frac{y}{z_0 - z}, \quad (9.38)$$

where V_l and V_r are constants that determine the maximum velocities in the arterial longitudinal and radial directions, respectively. The lateral, elevational, and vertical positions of a scatterer in the coordinate system in ultrasound imaging are denoted by x, y, and z, respectively, and the vertical position of the central axis of the cylinder is z_0. First, arterial motion was considered to occur only in its radial direction owing to an increase in internal pressure. However, it was later found that the arterial wall also moved in its longitudinal direction with the same order of magnitude as that of the radial motion [41]. Therefore, the effects in the arterial longitudinal direction should also be considered. In [40], only the radial strain or strain rate were considered, even when both lateral and vertical displacements or velocities were estimated, because the estimation accuracy of the lateral displacements or velocities was significantly lower than that of the vertical displacements or velocities.

The results of the numerical simulation of the cylindrical phantom are shown in figure 9.9. Ultrasonic echo signals acquired with a 7.5 MHz linear array composed of 192 elements at element pitches of 0.2 mm were simulated using the Field II software [13, 14]. The beamformed ultrasonic signal at each spatial position was obtained using a single emission of a nonsteered plane wave. To simulate an acquisition system with a limited number of transmit–receive channels (in this case, 96), the imaging

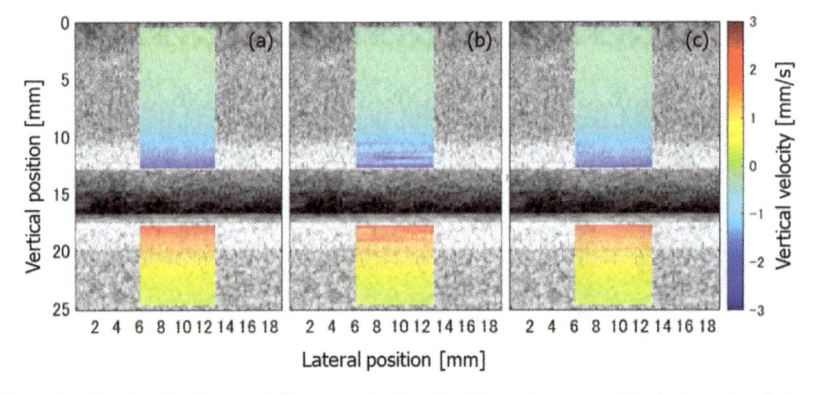

Figure 9.9. Velocity distributions of the numerical cylindrical phantom. (a) Assigned velocity values. (b) Velocities estimated by 1D estimator. (c) Velocities estimated by 2D estimator.

field of view was divided into four segments, and each segment, which had 24 receive lines at 0.2-mm intervals, was imaged using a single emission of a nonsteered plane wave. Consequently, an image frame composed of 96 receive lines was obtained using four emissions. The expected frame rate was 1302 Hz at a pulse repetition interval (PRI) of 192 μs.

The assigned radial (vertical) motion velocities of the phantom are shown in figure 9.9(a). The velocities were overlaid on the corresponding B-mode image of the phantom. The maximum phantom longitudinal motion velocity was set to 15 mm s^{-1}. The phantom radial velocities in figure 9.9(b) were estimated by a 1D phase-sensitive motion estimator [42]. As seen in figure 9.9(b), some fluctuations, which are not seen in the true velocity distribution in figure 9.9(a), occur in the estimated velocity distribution in the case of 1D estimation. Figure 9.9(c) shows the velocity distribution obtained by a 2D phase-sensitive motion estimator [30]. As a result of the use of 2D estimation, the undesirable fluctuations in the velocity distribution in figure 9.9(b) are largely suppressed.

Figures 9.10(a)–(c) show the phantom radial (vertical normal) strain distributions obtained from the true velocity distribution (figure 9.9(a)), the velocity distribution estimated by the 1D phase-sensitive motion estimator (figure 9.9(b)), and that estimated by the 2D phase-sensitive motion estimator (figure 9.9(c)), respectively. In the same way as for the estimation of velocities, more accurate strain estimates can be obtained from the 2D motion estimator when bidirectional motion exists. A 2D matrix array probe and a 3D motion estimator would be the ideal combination for a target exhibiting 3D motion.

The utilization of numerical simulations, such as finite-element analysis and computational fluid dynamics analysis, is one of the strategies used to evaluate ultrasonic motion estimators in more complex scenarios. A model consisting of a cylindrical shell with an atherosclerotic plaque model and the surrounding tissue model illustrated in figure 9.11 was analyzed via fluid–structure interaction analysis using COMSOL Multiphysics® software [43].

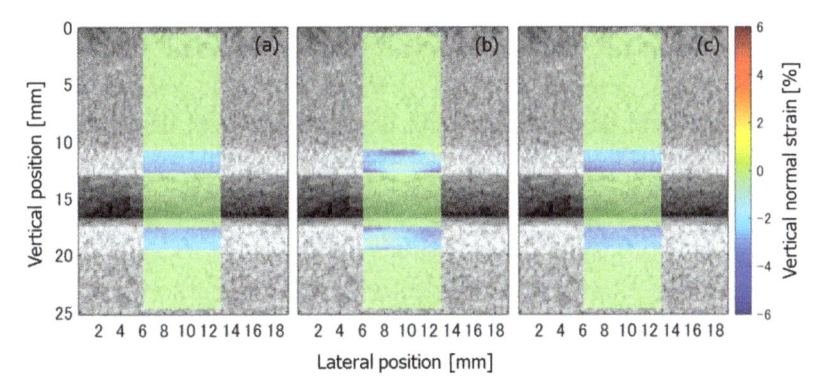

Figure 9.10. Radial (vertical normal) strains of the numerical cylindrical phantom obtained from assigned velocity values (a), velocities estimated by the 1D estimator (b), and velocities estimated by the 2D estimator. Adapted from [40]. Copyright 2019 The Japan Society of Applied Physics. All rights reserved.

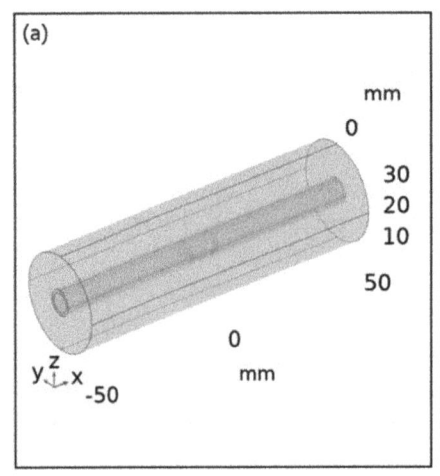

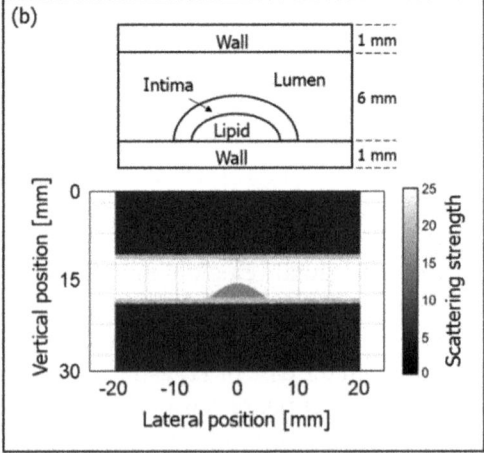

Figure 9.11. Arterial model that includes lesions mimicking atherosclerotic plaques. Adapted from [43]. © 2019 The Japan Society of Applied Physics. All rights reserved. (a) Model of the artery and surrounding tissue. (b) Longitudinal cross section of the model: (top) conceptual scheme; (bottom) distributed scatterers.

Table 9.1. Material properties of the arterial model. Adapted from [43]. Copyright 2021 The Japan Society of Applied Physics. All rights reserved.

Material properties	Values
Young's modulus of fibrous cap and wall	600 kPa
Young's modulus of lipids	50 kPa
Young's modulus of surrounding tissue	200 kPa
Densities of tissues	1000 kg m^{-3}
Poisson's ratio	0.49

To construct the arterial model, a cylindrical shell with internal and external diameters of 8 and 10 mm, respectively, was first generated. The cylindrical tube was surrounded by a tissue-mimicking material. The radius of the external surface of the tissue-mimicking material was 15 mm. An ellipsoid part was placed on the internal surface of the cylindrical tube as an atherosclerotic plaque model. The plaque model included lipids and covering intima with thicknesses of 1.0 and 1.5 mm, respectively. The models of the arterial wall and surrounding tissue were assumed to be homogeneous, isotropic, and incompressible Hooke's solids. The material properties of the model, i.e. the Young's moduli, densities, and Poisson's ratios of the arterial wall, intima, lipids, and surrounding tissue, are described in table 9.1. The densities and Poisson's ratios were set to constant values for the arterial wall, intima, lipids, and surrounding tissue. The density and viscosity of the fluid used to simulate blood were set to 1060 kg m^{-3} and 0.005 Pa • s, respectively. The applied pressure increment inside the arterial model was 40 mm Hg, which is a typical value under physiological conditions. Ultrasonic point scatterers were randomly distributed in the arterial model and surrounding tissue model, as shown in figure 9.11(c)(bottom). The point scatterers were moved based on the displacements obtained by fluid–structure interaction analysis using COMSOL software.

The ultrasonic echo signals from the arterial model were also simulated using Field II software. A 7.5 MHz linear array composed of 192 elements at pitches of 0.2 mm was simulated, and beamformed signals were obtained by a single emission of a nonsteered plane wave. In this simulation, a plane wave was emitted by all 192 elements, and 96 receive lines were created for each emission. The expected frame rate was 10 417 Hz at a PRI of 96 μs. Figures 9.12(a) and (b) show the assigned vertical velocity distribution in the plaque model and the velocity distribution estimated by the 2D phase-sensitive motion estimator, respectively, overlaid on the corresponding B-mode image. As shown in figure 9.12, the velocity distribution obtained by the 2D phase-sensitive motion estimator was in good agreement with the assigned velocity distribution. Figures 9.13(a) and (b) show the vertical normal

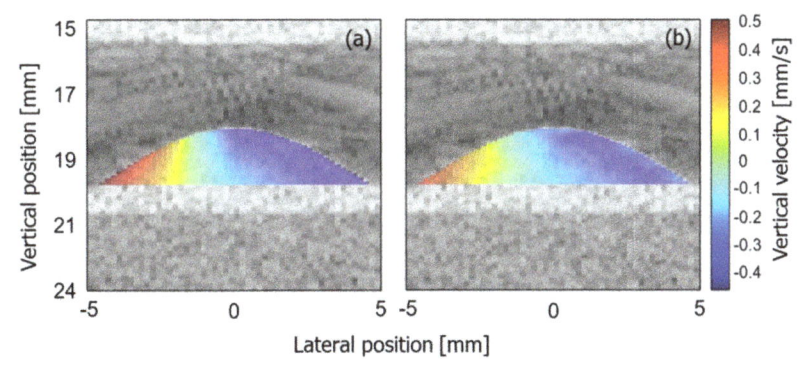

Figure 9.12. Velocity distributions in the atherosclerotic plaque model. Adapted from [43]. Copyright 2019 The Japan Society of Applied Physics. All rights reserved. (a) Assigned velocity values. (b) Velocities estimated by 2D estimator.

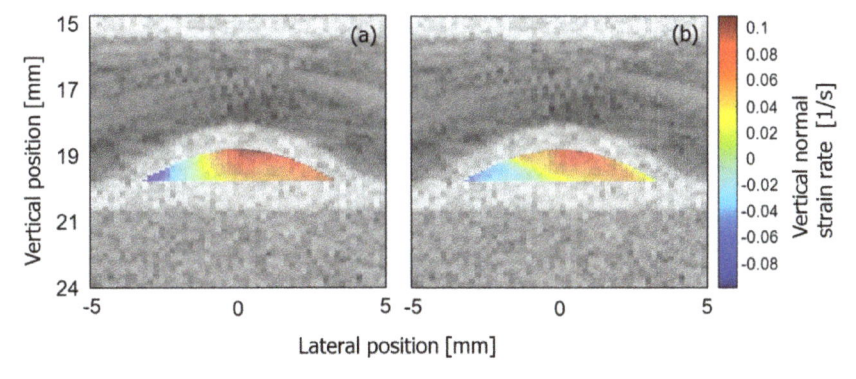

Figure 9.13. Strain rate distributions in the atherosclerotic plaque model obtained from the assigned velocity distribution (a) and the velocity distribution estimated by the 2D motion estimator (b). Adapted from [43]. Copyright 2019 The Japan Society of Applied Physics. All rights reserved.

(corresponding to phantom radial) strain-rate distributions obtained from the assigned velocity distribution and the velocity distribution estimated by the 2D phase-sensitive motion estimator. Although the strain distribution around the luminal edge of the plaque model could not be estimated accurately due to the irregular shape of the plaque model and the effect of a finite strain kernel size, the strain-rate distribution estimated by the 2D phase-sensitive motion estimator was also in good agreement with the assigned strain-rate distribution.

Figure 9.14(1) and (2) show examples of *in vivo* measurements of carotid artery atherosclerotic plaques. Ultrasonic echoes from the arteries were measured using a 7.5 MHz linear array probe (Fujifilm, UST-5412) composed of 192 elements at pitches of 0.2 mm. The echo signals received by individual elements were acquired with a custom-made ultrasound imaging system (RSYS0016, Microsonic) at a sampling frequency of 31.25 MHz. In the *in vivo* measurement of carotid atherosclerotic plaques, undesirable echoes from side lobes should be reduced compared with plane-wave imaging for better visualization of the plaques. Therefore, high-frame-rate imaging was realized by synthetic aperture imaging using a spherically diverging transmitted beam. A spherically diverging beam from a virtual point source at a distance of 40 mm behind the array was emulated using 72 active elements in a transmission aperture. Delay-and-sum (DAS) beamforming was performed on the received echo signals in each transmit–receive event to obtain low-resolution beamformed RF signals. The transmission aperture was translated laterally by six elements, and the same transmit–receive event was repeated.

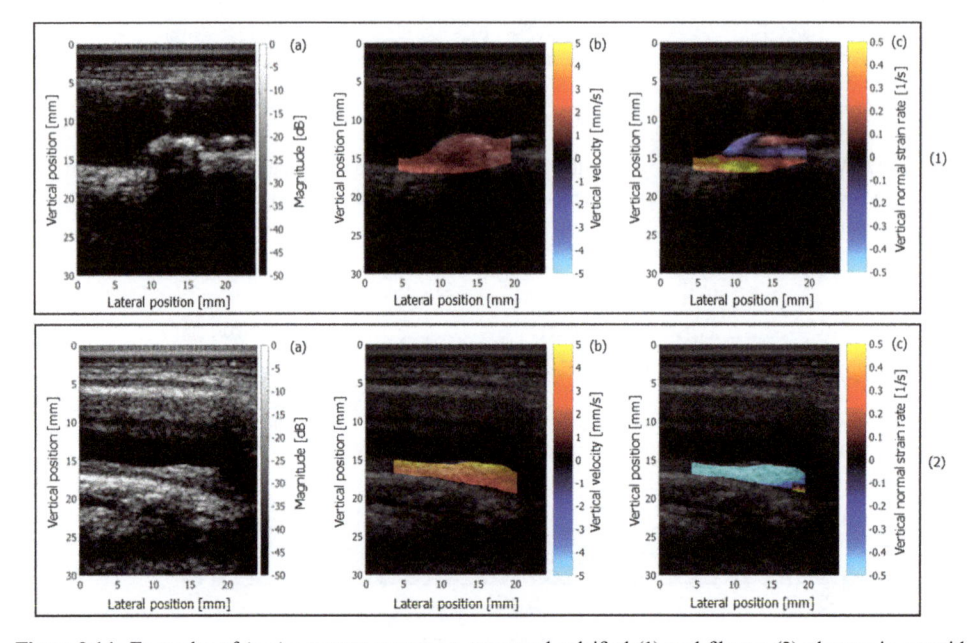

Figure 9.14. Examples of *in vivo* measurements on presumed calcified (1) and fibrous (2) plaques in carotid arteries. (a) B-mode image. (b) Estimated vertical velocity distribution. (c) Estimated vertical normal strain rates.

High-resolution RF signals were obtained by repeating the transmit–receive event 21 times and coherently compounding the resultant low-resolution beamformed RF signals. The frame rate was 496 Hz at a PRI of 96 μs. The B-mode images in figures 9.14(1-a) and (2-a) were obtained from the high-resolution RF signals, and the 2D phase-sensitive motion estimator was applied to the high-resolution RF signals. The strain-rate distributions in figures 9.14(1-c) and (2-c) were obtained by applying the least-squares strain estimator to the vertical velocity distributions in figures 9.14(1-b) and (2-b), respectively. Based on the observation of an expert, the atherosclerotic plaques in figures 9.14(1) and (2) were presumed to be calcified and fibrous plaques, respectively, because of the high brightness and homogeneous speckle patterns in figures 9.14(1-a) and (2-a), respectively. The calcified plaque showed significantly lower strain rates than the fibrous plaque. Tissue strain or strain-rate imaging can detect this type of difference in the deformability (mechanical property) of plaques due to the difference in their compositions.

9.4.2 Measurement of propagation of mechanical waves in tissue

As described in section 9.4.1, strain or strain-rate elastography is useful for the assessment of tissue mechanical properties. However, it can only evaluate a relative difference in elastic properties because the stress distribution in the tissue under deformation is generally unknown. Although some attempts have been made to estimate the stress distribution using the finite element method [44], the quantitative estimation of elastic properties based on strain or strain-rate elastography is ongoing. Shear-wave elastography measures the propagation speed of a shear wave propagating in tissue. The shear-wave speed c_s in an isotropic linear elastic medium is expressed as

$$c_s = \sqrt{\frac{\mu}{\rho}}, \qquad (9.39)$$

where μ and ρ denote the shear modulus and the density of the medium, respectively. Therefore, the shear modulus μ can be estimated by measuring the propagation speed c_s of a shear wave in tissue and assuming the density ρ. Consequently, shear-wave elastography is expected to serve as a quantitative method for the evaluation of tissue elastic properties. Initially, a shear wave was generated by an external oscillating force acting on the skin surface [45], and the penetration depth was limited. In the early 2000s, an innovative method emerged. In this method, a shear wave is generated by acoustic radiation forces produced by a focused ultrasonic beam, called a 'push beam,' and the generated shear wave is measured by high-frame-rate ultrasonic imaging [7]. By controlling the focal spot of the push beam, shear waves can be generated in an organ situated deep inside the body, such as the liver [46]. This method has also been applied to measure the elastic property of an arterial wall [47]. However, the generated mechanical wave would be a guided wave, such as a Lamb wave, in a layered structure and would exhibit significant dispersion, since its wavelength would be greater than the thickness of the arterial wall [48].

In arteries, pressure waves are spontaneously generated by the pulsation of the heart. This wave, called the pulse wave, was used to evaluate the elastic property of the arterial wall long ago. The relationship between the pulse-wave velocity (PWV) and Young's modulus E_w is expressed by

$$\text{PWV} = \sqrt{\frac{E_w h}{2\rho r_i}}, \tag{9.40}$$

where h and ρ denote the thickness and density of the arterial wall, respectively, and r_i denotes the inner radius of the artery. In a traditional PWV method, the pulsation of the artery is measured at two different positions along the arterial tree using tactile sensors placed on the skin surface above the artery. The PWV is obtained by estimating the time delay between the measured pulsation waveforms and assuming the length of the propagation path between the two positions. The two sensors are typically placed on the brachial and ankle arteries [49]. The sensing positions are several tens of centimetres apart from each other, and the average elastic property between the two positions can be evaluated. The traditional PWV method is useful for screening a long segment of artery between the two sensing positions. On the other hand, the stiffness of the artery differs depending on the position, i.e. peripheral arteries are stiffer than central arteries, and focal lesions are often generated during the progression of atherosclerosis. Therefore, more regional measurements of PWV are also needed.

An extremely high temporal resolution in high-frame-rate ultrasonic imaging is beneficial when analyzing the propagation of the pulse wave in a short segment of a few centimetres, because the pulse wave passes through such a short segment within a few milliseconds at a propagation speed of several meters per second [50]. The arterial wall motion caused by the pulse wave, which is in the arterial radial direction, can be detected by a 1D phase-sensitive motion estimator, i.e. the autocorrelation method described in section 9.3.1, when the artery is scanned in its longitudinal direction, because the directions of the ultrasonic beams almost coincide with the arterial radial direction. Let us define the arterial wall acceleration measured by a receive line as $a(x, t)$, where x is the lateral position of the receive line, and the arterial wall acceleration is obtained by temporal differentiation of the arterial wall velocity estimated by the autocorrelation method. It is preferable to use acceleration waveforms in the estimation of PWV because high-frequency components are enhanced in acceleration waveforms compared with velocity waveforms, and the phases of the high-frequency components of acceleration waveforms are more sensitive to small time delays than those of the low-frequency components. A Hilbert transform was applied to the acceleration waveform $a(x, t)$ to obtain the complex analytic signal $\tilde{a}(x, t)$ of $a(x, t)$ [51]. By assuming that the measured acceleration is a temporal waveform at a dominant frequency of $f_{\text{PWV}} = \omega_{\text{PWV}}/2\pi$ and that there is only a forward propagation wave from the upstream side to the downstream side, the complex acceleration waveform $a(x, t)$ can be modeled by

$$\tilde{a}(x, t) = \tilde{a}(0, 0) \cdot e^{j(\omega_{\text{PWV}} t - k_{\text{PWV}} x)}, \tag{9.41}$$

where l_x is the length of the propagation path from the point of interest on the arterial wall at a receive line position of 0 to that at x. The phase velocity can be estimated by determining the wave number k_{PWV} at the corresponding temporal frequency f_{PWV} of the acceleration waveform. As described in section 9.3.1,

$$\hat{\omega}_0 = \frac{\angle \gamma_a(T_{FR})}{T_{FR}}, \tag{9.42}$$

$$\gamma_a(\tau) = \frac{1}{2X_w} \int_{-X_w}^{X_w} \tilde{a}^*(x, t) \cdot \tilde{a}(x, t + \tau) dx, \tag{9.43}$$

where T_{FR} denotes the frame interval, which corresponds to the sampling interval of the acceleration waveforms, and X_w determines the number of receive lines used for the calculation of the complex correlation function $\gamma_a(\tau)$.

One of the methods used to estimate the wave number k_{PWV} is the Fourier transform applied to the complex acceleration waveforms $a(x, t)$ with respect to the receive line position x. However, the lateral length of the imaging field of view, which corresponds to the length of the spatial window for the Fourier transform, is generally limited to less than 50 mm. In this case, the frequency resolution of the Fourier transform is 20 m^{-1}. On the other hand, a typical wavelength of the pulse wave is 0.5 m (at a PWV of 5 m s^{-1} and a temporal frequency of 10 Hz), which corresponds to a spatial frequency of 2 m^{-1}. Therefore, a higher-frequency resolution is preferable for visualization of the wave number of the pulse wave in a short segment of less than 50 mm. The phases of the complex acceleration waveforms have been used for visualization of the wave number of the pulse wave [51, 52].

Let us consider the phase of the product of the measured complex acceleration waveform $a(x, t)$ and a wave model $\tilde{a}(0, 0) \cdot e^{j(\omega t - kl_x)}$ at temporal frequencies and wave numbers of $f = \omega/2\pi$ and k. Since the measured complex acceleration waveform is modeled by equation (9.41), the phase of the complex product $\tilde{a}(x, t) \cdot \{\tilde{a}(0, 0) \cdot e^{j(\omega t - kl_x)}\}^*$ becomes independent of the path length l_x, i.e. the phase variance along the propagation path is zero, when the wave number k coincides with that of the pulse wave k_{PWV}. Based on this consideration, a function can be defined, as follows [52]:

$$A_p(k, t) = \frac{|E[\tilde{a}(x, t)]_x|^2}{V\left[\angle\left\{\tilde{a}(x, t) \cdot \{\tilde{a}(0, 0) \cdot e^{j(\omega t - kl_x)}\}^*\right\}\right]_x}, \tag{9.44}$$

where $E[\cdot]_x$ and $V[\cdot]_x$ denote the mean and variance operations with respect to the received line position x. The proposed metric $A_p(k, t)$ becomes large when the temporal frequency f and the wave number k coincide with those of the pulse waves f_{PWV} and k_{PWV}, respectively, because the phase variance of the term $\tilde{a}(x, t) \cdot \{\tilde{a}(0, 0) \cdot e^{j(\omega t - kl_x)}\}^*$ becomes small in such a case. Additionally, the metric $A_p(k, t)$ includes the power of the averaged acceleration waveform in its numerator to emphasize the wave number of a component with a large amplitude (good signal-to-noise ratio). The PWV is estimated using

$$\text{PWV} = \frac{\hat{k}_{\text{PWV}}}{\hat{\omega}_{\text{PWV}}} = \frac{\angle \gamma_a(T_{\text{FR}})}{T_{\text{FR}} \cdot \underset{k}{\operatorname{argmax}}\, A_{\text{p}}(k, t)}. \qquad (9.45)$$

The fundamental characteristic of the proposed metric $A_{\text{p}}(k, t)$ was evaluated by simulations. The arterial wall acceleration waveform was modeled by a 1.5-cycle sinusoidal wave with a Gaussian envelope [51]. Figure 9.15(a) shows an example of a simulated acceleration waveform. Figure 9.15(b) shows the spatiotemporal distribution of simulated acceleration values, and figure 9.15(c) shows the spatiotemporal distribution of the corresponding phase values. The PWV was set to 2.5 m s^{-1} for figure 9.15.

Figure 9.16(1-a) shows the mean temporal frequency estimated by equation (9.42). The same figure is also shown in figure 9.16(2-a). A mean temporal frequency of approximately 10 Hz is obtained during the period that the acceleration waveform exists. Figure 9.16(1-b) shows the proposed metric $A_{\text{p}}(k, t)$ described in equation (9.44). The spatial frequency of the simulated acceleration wave can clearly be seen in figure 9.16(1-b), and the PWV is estimated to be 2.54 m s^{-1}, which is in good agreement with the assigned value. Figure 9.16(2-b) shows the power spectrum of the simulated acceleration waveform obtained by applying the Fourier transform with respect to the receive line position x. As shown in figure 9.16(2-b), it

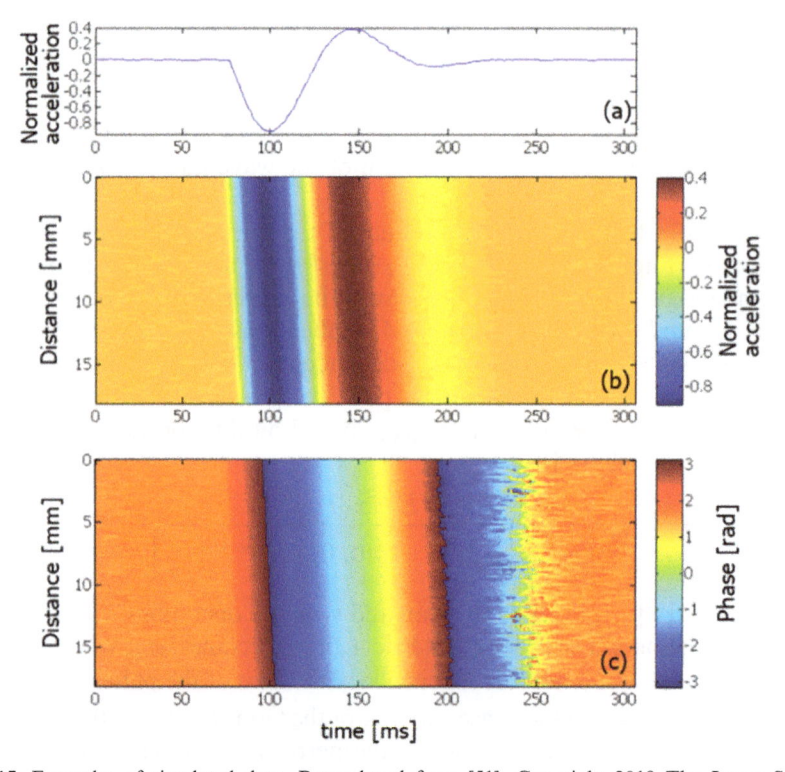

Figure 9.15. Examples of simulated data. Reproduced from [51]. Copyright 2019 The Japan Society of Applied Physics. All rights reserved. (a) Acceleration waveform. (b) Spatiotemporal distribution of acceleration. (c) Spatiotemporal distribution of the phases of the analytic signals of the acceleration waveforms.

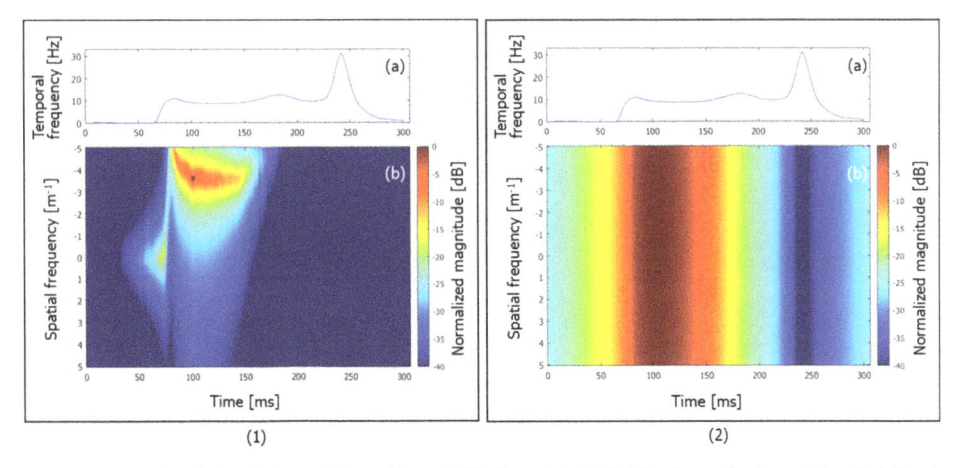

Figure 9.16. Results of simulations. Adapted from [51]. Copyright 2019 The Japan Society of Applied Physics. All rights reserved. (1) Proposed method. (2) Fourier transform. (a) Estimated mean temporal frequency. (b) Distribution of proposed metrics.

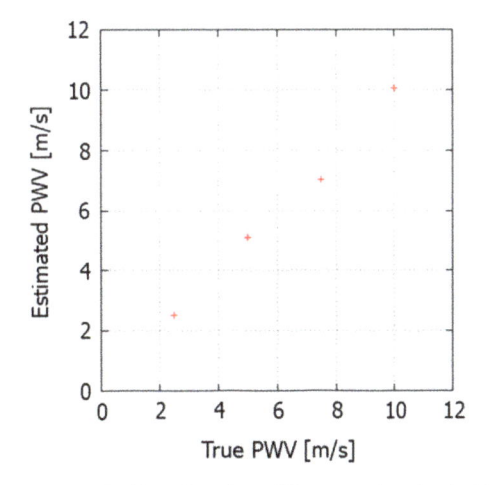

Figure 9.17. Estimated pulse-wave velocities plotted at different assigned velocities. Reproduced from [51]. Copyright 2019 The Japan Society of Applied Physics. All rights reserved.

is difficult to observe the peak position in the power spectrum due to the limited spatial frequency resolution in the Fourier transform. Figure 9.17 shows PWVs estimated using the proposed metric $A_p(k, t)$ for different assigned PWVs. The results shown in figure 9.17 show that the proposed metric $A_p(k, t)$ works well for different PWV values.

The feasibility of the proposed metric $A_p(k, t)$ was also evaluated using an *in vivo* measurement. Figure 9.18(a) shows a B-mode image of a human carotid artery obtained by plane-wave imaging, whose transmit–receive sequence is described in section 9.4.1. Figure 9.18(b) shows an example of the acceleration waveform of the

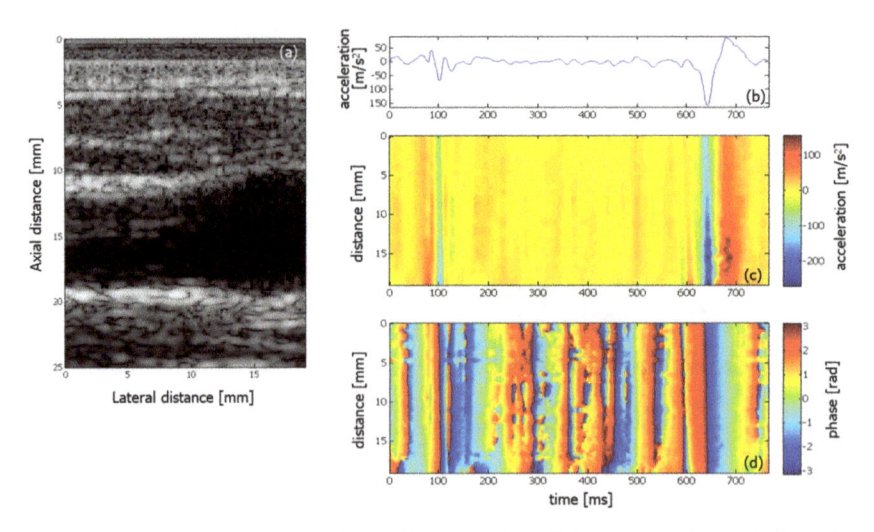

Figure 9.18. *In vivo* experimental data. Adapted from [51]. Copyright 2019 The Japan Society of Applied Physics. All rights reserved. (a) B-mode image of human carotid artery. (b) Acceleration waveform. (c) Spatiotemporal distribution of acceleration. (d) Spatiotemporal distribution of the phases of the analytic signals of the acceleration waveforms.

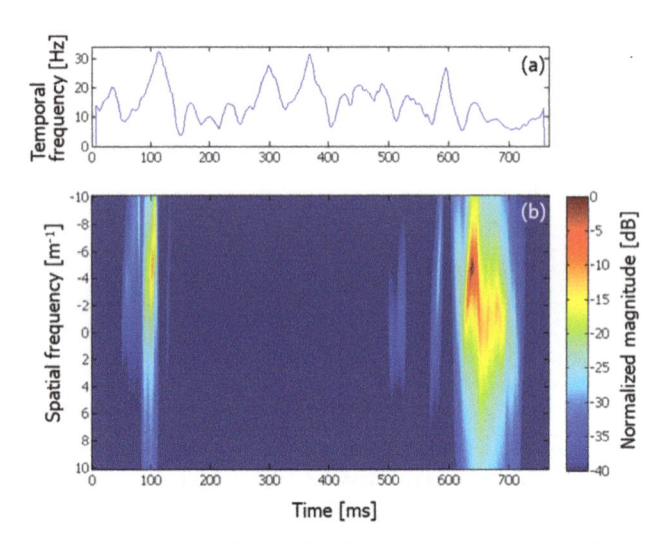

Figure 9.19. *In vivo* experimental results of the estimation of temporal and spatial frequencies. Reproduced from [51]. Copyright 2019 The Japan Society of Applied Physics. All rights reserved. (a) Estimated mean temporal frequency. (b) Distribution of proposed metrics.

arterial wall. The pulsive waveform between 600 and 700 ms is generated by heart ejection. Figures 9.18(c) and (d) show the spatiotemporal distribution of the accelerations and their phases. From the measured acceleration waveforms in figure 9.18, the mean temporal frequency and proposed metric $A_p(k, t)$ were obtained, as shown in figures 9.19(a) and (b), respectively. From the peak at approximately 630 ms in figure 9.19(b), the spatial frequency of the pulse wave was determined to be -5.05 m^{-1}. At the time of the peak in $A_p(k, t)$, the mean temporal frequency was identified to be 14.7 Hz in figure 9.19(a). The PWV was estimated to be 2.91 m s^{-1} from the identified mean temporal frequency and spatial frequency of the pulse wave, where the inverse of the identified spatial frequency corresponds to the wavelength of the pulse wave.

As can be seen in figure 9.19(b), the distribution of $A_p(k, t)$ is useful for observing temporal changes in the wavelengths of propagating waves, which can hardly be observed in the power spectrum obtained by Fourier transform, as shown in figure 9.16(2). Additionally, since $A_p(k, t)$ is weighted by the magnitude of the acceleration waveform, dominant waves propagating along the arterial wall can be identified. In figure 9.19(b), there is another propagating wave at approximately 100 ms. This component is thought to be generated by a rapid pressure decrement due to the closure of the aortic valve. As demonstrated in these results, the proposed metric $A_p(k, t)$ can be used to observe wave propagation phenomena at a high resolution. The group velocity can be estimated using the coefficient of variation of the measured acceleration waveforms [53], and the resolution of the identification of the wavelength is further improved. On the other hand, to estimate the exact phase velocity, each frequency component should be analyzed. Such an analysis can be realized using a short-period Fourier transform to obtain the complex acceleration waveform at each frequency [52].

9.4.3 Blood-flow imaging

Although color flow imaging is widely used in clinical situations, the frame rate in the color flow mode is significantly lower than that in B-mode imaging. CPWC also significantly improves the frame rate in color flow imaging [54]. Although CPWC realizes image quality in the B-mode similar to that obtained from line-by-line acquisition with a focused transmitted beam using multiple steered plane waves, the frame rate is reduced by increasing the number of steered plane waves. On the other hand, the frame rate can be significantly increased by decreasing the number of transmissions per frame at the expense of resolution and contrast. In [54], the number of transmissions per frame was set to nine for a fast flow, similar to that in a carotid artery, and 16 for a slow flow, similar to that in a thyroid artery. CPWC color flow imaging enables detailed observation of the dynamics of a fast flow by increasing the frame rate; it also enables highly sensitive visualization of a slow flow by increasing the number of transmissions (compounded plane waves). However, the aliasing limit is reduced by a factor corresponding to the number of transmissions. Figure 9.20(a) illustrates the transmission sequence for three transmissions per frame. In CPWC color flow imaging, beamformed ultrasonic signals obtained at different plane-wave steering angles are coherently compounded, and the coherently compounded RF signals are processed by the autocorrelation method. As a result, the frame rate is reduced, depending on the number of transmissions per frame. Additionally, the velocity component in the axial direction of the compounded ultrasonic field is estimated.

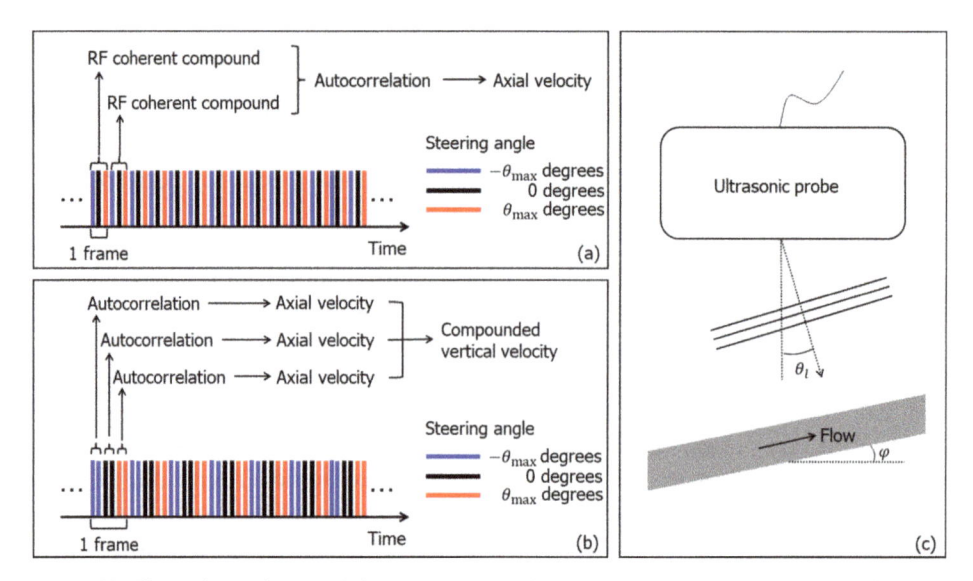

Figure 9.20. Illustrations of transmission sequences and measurement geometry. Adapted from [12]. Copyright 2022 The Japan Society of Applied Physics. All rights reserved. (a) Transmission sequence in conventional ultrafast compound Doppler. (b) Repeated transmission sequence. (c) Geometry in numerical simulation.

To keep the aliasing limit as high as possible and estimate 2D velocity vectors, the transmission sequence illustrated in figure 9.20(b) was examined [12, 55, 56]. In this sequence, plane waves are transmitted in the same direction twice before changing the steering angles, and the two resultant beamformed RF signals at the same steering angles are processed by the autocorrelation method to estimate axial velocities at the corresponding steering angle. By engaging in such a strategy, the time interval between the two beamformed RF signals is always the PRI, which means that the aliasing limit is the highest for a given PRI. Velocity vectors are estimated by processing the axial velocities obtained at different steering angles based on the principle described in section 9.3.2.

The proposed strategy was validated by numerical simulations performed using the Field II program [13, 14]. Ultrasonic point scatterers were randomly distributed in a cylinder with a radius r_0 of 2.5 mm. A parabolic flow profile was assigned by moving the distributed scatterers at velocities described by

$$v(r) = v_{max}\frac{(r_0 - r)^2}{r_0^2}, \qquad (9.46)$$

where r is the distance between the scatterer and the central axis of the cylinder, and v_{max} denotes the maximum flow velocity. The maximum flow velocity v_{max} was set to 100, 200, 400, and 800 mm s^{-1}. Additionally, the flow angle φ illustrated in figure 9.20(c) was set to 0, 10, 20, and 30°.

A 7.5 MHz linear array with 192 elements at pitches of 0.2 mm was simulated, and plane waves were emitted by all 192 elements. The number of steering angles

N_{angle} was set to three, and the sets of steering angles examined were (−5, 0, 5), (−10, 0, 10), (−15, 0, 15), and (−20, 0, 20) degrees (maximum steering angles θ_{max} of 5, 10, 15, and 20, respectively). The ultrasonic pulse emitted by each transducer element was a three-cycle sinusoidal wave at a central frequency of 7.5 MHz with a Hanning envelope. The echo signals received by the individual elements were sampled at 31.25 MHz.

Figure 9.21 shows an example of numerical simulations obtained using a steering angle set of (−10, 0, 10) degrees and a maximum flow velocity v_{max} of 100 mm s^{-1}. Figures 9.21(a), 9.21(b), and 9.21(c) show the B-mode image, lateral velocity distribution, and vertical velocity distribution, respectively. The errors in the estimated velocities are evaluated using the absolute bias error (ABE) given by

$$\text{ABE} = |\,\text{E}_{R_f}[\mathbf{v}_{est} - \mathbf{v}_{tru}]\,|, \quad (9.47)$$

where $\mathbf{v}_{est}$ and $\mathbf{v}_{tru}$ are the estimated and assigned true velocities, respectively, and $\text{E}_{R_f}[\,\cdot\,]$ denotes the averaging operation with respect to the region R_f where the flow exists. Additionally, by assuming that the fluctuating velocity components are independent of the ABE components, the root mean squared error, excluding bias error (RMSEexBE), can be defined as

$$\text{RMSEexBE} = \sqrt{\text{E}_{R_f}[|\,\mathbf{v}_{est} - \mathbf{v}_{tru}\,|^2] - \text{ABE}^2}. \quad (9.48)$$

Both errors were described using percentage values relative to the maximum assigned velocity v_{max}.

In figure 9.22, the plots and vertical bars show the ABEs and the RMSEexBEs, respectively, and the errors are evaluated at different maximum steering angles for a flow tilt angle and a maximum flow velocity of 10° and 100 mm s^{-1}, respectively. The errors increased significantly at steering angles larger than 10° due to the effects of grating lobes. The errors were further evaluated for maximum steering angles of 5 and 10°.

Figures 9.23(a) and (b) show the errors obtained at different flow tilt angles and maximum flow velocities, respectively. As shown in figure 9.23(a), the errors in the velocity vectors obtained at a maximum steering angle of 10° increase when the flow tilt

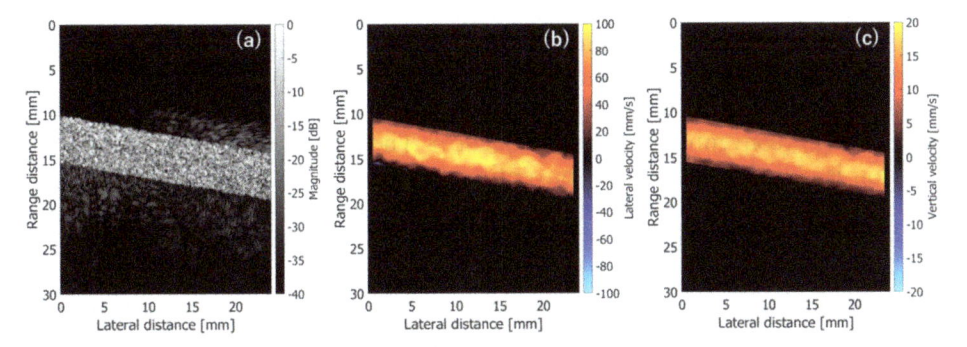

Figure 9.21. Examples of numerical simulations using a steering angle set of (−10, 0, 10) degrees and a maximum flow velocity of 100 mm s^{-1}. Reproduced from [12]. Copyright 2022 The Japan Society of Applied Physics. All rights reserved. (a) B-mode image. (b) Estimated lateral velocity. (c) Estimated axial velocity.

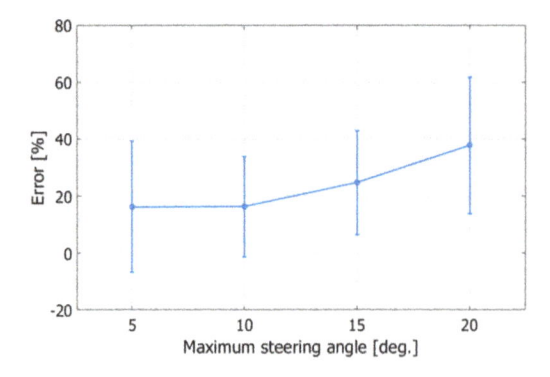

Figure 9.22. Errors in the estimated velocities at different maximum beam-steering angles. Adapted from [12]. Copyright 2022 The Japan Society of Applied Physics. All rights reserved.

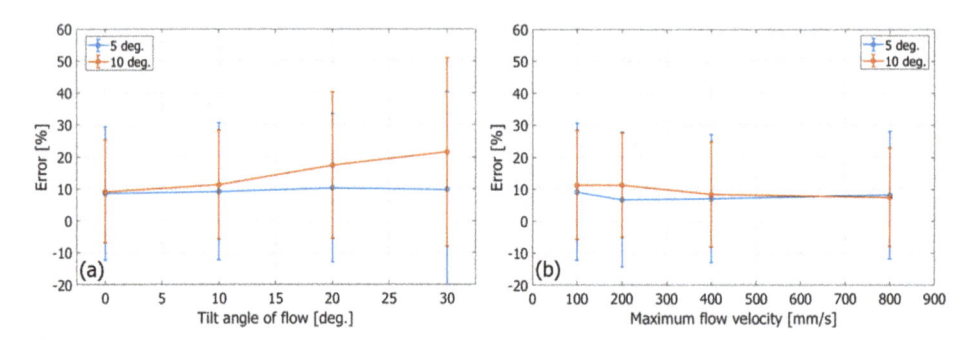

Figure 9.23. Errors in estimated velocities. Adapted from [12]. Copyright 2022 The Japan Society of Applied Physics. All rights reserved. (a) At different flow tilt angles with a maximum flow velocity of 100 mm s^{-1}. (b) At different maximum flow velocities with a maximum steering angle of 10°.

angle is larger than 10°. Therefore, the steering angle should be limited when the flow tilt angle is large. Figure 9.23(b) shows that the accuracies are not affected by maximum flow velocities of up to 800 mm s^{-1} and the estimations do not suffer from the aliasing effect.

In *in vivo* blood flow imaging, strong echoes from tissues and clutter overlap with weak echoes from blood cells. Therefore, a clutter filter is required to visualize weak echoes from blood cells. In conventional color flow imaging, ultrasonic pulses are transmitted several times in the same direction or scan line, as illustrated in figure 9.24(a) (conventional packet sequence). The group of transmissions in each direction is called a packet. In conventional color flow imaging, a clutter filter is applied to ultrasound signals within a packet. However, it is difficult to apply a clutter filter to signals within a packet when there are only two transmissions per angle, as illustrated in figure 9.24(b) (repeated transmission sequence). Therefore, a group of signals is composed of the signals in the first or second emissions in different packets in the sequence illustrated in figure 9.24(b). The performances of the clutter filters in the transmission sequences illustrated in figure 9.24 were compared, where the number of transmissions (Txs) per angle N_{packet} was set to 32 in the sequence illustrated in figure 9.24(a).

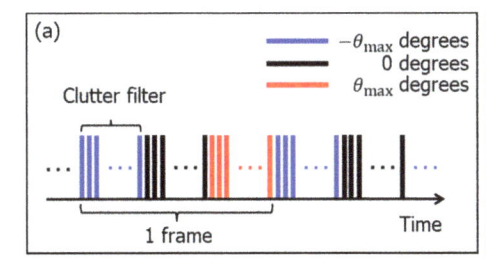

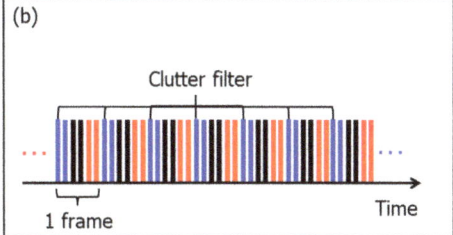

Figure 9.24. Illustration of strategies for clutter filtering in plane-wave imaging using a packet transmission sequence [56] (2021) (Copyright 2016, the author(s)). With permission of Springer. (a) Thirty-two transmissions per angle. (b) Two transmissions per angle.

Recently, a clutter filter based on singular value decomposition (SVD) has exhibited an excellent ability to separate the ultrasonic echoes produced by blood cells and tissues [57]. The feasibility of the SVD clutter filter was examined using a repeated transmission sequence. To utilize SVD in clutter filtering, $(M_x \times M_z)$ beamformed RF signals $g_k(m_x, m_z, \theta_l, n)$ ($k = 1, 2, \ldots, N_{\text{packet}}$; $l = 1, 2, \ldots, N_{\text{angle}}$; $n = 1, 2, \ldots, N_{\text{tap}}$) were formulated into a $(M_x M_z \times N_{\text{tap}})$ matrix $\mathbf{G}_k(\theta_l)$ in the repeated transmission sequence. The spatiotemporal matrix $\mathbf{G}_k(\theta_l)$ was decomposed by SVD into a product of three matrices using

$$\mathbf{G}_k(\theta_l) = \mathbf{U\Sigma V}^T, \qquad (9.49)$$

where $\mathbf{U}$ and $\mathbf{V}$ are matrices composed of spatial and temporal singular vectors, respectively, and $\mathbf{\Sigma}$ is a diagonal matrix composed of singular values arranged in descending order.

The SVD-filtered signal $\tilde{\mathbf{G}}_k(\theta_l)$ is obtained using

$$\tilde{\mathbf{G}}_k(\theta_l) = \mathbf{U\Sigma}_t \mathbf{V}^T, \qquad (9.50)$$

where $\mathbf{\Sigma}_t$ is a diagonal matrix obtained by replacing singular values, whose orders are higher than the upper threshold or lower than the lower threshold, with zeros. The magnitude of a singular value corresponds to the amplitude of the corresponding decomposed component. Components with large singular values (low-order singular values) correspond to echo signals from stationary or slowly moving tissues, and those with small singular values (high-order singular values) correspond to noise. Therefore, such components can be removed from the echo signal by setting the corresponding singular values to zero.

In order to permit a comparison, blood flow images were also obtained using the conventional packet transmission sequence. In the conventional packet sequence, an $(M_x M_z \times N_{\text{packet}})$ matrix $\mathbf{G}'(\theta_l, n)$ was composed of $g_k(m_x, m_z, \theta_l, n)$, and the SVD clutter filter was applied to $\mathbf{G}'(\theta_l, n)$ to obtain the clutter-filtered signal $\tilde{\mathbf{G}}'(\theta_l, n)$. Additionally, a polynomial regression clutter filter was used with the conventional packet sequence as the traditional strategy for clutter filtering.

A blood flow image, which is presented as a blood speckle image in this chapter, is obtained from the clutter-filtered signal $\tilde{\mathbf{G}}_k(\theta_l)$. When the repeated transmission sequence is used, a dataset for one frame can be acquired during a relatively short period, as illustrated in figure 9.24(b). Therefore, both coherent and incoherent compounding were examined, as follows:

$$I_{\text{coh}}(m_x, m_z, n) = \left| \frac{1}{N_{\text{packet}} N_{\text{angle}}} \sum_{k=1}^{N_{\text{packet}}} \sum_{l=1}^{N_{\text{angle}}} \tilde{g}_k(m_x, m_z, \theta_l, n) \right|, \tag{9.51}$$

$$I_{\text{inc}}(m_x, m_z, n) = \frac{1}{N_{\text{packet}} N_{\text{angle}}} \sum_{k=1}^{N_{\text{packet}}} \sum_{l=1}^{N_{\text{angle}}} | \tilde{g}_k(m_x, m_z, \theta_l, n) |. \tag{9.52}$$

On the other hand, the conventional packet transmission sequence requires a longer acquisition time than the repeated transmission sequence, as illustrated in figure 9.24(a), and the loss of coherence between the filtered signals $\tilde{g}_k(m_x, m_z, \theta_l, n)$ would be significant due to the motion of blood cells during the acquisition period required for one frame. Consequently, only incoherent compounding was examined for use with the conventional packet transmission sequence.

Figures 9.25(a)–(d) show blood speckle images of a common carotid artery obtained with the 32-Tx packet sequence and polynomial regression filter, the 32-Tx packet sequence and SVD filter, and coherent and incoherent compounding with the repeated transmission sequence and SVD filter, respectively. The maximum beam-steering angle θ_{max} was set to 10°. The red and yellow rectangles in figure 9.25 show the regions inside and outside the artery for contrast evaluation. Figure 9.26(a) shows the contrast values obtained using the polynomial regression and SVD filters with the conventional packet transmission sequence. The polynomial regression filter realized good contrast during a specific period when blood flow velocities were high during the cardiac systolic phase. On the other hand, the SVD filter achieved significantly better

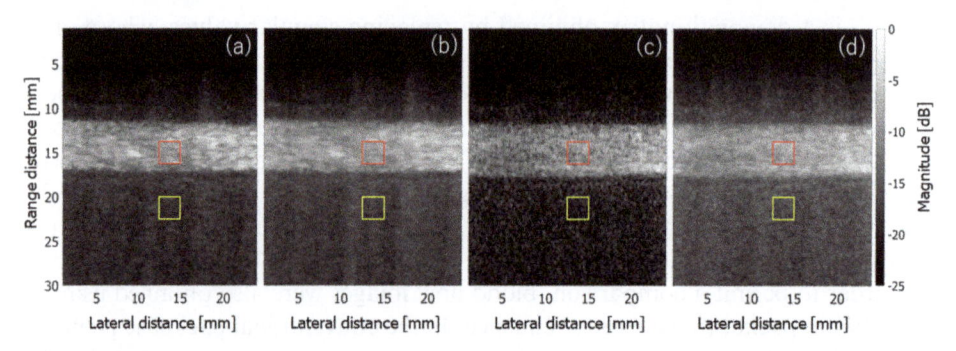

Figure 9.25. Clutter-filtered B-mode images [56] (2021) (Copyright 2016, the author(s)). With permission of Springer. The regions inside and outside the artery used for the evaluation of contrast are shown by red and yellow rectangles, respectively. (a) Thirty-two transmissions per packet with a polynomial regression filter and incoherent averaging. (b) Thirty-two transmissions per packet with an SVD filter and incoherent averaging. (c) Two transmission per packet with an SVD filter and coherent averaging. (d) Two transmissions per packet with an SVD filter and incoherent averaging.

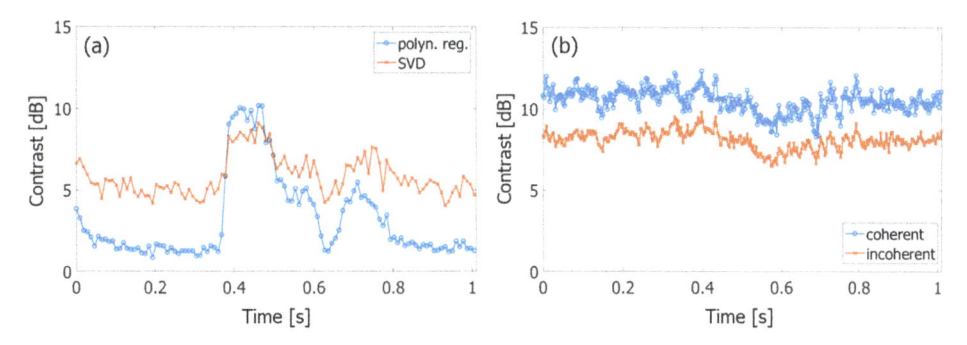

Figure 9.26. Contrast of brightness in regions inside and outside the artery obtained by (a) a polynomial regression filter and SVD filter with incoherent averaging at 32 Txs per packet and (b) an SVD filter with coherent and incoherent averaging at 2 Txs per packet [56] (2021) (Copyright 2016, the author(s)). With permission of Springer.

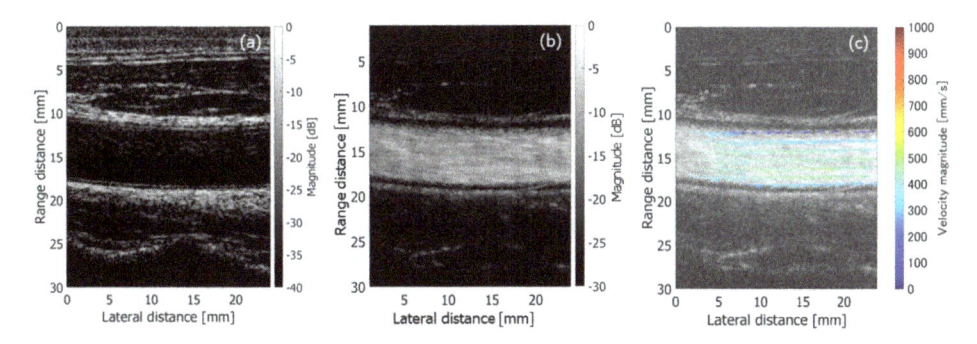

Figure 9.27. *In vivo* measurements of flow velocity vectors in the carotid artery. Adapted from [12]. Copyright 2022 The Japan Society of Applied Physics. All rights reserved. (a) B-mode images. (b) Blood speckle image obtained with coherent compounding. (c) Flow velocity vectors in cardiac systole.

contrast than the polynomial regression filter in slow flow phases, while its maximum contrast was slightly worse than that of the polynomial regression filter.

Figure 9.26(b) shows the contrast values obtained by coherent and incoherent compounding of the filtered echo signals with the repeated transmission sequence and SVD filter. The number of temporal samples N_{tap} was set to 300. As shown in figure 9.26(b), the contrast values obtained using the repeated transmission sequence are consistently higher than those obtained with the conventional packet sequence. Additionally, coherent compounding of the filtered echo signals further improves the contrast. The SVD clutter filter implemented in the repeated transmission sequence enables the visualization of weak echoes from blood cells with high contrast.

Figure 9.27 shows an *in vivo* experimental result for the measurement of blood flow velocity vectors. Figure 9.27(a) shows a B-mode image of a common carotid artery. The maximum beam-steering angle θ_{max} was set to 10°. Figure 9.27(b) shows a blood speckle image obtained using the repeated transmission sequence and the SVD clutter filter. As shown in figure 9.27(b), weak echoes from blood cells were clearly visualized. By applying the vector Doppler method described in section 9.3.2, the blood flow velocity vectors were estimated, as shown in figure 9.27(c). The estimated flow velocity vectors in the cardiac systolic phase are overlaid on the blood speckle image. As shown in figure 9.27(c), physiologically convincing flow velocity vectors can be obtained by high-frame-rate ultrasonic imaging using the vector Doppler method.

High-frame-rate ultrasonic imaging also enables the blood flow velocity vectors in a cardiac ventricle to be measured. In cardiac ultrasound imaging, an ultrasonic beam should be insonified from a narrow acoustic window between the ribs. In high-frame-rate cardiac imaging, a transmitted wave, which emulates a spherically diverging wave from a virtual point source behind an array, is frequently used to illuminate a wide region with one or a few emissions [17, 18]. Since a wide region is illuminated at once, a receiving focal point can be placed at an arbitrary position in the illuminated region. In conventional cardiac ultrasound imaging, a beamforming grid is generated based on the polar coordinate system (sector format), as illustrated in figure 9.28(a). Under these conditions, the lateral sampling interval of the beamformed signal increases with the range distance, and such an unfixed sampling interval may affect the accuracy of motion estimation. Therefore, echo signals beamformed in the Cartesian coordinate system were also created, as shown in figure 9.28(b) [58]. A sponge phantom, whose B-mode images are shown in figure 9.28, was measured with a 3 MHz phased array probe (PU-0541, Ueda Japan Radio) composed of 96 elements at pitches of 0.2 mm. A spherically diverging wave was produced using all 96 elements to illuminate the field of view at once. The virtual point source was placed 30 mm behind the array, and the PRF was set to 6250 Hz. The angle and lateral intervals of the beamformed signals in the polar and Cartesian coordinate systems were 0.375° and 0.2 mm, respectively. The ultrasonic probe were moved by an automatic stage at constant lateral and vertical speeds of 2 and 1 mm s^{-1}, respectively, to produce relative motion between the phantom and the ultrasonic probe.

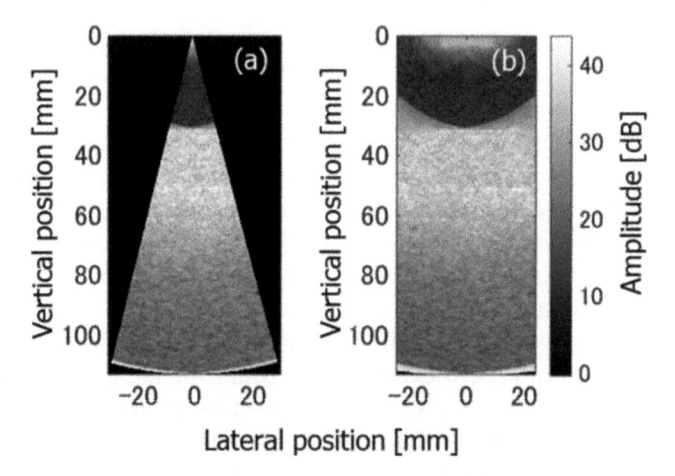

Figure 9.28. B-mode images of the phantom. (a) In polar coordinate system (sector format). (b) In Cartesian coordinate system.

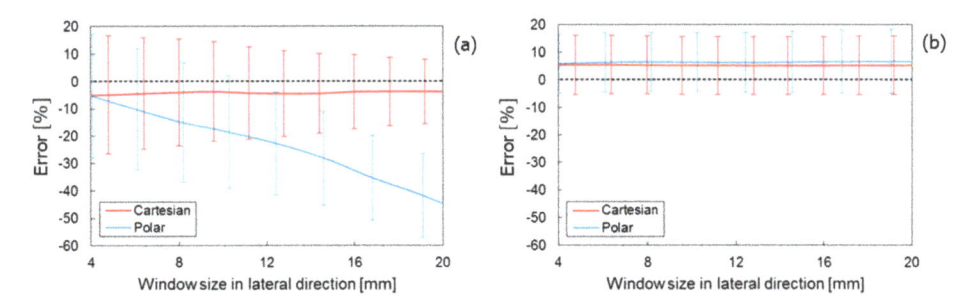

Figure 9.29. Errors in estimated velocities. Adapted from [58]. Copyright 2018 The Japan Society of Applied Physics. All rights reserved. (a) Lateral direction. (b) Vertical direction.

The plots and vertical bars in figure 9.29 show the bias errors and standard deviations in the velocities estimated by the 2D phase-sensitive motion estimator described in section 9.3.4. Figures 9.29(a) and (b) show the errors in the estimated lateral and vertical velocities, respectively, obtained at different lateral window sizes in the Fourier transform. The vertical window size was fixed at 14.79 mm. As shown in figure 9.29(a), the velocities obtained using RF signals beamformed in the polar coordinate system are influenced by the lateral window size. This dependency can be avoided using RF signals beamformed in the Cartesian coordinate system. On the other hand, the estimation of vertical velocities is not significantly dependent on the coordinate system used for beamforming, as shown in figure 9.29(b). These results indicate that beamforming in the Cartesian coordinate system is preferable in phased array imaging.

As described above, a human heart can only be imaged by insonifying an ultrasound beam from a narrow acoustic window between the ribs. Therefore, an ultrasonic probe with a large footprint is not feasible. In such a situation, it is difficult to use the vector Doppler method because the difference between the angles of the ultrasonic beams insonifying each spatial position would be small. Additionally, in cardiac motion imaging, it has been found that motion tracking based on the amplitude envelope of the ultrasonic RF signal is preferable compared with that based on the RF signal [59, 60]. This phenomenon is also reported in measurements of heart wall motion [29]. This mechanism should be investigated further, but a possible explanation is the decorrelation of ultrasonic echo signals due to the rapid motions of the blood cells and the heart wall. Therefore, the block-matching method described in section 9.3.3 was applied to the envelope signals of the beamformed RF echoes obtained from a human heart. Figure 9.30(a) shows a blood speckle image of a left ventricle obtained at a frame rate of 6250 Hz, which corresponds to the PRF. The SVD clutter filter described in this section was used to visualize weak echoes from blood cells. Blood flow velocity vectors were estimated by applying the block-matching method to the visualized echo signals, as shown in figure 9.30(b). This method noninvasively enables both qualitative observation of complex cardiac blood flow without using contrast agents and quantitative estimation of blood flow velocity vectors.

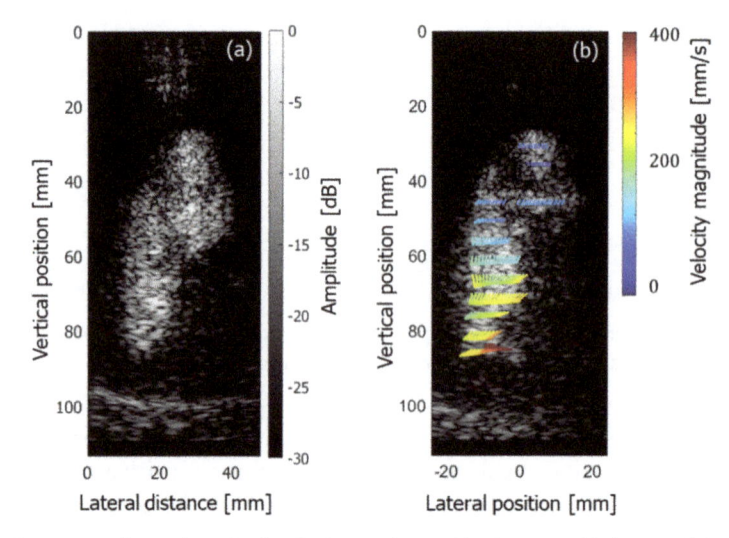

Figure 9.30. *In vivo* experimental results for the human heart. (a) Blood speckle image of the left ventricle. (b) Blood flow velocity vectors overlaid on blood speckle images.

References

[1] Kikuchi K, Uchida R, Tanaka K and Wagai T 1957 Early cancer diagnosis through ultrasonics *J. Acoust. Soc. Am.* **29** 111–12

[2] Chilowsky C and Langevin P 1920 Procedes et appareils pour la production de signaux sous-marins diriges et pour la localisation a distance d'obstacles sous-marins *French Patent* **502** 913

[3] Uchida R, Hagiwara Y and Irie T 1971 Electro-scanning ultrasonic equipment *Jpn. J. Med. Ultrason.* **18** 65–6

[4] Bom M, Roelandt J, Kloster F E, Lancee C T and Hugenholtz P G 1973 A multi element system and its application to cardiology *Proc. of the second World Congress on Ultrasonics in Medicine, Rotterdam, 4–8 June 1973, Int. Congress series* 309 (New York: Elsevier) pp 297–9

[5] Delannoy B, Torguet R, Bruneel C, Bridoux E, Rouaven J M and Lasota 1979 Acoustic image reconstruction in parallel-processing analog electronic systems *J. Appl. Phys.* **50** 3153–9

[6] Shattuck D, Weinshenker M, Smith S and von Ramm O 1984 Explososcan: a parallel processing technique for high speed ultrasound imaging with linear phased arrays *J. Acoust. Soc. Am.* **75** 1273–82

[7] Tanter M, Bercoff J, Sandrin L and Fink M 2002 Ultrafast compound imaging for 2-D motion vector estimation: application to transient elastography *IEEE Trans. Ultrason. Ferroelectr. Freq. Control* 1363–74

[8] Tanter M and Fink M 2014 Ultrafast imaging in biomedical ultrasound *IEEE Trans. Ultrason. Ferroelectr. Freq. Control* **61** 102–19

[9] Montaldo G, Tanter M, Bercoff J, Benech N and Fink M 2009 Coherent plane-wave compounding for very high frame rate ultrasonography and transient elastography *IEEE Trans. Ultrason. Ferroelectr. Freq. Control* **56** 489–506

[10] Yiu B Y S and Yu A C H 2016 Least-squares multi-angle Doppler estimators for plane wave vector fow imaging *IEEE Trans. Ultrason. Ferroelectr. Freq. Control* **63** 1733–44

[11] Karageorgos G M, Apostolakis I Z, Nauleau P, Gatti V, Weber R, Kemper P and Konofagou E E 2021 Pulse wave imaging coupled with vector flow mapping: a phantom, simulation, and *in vivo* study *IEEE Trans. Ultrason. Ferroelectr. Freq. Control* **68** 2516–31

[12] Hasegawa H, Mozumi M, Omura M, Nagaoka R and Saito K 2021 Preliminary study on estimation of flow velocity vectors using focused transmit beams *J. Med. Ultrason.* **48** 417–27

[13] Jensen J A 1991 A model for the propagation and scattering of ultrasound in tissue *J. Acoust. Soc. Am.* **89** 182–90

[14] Jensen J A and Svendsen N B 1992 Calculation of pressure fields from arbitrarily shaped, apodized, and excited ultrasound transducers *IEEE Trans. Ultrason. Ferroelectr. Freq. Control* **39** 262–7

[15] Porée J, Posada D, Hodzic A, Tournoux F, Cloutier G and Garcia D 2016 High-frame-rate echocardiography using coherent compounding with Doppler-based motion-compensation *IEEE Trans. Med. Imaging* **35** 1647–57

[16] Jensen J A, Nikolov S I, Gammelmark K L and Pedersen M H 2006 Synthetic aperture ultrasound imaging *Ultrasonics* **44** e5–15

[17] Couade M, Pernot M, Tanter M, Messas E, Bel A, Ba M, Hagège A-A and Fink M 2009 Ultrafast imaging of the heart using circular wave synthetic imaging with phased arrays *2009 IEEE Int. Ultrasonics Symp.* (Piscataway, NJ: IEEE) 515–8

[18] Hasegawa H and Kanai H 2011 High-frame-rate echocardiography using diverging transmit beams and parallel receive beamforming *J. Med. Ultrason.* **38** 129–40

[19] Satomura S 1957 Ultrasonic Doppler method for the inspection of cardiac functions *J. Acoust. Soc. Am.* **29** 1181–5

[20] Kasai C, Namekawa K, Koyano A and Omoto R 1985 Real-time two-dimensional blood flow imaging using an autocorrelation technique *IEEE Trans. Sonics Ultrason.* **32** 458–64

[21] Dunmire B, Beach K W, Labs K-H, Plett M and Strandness D R Jr 2000 Cross-beam vector Doppler ultrasound for angle-independent velocity measurements *Ultrasound Med. Biol.* **26** 1213–35

[22] Langeland S, D'hooge J, Torp H, Bijnens B and Suetens P 2003 Comparison of time-domain displacement estimators for two-dimensional RF tracking *Ultrasound Med. Biol.* **29** 1177–86

[23] Céspedes I, Huang Y, Ophir J and Spratt S 1995 Methods for estimation of subsample time delays of digitized echo signals *Ultrason. Imaging* **17** 142–71

[24] Konofagou E E, D'hooge J and Ophir J 2002 Myocardial elastography—a feasibility study *in vivo Ultrasound Med. Biol.* **28** 475–82

[25] de Korte C L, Pasterkamp G, van der Steen A F, Woutman H A and Bom N 2000 Characterization of plaque components with intravascular ultrasound elastography in human femoral and coronary arteries *in vitro Circulation* **102** 617–23

[26] Maurice R L, Soulez G, Giroux M F and Cloutier G 2008 Noninvasive vascular elastography for carotid artery characterization on subjects without previous history of atherosclerosis *Med. Phys.* **35** 3436–43

[27] Takahashi H, Hasegawa H and Kanai H 2014 Echo speckle imaging of blood particles with high-frame-rate echocardiography *Jpn. J. Appl. Phys.* **53** 07KF08-1-7

[28] Fadnes S, Nyrnes S A, Torp H and Lovstakken L 2014 Shunt flow evaluation in congenital heart disease based on two-dimensional speckle tracking *Ultrasound Med. Biol.* **40** 2379–91

[29] Orlowska M, Ramalli A, Petrescu A, Cvijic M, Bézy S, Santos P, Pedrosa J, Voigt J-U and D'hooge J 2020 In-vivo comparison of multiline transmission and diverging wave imaging for high frame rate speckle tracking echocardiography *IEEE Trans. Ultrason. Ferroelectr. Freq. Control* **67** 1764–75

[30] Hasegawa H 2016 Phase-sensitive 2D motion estimators using frequency spectra of ultrasonic echoes *Appl. Sci.* **6** 195

[31] Nunome S, Nagaoka S and Hasegawa H 2020 Accuracy evaluation of 3D velocity estimation by multi-frequency phase-sensitive motion estimator under various specifications of matrix array probe *Jpn. J. Appl. Phys.* **59** SKKE01-1-6

[32] Suzuki K, Iwasaki R, Takagi R, Yoshizawa S and Umemura S 2017 Simultaneous observation of cavitation bubbles generated in biological tissue by high-speed optical and acoustic imaging methods *Jpn. J. Appl. Phys.* **56** 07JF27-1-7

[33] Bonithon-Kopp C, Touboul P-J, Berr C, Leroux C, Mainard F, Courbon D and Ducimetière P 1996 Relation of intima-media thickness to atherosclerotic plaques in carotid arteries. The Vascular Aging (EVA) Study *Arterioscler. Thromb. Vasc. Biol.* **16** 310–6

[34] Casscells W, Naghavi M and Willerson J T 2003 Vulnerable atherosclerotic plaque: a multifocal disease *Circulation* **107** 2072–5

[35] Hasegawa H, Kanai Y, Koiwa and Chubachi N 1997 Noninvasive evaluation of Poisson's ratio of arterial wall using ultrasound *Electron. Lett.* **33** 340–2

[36] de Korte C L, Céspedes E I, van der Steen A F W and Lanée C T 1997 Intravascular elasticity imaging using ultrasound: feasibility studies in phantoms *Ultrasound Med. Biol.* **23** 735–46

[37] Kallel F and Ophir J 1997 A least-squares strain estimator for elastography *Ultrason. Imaging* **19** 195–208

[38] Miyajo A and Hasegawa H 2018 Comparison of method using phase-sensitive motion estimator with speckle tracking method and application to measurement of arterial wall motion *Jpn. J. Appl. Phys.* **57** 07LF11-1-8

[39] Fekkes S, Swillens A E S, Hansen H H G, Saris A E C, Nillesen M M, Iannaccone F, Segers P and de Korte C L 2016 2-D versus 3-D cross-correlation-based radial and circumferential strain estimation using multiplane 2-D ultrafast ultrasound in a 3-D atherosclerotic carotid artery model *IEEE Trans. Ultrason. Ferroelectr. Freq. Control* **63** 1543–53

[40] Miyajo A, Nagaoka R and Hasegawa H 2019 Comparison of ultrasonic motion estimators for vascular applications *Jpn. J. Appl. Phys.* **58** SGGE16-1-7

[41] Cinthio M, Ahlgren A R, Jansson T, Eriksson A, Persson H W and Lindstrom K 2005 Evaluation of an ultrasonic echo-tracking method for measurements of arterial wall movements in two dimensions *IEEE Trans. Ultrason. Ferroelectr. Freq. Control* **52** 1300–11

[42] Hasegawa H and Kanai H 2008 Reduction of influence of variation in center frequencies of RF echoes on estimation of artery-wall strain *IEEE Trans. Ultrason. Ferroelectr. Freq. Control* **55** 1921–34

[43] Ishikawa K, Mozumi M, Omura M, Nagaoka R and Hasegawa H 2021 Evaluation of accuracy of phase-sensitive method in estimation of axial motion and deformation with fluid-structure interaction analysis *Jpn. J. Appl. Phys.* **60** SDDE01-1-3

[44] Poree J, Chayer B, Soulez G, Ohayon J and Cloutier G 2017 Noninvasive vascular modulography method for imaging the local elasticity of atherosclerotic plaques: simulation and *in vitro* vessel phantom study *IEEE Trans. Ultrason. Ferroelctr. Freq. Control* **64** 1805–17

[45] Yamakoshi Y, Sato J and Sato T 1990 Ultrasonic imaging of internal vibration of soft tissue under forced vibration *IEEE Trans. Ultrason. Ferroelectr. Freq. Control* **37** 45–53

[46] Bavu E *et al* 2011 Noninvasive *in vivo* liver fibrosis evaluation using supersonic shear imaging: a clinical study on 113 hepatitis C virus patients *Ultrasound Med. Biol.* **37** 1361–73

[47] Couade M, Pernot M, Prada C, Messas E, Emmerich J, Bruneval P, Criton A, Fink M and Tanter M 2010 Quantitative assessment of arterial wall biomechanical properties using shear wave imaging *Ultrasound Med. Biol.* **36** 1662–76

[48] Guo Y, Wang Y, Chang E J-H and Lee W-N 2018 Multidirectional estimation of arterial stiffness using vascular guided wave imaging with geometry correction *Ultrasound Med. Biol.* **44** 1344–54

[49] Ohkuma T *et al* 2017 Brachial-ankle pulse wave velocity and the risk prediction of cardiovascular disease: an individual participant data meta-analysis *Hypertension* **69** 1045–52

[50] Hasegawa H, Hongo K and Kanai H 2013 Measurement of regional pulse wave velocity using very high frame rate ultrasound *J. Med. Ultrason.* **40** 91–8

[51] Hasegawa H 2018 Analysis of arterial wall motion for measurement of regional pulse wave velocity *Jpn. J. Appl. Phys.* **57** 07LF01-1-6

[52] Hasegawa H, Sato M and Irie T 2016 High resolution wavenumber analysis for investigation of arterial pulse wave propagation *Jpn. J. Appl. Phys.* **55** 07KF01-1-7

[53] Nagaoka R and Hasegawa H 2020 Basic study on estimation method of wall shear stress in common carotid artery using blood flow imaging *J. Med. Ultrason.* **47** 167–77

[54] Bercoff J, Montaldo G, Loupas T, Savery D, Mézière F, Fink M and Tanter M 2011 Ultrafast compound Doppler imaging: providing full blood flow characterization *IEEE Trans. Ultrason. Ferroelectr. Freq. Control* **58** 134–47

[55] Podkowa A S, Oelze M L and Ketterling J A 2018 High-frame-rate Doppler ultrasound using a repeated transmit sequence *Appl. Sci.* **8** 227

[56] Hasegawa H, Nagaoka R, Omura M, Mozumi M and Saito K 2021 Investigation of feasibility of singular value decomposition clutter filter in plane wave imaging with packet transmission sequence *J. Med. Ultrason.* **48** 13–20

[57] Demené C *et al* 2015 Spatiotemporal clutter filtering of ultrafast ultrasound data highly increases Doppler and fultrasound sensitivity *IEEE Trans. Med. Imaging* **34** 2271–85

[58] Kaburaki K, Mozumi M and Hasegawa H 2018 Estimation of two-dimensional motion velocity using ultrasonic signals beamformed in Cartesian coordinate for measurement of cardiac dynamics *Jpn. J. Appl. Phys.* **57** 07LF03-1-6

[59] Mozumi M, Nagaoka R and Hasegawa H 2020 Noise suppression in blood speckle imaging by estimation of point spread function of imaging system *IEEE Int. Ultrason. Symp.* 1382

[60] Mozumi M, Nagaoka N and Hasegawa H 2022 Improving image contrast and accuracy in velocity estimation by convolution filters for intracardiac blood flow imaging *Ultrasonics* **120** 106650

IOP Publishing

Ultrasonics

Mami Matsukawa, Pak-Kon Choi, Kentaro Nakamura, Hirotsugu Ogi and Hideyuki Hasegawa

Chapter 10

High-intensity focused ultrasound

Shin Yoshizawa and Shin-ichiro Umemura

High-intensity focused ultrasound (HIFU) is a noninvasive treatment modality which is being clinically applied in the treatment of many diseases. In this chapter, an overview of HIFU is given, and then studies of the transducers and drive circuits used for HIFU, which are the main components of HIFU transmission systems, are introduced. This is followed by a description of studies of the measurement methods and visualization techniques used with HIFU pressure fields, a treatment method that uses cavitation bubbles induced by HIFU, and the use of ultrasound imaging to guide HIFU treatment.

10.1 Introduction

Ultrasound with much higher energy than that used for diagnostic purposes can cause irreversible changes to biological tissues. High-intensity focused ultrasound (HIFU) can be used to induce irreversible changes for therapeutic purposes. Although unfocused ultrasound (known as high-intensity therapeutic ultrasound (HITU)) is also used, only focused ultrasound is discussed in this chapter.

HIFU is a noninvasive treatment modality. Today, HIFU treatment is applied clinically in the treatment of many diseases, such as prostate cancer [1, 2], liver cancer [3, 4], pancreatic cancer [5, 6], and essential tremor [7, 8]. Figure 10.1 shows a schematic of a typical HIFU treatment setup. Focused ultrasound is generated outside the body by a spherical HIFU transducer. The ultrasound is focused onto a target tissue inside the body through water. The water acts as a coupler for the ultrasound and as a coolant for the tissue surface and the transducer. Figure 10.2 shows an example of an HIFU pressure field around the focal region obtained using a numerical simulation that neglects the nonlinear propagation of ultrasound. A continuous wave at a frequency of 1 MHz generated by a spherical transducer with an f-number of one propagates from left to right in figure 10.2. The full widths at half maximum of the focal region are about 13 and 2 mm in the directions parallel

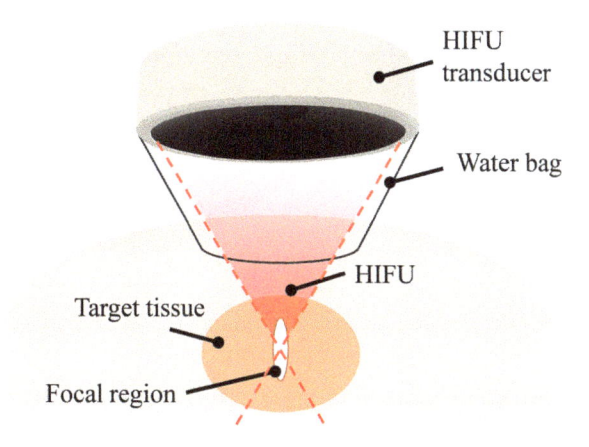

Figure 10.1. Schematic of HIFU treatment.

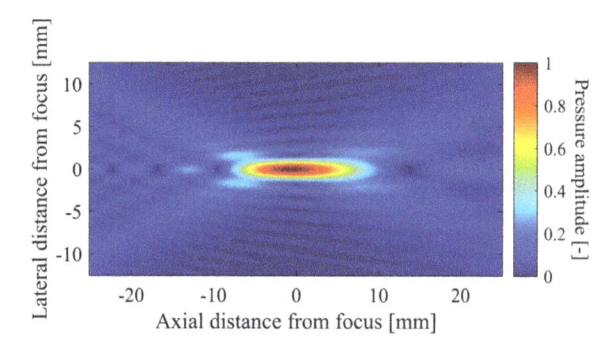

Figure 10.2. Example of an HIFU pressure field.

and perpendicular to HIFU propagation (the horizontal and vertical directions), respectively. If the f-number is fixed, the size of the focal region is approximately proportional to the wavelength. The acoustic intensity in the focal region of HIFU is much higher than that used for diagnostic purposes. When a tissue is continuously exposed to high-intensity ultrasound, the temperature in the tissue increases due to ultrasonic absorption by the tissue, resulting in thermal coagulation of the tissue. Figure 10.3 conceptually shows the bioeffect and safety areas of medical ultrasound. A metric called 'cumulative equivalent minutes at 43 °C' (CEM43) [9] is used to quantify the thermal bioeffect caused by HIFU treatment. CEM43 (t_{43}) is calculated by

$$t_{43} = \int R^{(T-43)} dt,$$

where T is the temperature in degrees Celsius and R is equal to two and four above and below 43°, respectively. A CEM43 of more than 240 min is often used as a measure of the efficacy of HIFU thermal therapy. For example, if the temperature is kept at 57° for 1 s, the CEM43 is calculated to be 273 min.

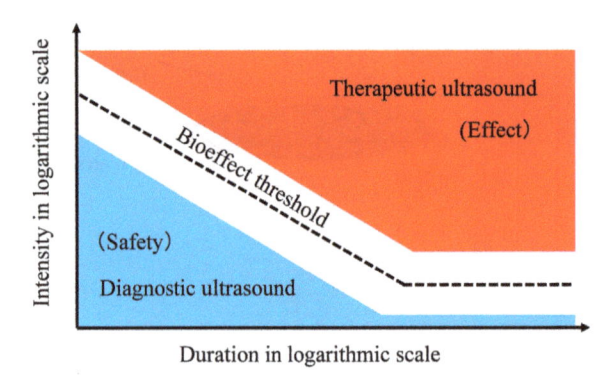

Figure 10.3. Bioeffect and safety areas of medical ultrasound.

10.2 HIFU devices

The main components of an HIFU transmission system are an HIFU transducer and a drive circuit. The focal region of HIFU has the shape of a spheroid, as shown in figure 10.2, and the surface area-to-volume (S/V) ratio of the treatment region is large, which lowers the efficiency of HIFU as a thermal treatment. To improve the efficiency of such ultrasound thermal treatments, Cain and Umemura developed a method and system that generated a ring-shaped focal region using a sector-vortex phased array [10, 11]. Köhler *et al* proposed a volumetric sonication method that electronically steered the HIFU focus along a predetermined trajectory consisting of multiple concentric outward-moving circles, which was tested *in vivo* on swine thigh muscle [12]. Inaba *et al* generated multiple cavitation clouds by electronic focus scanning to coagulate a large tissue region [13]. As seen in these examples, two-dimensional matrix array transducers are important for high-efficiency HIFU treatment. They are also needed to focus through very heterogeneous media, such as the skull or ribs. Kobayashi *et al* numerically estimated the appropriate phase of each element of a transducer using a skull model of a monkey based on computed tomography (CT) images and performed experiments using a 64-channel array transducer [14].

Piezoelectric composites are used as the electromechanical conversion material for many such array transducers. Cathignol *et al* compared the acoustic fields produced by piezoceramic and piezocomposite focused transducers and reported that Lamb waves were eliminated in the piezocomposite transducer, with the result that its pressure field agreed well with a simulation that assumed a uniform distribution of the normal velocity along the transducer surface [15]. Figure 10.4 shows a photograph and the element configuration of a 128-channel piezocomposite transducer which has an outer diameter of 147.8 mm and a focal length of 120 mm. Since the transducer is made of 1–3 piezocomposite consisting of small piezoelectric columns, arrays are constructed using electrode patterns. One type of array transducer is the capacitive micromachined ultrasonic transducer (CMUT). Yoon *et al* successfully coagulated *ex vivo* bovine muscle and liver tissues using a CMUT array with 1024 elements [16].

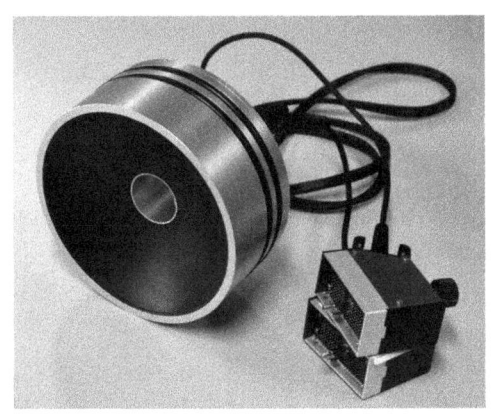

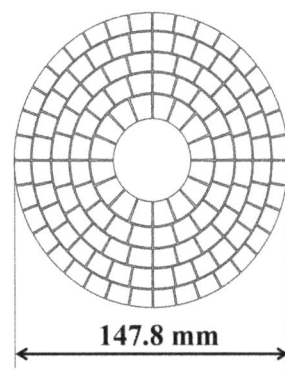

Figure 10.4. Piezocomposite array transducer with 128 channels.

One of the problems with array transducers, including piezocomposite arrays, is that they require a large number of high-voltage drive circuits. The drive voltage can be reduced by lowering the electrical impedance of each transducer element. Song and Hynynen developed an ultrasound phased array consisting of 1372 cylindrical piezoelectric transducers for transcranial treatments [17]. The transducer was designed to be used with lateral coupling to reduce the electric impedance and driven at 306 or 840 kHz. Otsu *et al* numerically investigated a piezoceramic transducer using a breathing mode [18]. They reported that a low electric impedance could be achieved by a concave hemispherical piezoceramic shell with a diameter slightly larger than its wavelength in water. Also, it was shown that a concave transducer with a convergence angle of 130° resonates at the second harmonic [18].

The superimposition of the second harmonic onto the fundamental has been investigated for the effective use of microbubbles and cavitation [19–21]. Since the conventional design for an air-backed transducer is ineffective in generating both the second harmonic and the fundamental at the same time, Zain *et al* numerically investigated a piezocomposite transducer with a heavy matching layer in order to produce both the fundamental and the second harmonic at high efficiency [22].

A multi-channel driving system is required to drive array transducers. The number of channels ranges from tens to sometimes more than 1000. High efficiency is important for compact multi-channel driver systems. Moro *et al* developed a staircase-voltage driver circuit using metal–oxide–semiconductor field-effect transistors (MOSFETs) [23]. Figure 10.5 shows the driving waveform. The values of a and b in figure 10.5 are selected so that the third harmonic is sufficiently suppressed. Tamano *et al* improved the circuit through the use of both N and P MOSFETs for each staircase-voltage level instead of only one of them, resulting in a reduction in the power consumption [24]. The circuit was implemented in an HIFU drive system with 128 channels [25]. Adams *et al* developed an HIFU drive system using a similar waveform and coagulated *ex vivo* chicken breast [26]. An ultrasound driver using gallium nitride (GaN) has been studied [27], which will lead to a further reduction of in power consumption of HIFU driving systems.

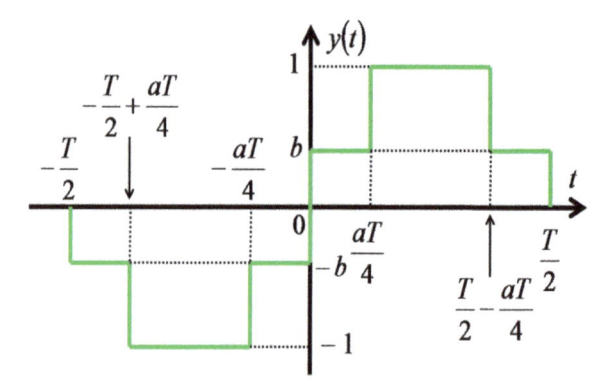

Figure 10.5. Staircase-voltage driving waveform.

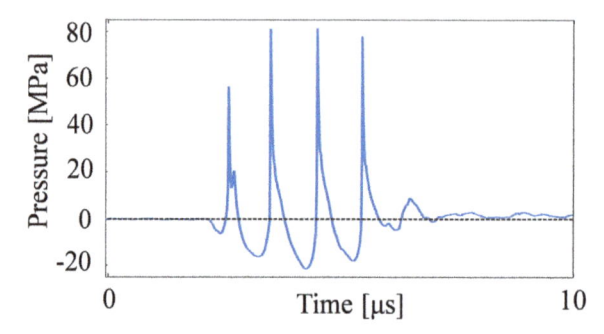

Figure 10.6. Pressure at an HIFU focus measured using a fiber-optic hydrophone.

10.3 Measurement and visualization of HIFU fields

The three-dimensional pressure field of diagnostic ultrasound is typically measured by scanning a hydrophone. Various evaluation methods have been studied with the aim of measuring the HIFU pressure field [28]. One of the reasons for this is that the risk of hydrophone damage due to cavitation is non-negligible in hydrophone measurements. Another reason is that the HIFU pressure field contains many higher harmonic components due to the effects of nonlinear propagation.

Staudenraus and Eisenmenger developed a fiber-optic probe hydrophone for ultrasonic and shock-wave measurements in water [29]. The measurements made by this type of hydrophone are based on the principle that the reflection coefficient of light at the water–fiber interface depends on the pressure of the water. A fiber-optic hydrophone generally has a broadband response. In addition, if the fiber is damaged, it can be reused by re-cleaving it. These characteristics are suitable for the measurement of high acoustic pressure in an HIFU focal region. Figure 10.6 shows an example of a pressure waveform at an HIFU focus measured using a fiber-optic hydrophone. The sharp rise and fall of the positive pressure are captured. The disadvantage of this type of fiber-optic hydrophone is its low sensitivity. A Fabry–Pérot type hydrophone with high sensitivity has been developed [30].

However, this type of hydrophone has the disadvantage of a lack of reusability when it is damaged.

Another approach is to use a robust hydrophone. Shiiba et al developed a robust hydrophone by depositing a hydrothermally synthesized lead zirconate titanate polycrystalline film on the back of a titanium plate for pressure measurement in the presence of acoustic cavitation bubbles [31, 32]. Wilkens et al developed a robust membrane hydrophone with a steel-foil front protection layer [33].

One of the challenges of HIFU pressure-field measurement is to calibrate the hydrophone over a wide frequency range. Igarashi et al developed an ultrasound source which could generate high-intensity ultrasound using a cylindrical acoustic waveguide for the calibration of hydrophones [34]. Chiba and Yoshioka investigated the effectiveness of sensitivity extrapolation to the frequency range of certificated sensitivities, although the pressure range was limited to diagnostic use [35].

The combination of measurement in a low-intensity field and nonlinear propagation simulation is one of the promising candidates for HIFU pressure-field evaluation. Kreider et al calculated the strength of an HIFU pressure field, including the effects of nonlinear propagation, using acoustic sources reconstructed and scaled from the measurement of the pressure field before it was focused, both (i) at a low intensity [36] and (ii) by acoustic holography [37].

Non-contact measurement methods of a pressure field using only an optical system (i.e. without a hydrophone) have also been studied. Kudo used a simple optical system for shadowgraphs to visualize an instantaneous pressure field by subtracting images with and without ultrasound exposure [38]. Using this technic with collimated light, ultrasound attenuation in a transparent medium was measured [39], and the interference between ultrasound waves in small containers was visualized [40]. Pitts and Greenleaf recovered the distribution of the optical phase shift induced by ultrasound from images obtained using a shadowgraph system. The optical phase shifts were obtained by rotating the transducer and then the three-dimensional pressure field was reconstructed [41]. Similarly, focused ultrasound pressure fields were also reconstructed using a shadowgraph system [42–45]. A phase-contrast method using the principle of phase-contrast microscopy has also been studied with the intention of recovering the optical phase shifts. Torikai and Negishi applied the method of phase-contrast microscopy to an acoustic field for visualization [46]. Pitts et al reconstructed a three-dimensional ultrasound field using the phase-contrast method [47]. Similarly, Harigane et al reconstructed a three-dimensional focused ultrasound field [48]. Figure 10.7 shows an example of the distribution of an optical phase shift caused by 1 MHz focused ultrasound, which exhibits phase wrapping in the region around the focus. Syahid et al reconstructed a higher-intensity pressure field using a phase plate that had two phase columns and a phase unwrapping technic [49]. Nakamura et al reconstructed a diagnostic ultrasound field using a combination of optical phase contrast and nonlinear acoustic holography methods [50]. Ishikawa et al recovered optical phase shifts using parallel phase-shifting interferometry with a high-speed polarization camera [51].

The visualization of HIFU using a tissue-mimicking phantom has been studied as well. Lafon et al developed a phantom which was made of polyacrylamide hydrogel

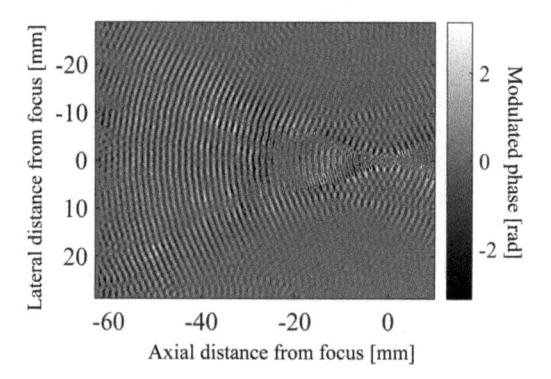

Figure 10.7. Distribution of optical phase shift showing phase wrapping (obtained using the phase-contrast method).

containing bovine serum albumin [52]. This type of phantom becomes optically opaque when exposed to HIFU and denatured. Kim *et al* embedded a thermochromic film into a polyvinyl alcohol gel phantom [53]. Maxwell *et al* developed an agarose phantom which had three layers. The middle layer contained red blood cells to permit an investigation of the tissue damage induced by acoustic cavitation [54]. Ueda *et al* inserted a thin slice of excised tissue into an agarose gel phantom in order to observe acoustic cavitation in the tissue [55].

10.4 Cavitation

When HIFU propagates, it can cause cavitation due to its high intensity. Since cavitation bubbles reflect and scatter ultrasound and may cause unintended tissue damage, it is important to monitor the generation of cavitation bubbles during HIFU treatments. On the other hand, cavitation bubbles in an ultrasound field are known to have a role in accelerating ultrasonic heating [56]. Therefore, if cavitation bubbles are generated only in the treatment region, the therapeutic effect of HIFU can be enhanced by cavitation without producing side effects. There are two main approaches to controlling the cavitation generation region: one is to apply feedback to the HIFU irradiation, and the other is to use pulsed or short burst waves of HIFU.

Hockham *et al* modulated the amplitude of HIFU according to the acoustic emission from cavitation bubbles measured using a passive cavitation detector (PCD) in order to achieve sustained cavitation [57]. Patel *et al* developed a controller using frequency-selective passive acoustic mapping (PAM) for the spatial and temporal controls of cavitation [58] using an ultrasound imaging probe.

Sokka *et al* proposed an HIFU exposure sequence consisting of a high-power burst followed by a moderate-power continuous wave [59]. The acoustic power and duration of the burst were 300 W and 0.5 s, respectively. Those of the continuous wave were 7–28 W and 19.5 s, respectively. Ultrasonic frequencies of 1.1 and 1.7 MHz were used. In the study, the lesions created by the proposed sequence were two to three times larger in volume than those created by the sequence without the high-power burst. Elbes *et al* investigated the effect of a high-power burst at powers from 250 W to 800 W with a duration of 0.5 s on the results obtained using magnetic resonance acoustic radiation force imaging (MR-ARFI) and MR thermometry [60]. Takagi *et al* proposed a sequence consisting of a high-intensity pulse (called the 'trigger pulse') at 14 kW cm^{-2} with a duration of 0.1 ms followed by a continuous wave (called the 'heating burst') at 400–800 W cm^{-2} with a duration of 5 s [61]. The sequence, which was called the 'trigger HIFU sequence' [62], was combined with electric focus scanning to obtain a large coagulation volume [13, 63].

The durations used for the high-power ultrasound, namely 500 and 0.1 ms, may have made a difference to the temperature-increase and standing-wave effects. Since bubbles migrate toward the nodes and antinodes of standing waves and coalesce, the cavitation threshold tends to decrease due to the presence of standing-wave components [64]. Conversely, if the effect of the standing waves is small, the cavitation threshold is very high. Maxwell *et al* investigated the probability of cavitation generation using a two-cycle pulse [65]. In their study, the statistical cavitation threshold range of the peak negative pressure was from −26 to −30 MPa in media with a high water content. This is called the 'intrinsic threshold.' Using a slightly longer pulse, another mechanism has been proposed to form clusters of cavitation bubbles or cavitation clouds, which is called 'shock scattering' [66]. The ultrasound waveform in a high-intensity focal region has a steep and large peak in the positive pressure and a relatively small peak in the negative pressure, as shown in figure 10.6, due to the focusing of nonlinearly propagated ultrasound. Once cavitation bubbles are generated, they provide a pressure release surface that converts positive pressure into negative pressure, which exceeds the intrinsic threshold. Cavitation clouds are generated through shock-scattering cycles. Since the cavitation clouds formed through shock scattering tend to grow backward from the focal point, as shown in figure 10.8, a trigger HIFU sequence with an intentional focal shift of the

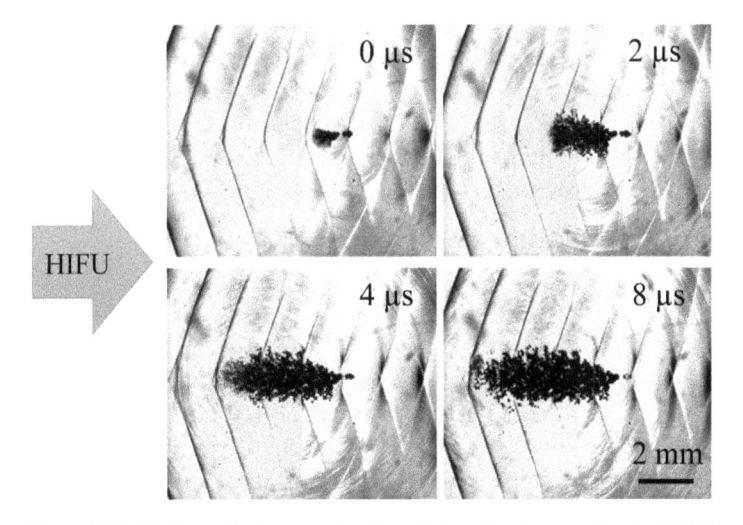

Figure 10.8. High-speed photographs of cavitation cloud generation by HIFU.

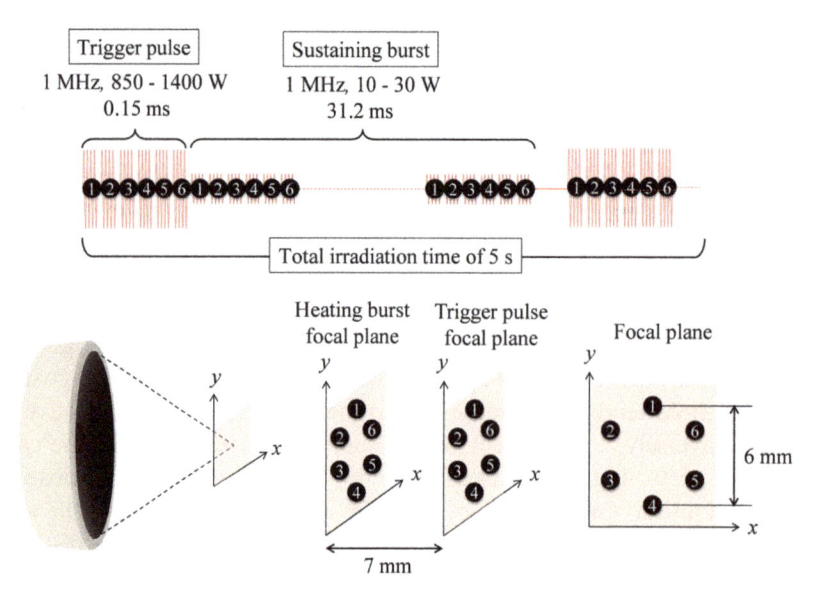

Figure 10.9. Example of a trigger HIFU sequence with electric scanning.

trigger pulses was investigated to match the axial position of the generated cavitation clouds to that of the focus of the heating waves [67].

Acoustic cavitation bubbles not only enhance HIFU heating, but also make nonthermal treatments such as mechanical and chemical treatments possible. Histotripsy is a mechanical treatment method that uses acoustic cavitation [68]. The surrounding soft tissues are mechanically destroyed through the collapses of cavitation bubbles. Qu *et al* investigated abscopal immune responses to histotripsy [69]. Sonodynamic therapy (SDT) is a treatment method that utilizes the chemical effects caused by oscillating bubbles in an ultrasound field and is often used in conjunction with sonosensitizers [70]. Figure 10.9 shows an example of a trigger HIFU sequence applied to SDT, which was used with anticancer micelles for canine cancer treatments [71]. The focal plane of the trigger pulses was shifted forward from the geometric focal plane by 7 mm and six foci were electronically scanned during irradiation by the trigger pulses and the following sustained bursts.

Methods have also been developed in which the blood–brain barrier (BBB) is temporarily opened for drug delivery by oscillating bubbles, although stabilized microbubbles need to be injected [72, 73].

10.5 Ultrasound image guidance

Since HIFU is a noninvasive treatment modality, it is used in conjunction with noninvasive image guidance, such as magnetic resonance imaging (MRI) and ultrasound imaging systems. The greatest advantage of using MRI is the availability of MR temperature mapping, while its main disadvantages are its relatively low frame rate and high cost. The main advantages of ultrasound imaging are its relatively high frame rate and relatively low cost. Another advantage is the self-compensating effect on targeting, because imaging ultrasound is refracted in the same way as HIFU. On the other hand, the ultrasound imaging of organs surrounded by air and bone, such as the brain, is difficult. In this section, studies of ultrasound image guidance are introduced.

An image guidance system is required to have the ability to perform targeting, real-time monitoring during HIFU exposure, and the evaluation of treatment effects. In ultrasound imaging, two approaches are used to achieve these functions: one is to use the brightness change in ultrasound B-mode images, and the other is to use the ultrasonically obtained displacement or strain of tissues. In HIFU therapy that uses cavitation, the monitoring of cavitation bubbles is also an important function.

When the temperature of a biological tissue changes, the backscattered ultrasound signal shifts due to thermal expansion and a change in the speed of sound. The time shift of echo signals caused by temperature change is observed as strain in an ultrasound image, and is thus called thermal strain imaging. For small temperature changes, the temperature change and the thermally induced strain have a linear relationship via tissue-dependent coefficients. Simon *et al* estimated a two-dimensional temperature distribution by thermal strain imaging [74]. Sharp gradients in the temperature distribution introduce ripples in the strain distribution due to a thermo-acoustic lens effect. Pernot *et al* used multiple transmissions of steered plane waves in thermal strain imaging to reduce the effect of thermo-acoustic lensing on the strain map [75]. It is still challenging to estimate a temperature distribution over a wide temperature range, in which a linear relationship between temperature and thermal strain can be not assumed.

When the tissue temperature changes, the shear-wave speed and shear modulus of the tissue also change. Arnal *et al* proposed shear-wave thermometry based on measuring changes in the shear modulus, which was obtained by shear-wave imaging of tissues [76]. When tissue is thermally coagulated, the shear modulus increases due to denaturation. Arnal *et al* obtained a strain map every 3 s using *ex vivo* tissues and showed that the tissue stiffness increased by up to four times [77]. Iwasaki *et al* showed that changes in shear-wave velocity can be used to detect a coagulation region produced by HIFU exposure using cavitation bubbles [78]. It was also shown that the acoustic radiation force induced by a HIFU burst was suitable for use as the shear-wave source [79].

During HIFU exposure, the acoustic radiation force (ARF) induced by HIFU acts on the tissue in the HIFU propagation direction. Maleke and Konofagou modulated the amplitude of HIFU and obtained the amplitude of the induced harmonic motion in the tissue [80]. The ability to perform harmonic motion imaging (HMI) was demonstrated by detecting the formation of a protein-denatured lesion in bovine liver samples. Sugiyama *et al* developed a real-time feedback control system using localized motion imaging (LMI), which was developed to improve the detection sensitivity of HMI [81]. The coagulation size was measured every 1 s and the HIFU exposure was controlled so that it matched the target size.

The acoustic radiation force is caused by ultrasound attenuation, and ultrasound absorption generates heat. Since ultrasound absorption is the major cause of the

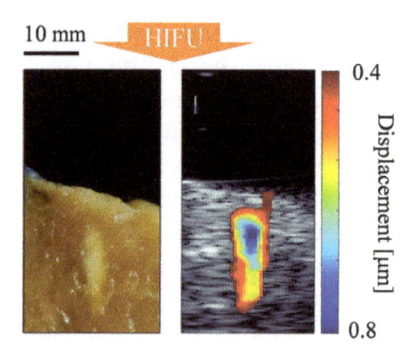

Figure 10.10. Gross pathology of coagulated chicken breast tissue (left) and tissue displacement distribution superimposed on a B-mode image (right).

attenuation in tissue, it is assumed that the distribution of tissue displaced by the HIFU radiation force and that of the HIFU heat source are closely related. Iwasaki *et al* measured the distribution of tissue displacement during and immediately after a HIFU burst [82]. The displacement distribution showed good agreement with the coagulation region produced by continuous HIFU exposure. Yabata *et al* investigated the effects of the timing of displacement distribution acquisition and shear modulus on the displacement distribution induced by a HIFU burst [83, 84]. Figure 10.10 shows an example of the gross pathology of excised chicken breast tissue after coagulation caused by a continuous HIFU exposure and the tissue displacement distribution induced by a short HIFU burst before the continuous HIFU exposure. The displacement distribution for values greater than half of the maximum is superimposed on the B-mode image. Obara *et al* compared the displacement distribution caused by the HIFU radiation force and the strain distribution using thermal strain imaging [85].

Some studies of ultrasound image guidance have used the change in the texture of biological tissue exposed to HIFU apparent in a B-mode image. Zheng and Vaezy showed that the coagulated region was visualized in two-dimensional (2D) images of the decay rate of the echo amplitude after HIFU exposure [86]. Mast *et al* showed that the decorrelation between ultrasound images during radio-frequency ablation experiments corresponded with the local tissue temperature and ablation effects [87]. Matsuzawa *et al* showed that the region coagulated by HIFU could be also monitored by the echo decorrelation method [88]. Sasaki *et al* showed that high-speed ultrasound imaging by parallel beamforming could be effective for the detection of coagulated regions in echo decorrelation maps [89]. Yoshizawa *et al* showed that the decorrelation method could be applied to coagulation detection by HIFU exposure using cavitation bubbles [90]. Shishitani *et al* investigated changes in the backscatter of *ex vivo* liver tissues exposed to HIFU in relation to the histological change in the concentration of hepatic cells [91]. Yamamoto and Yoshizawa investigated thermally induced strain in a tissue during HIFU exposure and showed that the strain caused echo decorrelation [92]. Takeuchi *et al* used Nakagami's shape parameter m to measure the temperature elevation in a living rat induced by capacitively coupled radio-frequency heating [93].

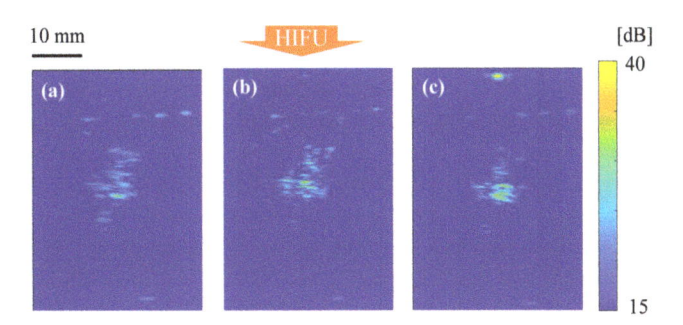

Figure 10.11. B-mode images during trigger HIFU exposure obtained by (a) single-transmission (b) pulse-inversion, and (c) triplet pulse sequences.

Considering the resonant size of the bubbles, most of the cavitation bubbles induced by HIFU at a frequency of around 1 MHz are expected to be less than a few μm in size. The dissolution time of such free microbubbles is on the order of, or shorter than, the typical frame time of conventional ultrasound imaging. Gateau *et al* used a combination of passive detection and high-speed ultrasound imaging with plane-wave transmission to monitor cavitation bubbles induced by short pulses of HIFU [94]. Iwasaki *et al* combined high-speed ultrasound imaging with plane-wave transmission and a triplet pulse sequence [95]. In the triplet pulse sequence, three ultrasound pulses with the same envelope but with phases shifted by 120° were used to extract nonlinear echo signals from bubbles. Shiozaki *et al* investigated the contrast ratio between the bubbles and tissue using the triplet pulse sequence in various HIFU exposure sequences [96]. Figure 10.11 shows an example of B-mode images of excised chicken tissue during trigger HIFU exposure obtained using single-transmission, pulse-inversion, and triplet pulse sequences. The highest contrast ratio is seen in the result obtained using the triplet pulse sequence. The use of spatiotemporal filters for monitoring cavitation has also been investigated. Arnal *et al* investigated a spatiotemporal singular value decomposition (SVD) of the RF echo data obtained from diverging wave transmissions [97]. Their method provided higher bubble-to-tissue contrast than that obtained using standard temporal filtering techniques in a moving phantom and liver tissue. Ikeda *et al* used an SDV filter to separate tissue, blood flow, and cavitation signals [98].

10.6 Concluding remarks

Clinical trials of HIFU treatments utilizing ultrasonically generated cavitation and also those utilizing cavitation initiated with stabilized microbubbles, which were explained in this review, are now underway. Cavitation has been regarded as a phenomenon to be avoided in medical applications of ultrasound, not only in diagnostics but even in therapeutic procedures, for more than several decades, but it will become an important tool of medical ultrasound when such trials are successful.

References

[1] Murat F L and Gelet A 2008 Current status of high-intensity focused ultrasound for prostate cancer: technology, clinical outcomes, and future *Curr. Urol. Rep.* **9** 113–21

[2] Shoji S, Hiraiwa S, Uemura K, Nitta M, Hasegawa M, Kawamura Y, Hashida K, Hasebe T, Tajiri T and Miyajima A 2020 Focal therapy with high-intensity focused ultrasound for the localized prostate cancer for Asian based on the localization with MRI-TRUS fusion image-guided transperineal biopsy and 12-cores transperineal systematic biopsy: prospective analysis of oncological and functional outcomes *Int. J. Clin. Oncol.* **25** 1844–53

[3] Kennedy J E, Wu F, ter Haar G R, Gleeson F V, Phillips R R, Middleton M R and Cranston D 2004 High-intensity focused ultrasound for the treatment of liver tumours *Ultrasonics* **42** 931–5

[4] Numata K, Fukuda H, Ohto M, Itou R, Nozaki A, Kondou M, Morimoto M, Karasawa E and Tanaka K 2010 Evaluation of the therapeutic efficacy of high-intensity focused ultrasound ablation of hepatocellular carcinoma by three-dimensional sonography with a perflubutane-based contrast agent *Eur. J. Radiol.* **75** e67–75

[5] Marinova M *et al* 2021 Improving quality of life in pancreatic cancer patients following high-intensity focused ultrasound (HIFU) in two European centers *Eur. Radiol.* **31** 5818–29

[6] Sofuni A *et al* 2021 Novel therapeutic method for unresectable pancreatic cancer-the impact of the long-term research in therapeutic effect of high-intensity focused ultrasound (HIFU) therapy *Curr. Oncol.* **28** 4845–61

[7] Giordano M, Caccavella V M, Zaed I, Manzillo L F, Montano N, Olivi A and Polli F M 2020 Comparison between deep brain stimulation and magnetic resonance-guided focused ultrasound in the treatment of essential tremor: a systematic review and pooled analysis of functional outcomes *J. Neurol. Neurosurg. Psychiatry* **91** 1270–8

[8] Abe K *et al* 2021 Focused ultrasound thalamotomy for refractory essential tremor: a Japanese multicenter single-arm study *Neurosurgery* **88** 751–7

[9] Sapareto S A and Dewey W C 1984 Thermal dose determination in cancer therapy *Int. J. Radiat. Oncol. Biol. Phys.* **1** 787–800

[10] Cain C A and Umemura S 1986 Concentric-ring and sector-vortex phased-array applicators for ultrasound hyperthermia *IEEE Trans. Microw. Theory Tech.* **34** 542–51

[11] Umemura S and Cain C A 1992 Acoustical evaluation of a prototype sector-vortex phased-array applicator *IEEE Trans. Ultrason. Ferroelectr. Freq. Control* **39** 32–8

[12] Köhler M O, Mougenot C, Quesson B, Enholm J, Le Bail B, Laurent C, Moonen C T W and Ehnholm G J 2009 Volumetric HIFU ablation under 3D guidance of rapid MRI thermometry *Med. Phys.* **36** 3521–35

[13] Inaba Y, Moriyama T, Yoshizawa S and Umemura S 2011 Ultrasonic coagulation of large tissue region by generating multiple cavitation clouds in direction perpendicular to ultrasound propagation *Jpn. J. Appl. Phys.* **50** 07HF13

[14] Kobayashi Y, Azuma T, Shimizu K, Koizumi M, Oya T, Suzuki R, Maruyama K, Seki K and Takagi S 2018 Development of focus controlling method with transcranial focused ultrasound aided by numerical simulation for noninvasive brain therapy *Jpn. J. Appl. Phys.* **57** 07LF22

[15] Cathignol D, Sapozhnikov O A and Theillère Y 1999 Comparison of acoustic fields radiated from piezoceramic and piezocomposite focused radiators *J. Acoust. Soc. Am.* **105** 2612–7

[16] Yoon H S, Chang C, Jang J H, Bhuyan A, Choe J W, Nikoozadeh A, Watkins R D, Stephens D N, Pauly K B and Khuri-Yakub B T 2016 Ex-vivo HIFU experiments using a 32 × 32-element CMUT array *IEEE Trans. Ultrason. Ferroelectr. Freq. Control* **63** 2150–8

[17] Song J and Hynynen K 2010 Feasibility of using lateral mode coupling method for a large scale ultrasound phased array for noninvasive transcranial therapy *IEEE Trans. Biomed. Eng.* **57** 124–33

[18] Otsu K, Yoshizawa S and Umemura S 2011 Breathing-mode ceramic element for therapeutic array transducer *Jpn. J. Appl. Phys.* **50** 07HC02

[19] Umemura S, Kawabata K and Sasaki K 1996 Enhancement of sonodynamic tissue damage production by second-harmonic superimposition: theoretical analysis of its mechanism *IEEE Trans. Ultrason. Ferroelectr. Freq. Control.* **43** 1054–62

[20] Takagi R, Yoshizawa S and Umemura S 2011 Cavitation inception by dual-frequency excitation in high-intensity focused ultrasound treatment *Jpn. J. Appl. Phys.* **50** 07HF14

[21] Sasaki H, Yasuda J, Takagi R, Miyashita T, Goto K, Yoshizawa S and Umemura S 2014 Highly efficient cavitation-enhanced heating with dual-frequency ultrasound exposure in high-intensity focused ultrasound treatment *Jpn. J. Appl. Phys.* **53** 07KF11

[22] Zaini Z, Osuga M, Jimbo H, Yasuda J, Takagi R, Yoshizawa S and Umemura S 2016 Study on heavy matching layer transducer towards producing second harmonics *Jpn. J. Appl. Phys.* **55** 07KF15

[23] Moro K, Yoshizawa S and Umemura S 2010 Staircase-voltage metal–oxide–semiconductor field-effect transistor driver circuit for therapeutic ultrasound *Jpn. J. Appl. Phys.* **49** 07HF02

[24] Tamano S, Jimbo H, Azuma T, Yoshizawa S, Fujiwara K, Itani K and Umemura S 2016 Improvement of high-voltage staircase drive circuit waveform for high-intensity therapeutic ultrasound *Jpn. J. Appl. Phys.* **55** 07KF15

[25] Tamano S, Yoshizawa S and Umemura S 2017 Multifunctional pulse generator for high-intensity focused ultrasound system *Jpn. J. Appl. Phys.* **56** 07JF21

[26] Adams C, Carpenter T M, Cowell D, Freear S and McLaughlan J R 2018 HIFU drive system miniaturization using harmonic reduced pulsewidth modulation *IEEE Trans. Ultrason. Ferroelectr. Freq. Control.* **65** 2407–17

[27] Peng H, Sabate J, Wall K A and Glaser J S 2018 GaN-based high-frequency high-energy delivery transformer push–pull inverter for ultrasound pulsing application *IEEE Power Electron. Mag.* **33** 6794–806

[28] Xing G, Wilkens V and Yang P 2021 Review of field characterization techniques for high intensity therapeutic ultrasound *Metrologia* **58** 022001

[29] Staudenraus J and Eisenmenger W 1993 Fibre-optic probe hydrophone for ultrasonic and shock-wave measurements in water *Ultrasonics* **31** 267–73

[30] Morris P, Hurrell A, Shaw A, Zhang E and Beard P 2009 A Fabry–Pérot fiber-optic ultrasonic hydrophone for the simultaneous measurement of temperature and acoustic pressure *J. Acoust. Soc. Am.* **125** 3611–22

[31] Shiiba M, Okada N, Uchida T, Kikuchi T, Kurosawa M and Takeuchi S 2014 Frequency characteristics of receiving sensitivity and waveform of an anti-acoustic cavitation hydrophone *Jpn. J. Appl. Phys.* **53** 07KE06

[32] Shiiba M, Okada N, Kurosawa M and Takeuchi S 2016 Development of anticavitation hydrophone using a titanium front plate: effect of the titanium front plate in high-intensity acoustic field with generation of acoustic cavitation *Jpn. J. Appl. Phys.* **55** 07KE16

[33] Wilkens V, Sonntag S and Georg O 2016 Robust spot-poled membrane hydrophones for measurement of large amplitude pressure waveforms generated by high intensity therapeutic ultrasonic transducers *J. Acoust. Soc. Am.* **139** 1319–32

[34] Igarashi S, Morishita T, Uchida T and Takeuchi S 2017 Experimental evaluation of high-intensity ultrasound source system using acoustic waveguide for calibration of hydrophone *Jpn. J. Appl. Phys.* **56** 07JF19

[35] Chiba Y and Yoshioka M 2021 Effectiveness evaluation of extrapolation to frequency response of hydrophone sensitivity for measuring instantaneous acoustic pressure of diagnostic ultrasound *Jpn. J. Appl. Phys.* **60** SDDE14

[36] Kreider W, Yuldashev P V, Sapozhnikov O A, Farr N, Partanen A, Bailey M R and Khokhlova V A 2013 Characterization of a multi-element clinical HIFU system using acoustic holography and nonlinear modeling *IEEE Trans. Ultrason. Ferroelectr. Freq. Control.* **60** 1683–98

[37] Sapozhnikov O A, Pishchal'nikov Y A and Morozov A V 2003 Reconstruction of the normal velocity distribution on the surface of an ultrasonic transducer from the acoustic pressure measured on a reference surface *Acoust. Phys.* **49** 354–60

[38] Kudo N 2015 A simple technique for visualizing ultrasound fields without schlieren optics *Ultrasound Med. Biol.* **41** 2071–81

[39] Iijima Y and Kudo N 2017 Evaluation of frequency-dependent ultrasound attenuation in transparent medium using focused shadowgraph technique *Jpn. J. Appl. Phys.* **56** 07JF13

[40] Aikawa T and Kudo N 2019 Visualization of wall propagation and surface reflection effects on ultrasound fields generated inside a small container *Jpn. J. Appl. Phys.* **58** SGGE11

[41] Pitts T A and Greenleaf J F 2000 Three-dimensional optical measurement of instantaneous pressure *J. Acoust. Soc. Am.* **125** 3611–22

[42] Omura R, Shimazaki Y, Yoshizawa S and Umemura S 2011 Quantitative measurement of focused ultrasound pressure field using subtraction shadowgraph *Jpn. J. Appl. Phys.* **50** 07HC07

[43] Shimazaki Y, Yoshizawa S and Umemura S 2012 Three-dimensional quantitative optical measurement of asymmetrically focused ultrasound pressure field *Jpn. J. Appl. Phys.* **51** 07GF25

[44] Miyasaka R, Yasuda J, Syahid M, Yoshizawa S and Umemura S 2014 Quantitative measurement of focused ultrasound pressure field by background-subtracted shadowgraph using holographic diffuser as screen *Jpn. J. Appl. Phys.* **53** 07KF24

[45] Hanayama H, Nakamura T, Takagi R, Yoshizawa S and Umemura S 2017 Simulation of optical propagation based on wave optics for phase retrieval in shadowgraph of ultrasonic field *Jpn. J. Appl. Phys.* **56** 07JC13

[46] Torikai Y and Negishi K 1952 The application of the phase method in visualizing ultrasonic waves *J. Phys. Soc. Japan* **8** 119–24

[47] Pitts T A, Sagers A and Greenleaf J F 2001 Optical phase contrast measurement of ultrasonic fields *IEEE Trans. Ultrason. Ferroelectr. Freq. Control.* **48** 1686–94

[48] Harigane S, Miyasaka R, Yoshizawa S and Umemura S 2013 Optical Phase Contrast mapping of highly focused ultrasonic fields *Jpn. J. Appl. Phys.* **52** 07HF07

[49] Syahid M, Oyama S, Yasuda J, Yoshizawa S and Umemura S 2015 Quantitative measurement of high intensity focused ultrasound pressure field by optical phase contrast method applying non-continuous phase unwrapping algorithm *Jpn. J. Appl. Phys.* **54** 07HC09

[50] Nakamura T, Iwasaki R, Yoshizawa S and Umemura S 2018 Quantitative measurement of ultrasonic pressure field using combination of optical phase contrast and nonlinear acoustic holography methods *Jpn. J. Appl. Phys.* **57** 07LB13

[51] Ishikawa K, Yatabe K, Chitanont N, Ikeda Y, Oikawa Y, Onuma T, Niwa H and Yoshii M 2016 High-speed imaging of sound using parallel phase-shifting interferometry *Opt. Express* **24** 12922–32

[52] Lafon C, Zderic V, Noble M L, Yuen J C, Kaczkowski P J, Sapozhnikov O A, Chavrier F, Crum L A and Vaezy S 2005 Gel phantom for use in high-intensity focused ultrasound dosimetry *Ultrasound Med. Biol.* **31** 1383–9

[53] Kim M, Kim J, Choi P and Lee H 2020 Phantom made of polyvinyl alcohol for visualization of temperature rising area due to ultrasound *Jpn. J. Appl. Phys.* **59** SKKB08

[54] Maxwell A D, Wang T, Yuan L, Duryea A P, Xu Z and Cain C A 2010 A tissue phantom for visualization and measurement of ultrasound-induced cavitation damage *Ultrasound Med. Biol.* **36** 2132–43

[55] Ueda K, Ito S, Umemura S and Yoshizawa S 2021 Effect of focal spot scanning method in agarose gel and chicken breast on heating efficiency in cavitation-enhanced ultrasonic heating *Jpn. J. Appl. Phys.* **60** SDDE13

[56] Holt R G and Roy R A 2001 Measurements of bubble-enhanced heating from focused, MHz-frequency ultrasound in a tissue-mimicking material *Ultrasound Med. Biol.* **27** 1399–412

[57] Hockham N, Coussios C C and Arora M 2010 A real-time controller for sustaining thermally relevant acoustic cavitation during ultrasound therapy *IEEE Trans. Ultrason. Ferroelectr. Freq. Control.* **57** 2685–94

[58] Patel A, Schoen S J Jr and Arvanitis C D 2019 Closed loop spatial and temporal control of cavitation activity with passive acoustic mapping *IEEE Trans. Biomed. Eng.* **66** 2022–31

[59] Sokka S D, King R and Hynynen K 2003 MRI-guided gas bubble enhanced ultrasound heating in *in vivo* rabbit thigh *Phys. Med. Biol.* **48** 223–41

[60] Elbes D, Denost Q, Robert B, Köhler M O, Tanter M and Bruno Q 2014 Magnetic resonance imaging for the exploitation of bubble-enhanced heating by high-intensity focused ultrasound: a feasibility study in *ex vivo* liver *Ultrasound Med. Biol.* **40** 956–64

[61] Takagi R, Yoshizawa S and Umemura S 2010 Enhancement of localized heating by ultrasonically induced cavitation in high intensity focused ultrasound treatment *Jpn. J. Appl. Phys.* **49** 07HF21

[62] Yoshizawa S, Takagi R and Umemura S 2017 Enhancement of high-intensity focused ultrasound heating by short-pulse generated cavitation *Appl. Sci.* **7** 288

[63] Nakamura K, Asai A, Sasaki H, Yoshizawa S and Umemura S 2013 Large volume coagulation utilizing multiple cavitation clouds generated by array transducer driven by 32 channel drive circuits *Jpn. J. Appl. Phys.* **52** 07HF10

[64] Azuma T, Kawabata K, Umemura S, Ogihara M, Kubota J, Sasaki A and Furuhata H 2005 Bubble generation by standing wave in water surrounded by cranium with transcranial ultrasonic beam *Jpn. J. Appl. Phys.* **44** 4625–30

[65] Maxwell A D, Cain C A, Hall T L, Fowlkes J B and Xu Z 2013 Probability of cavitation for single ultrasound pulses applied to tissues and tissue-mimicking materials *Ultrasound Med. Biol.* **39** 449–65

[66] Maxwell A D, Wang T, Cain C A, Fowlkes J B, Sapozhnikov O A, Bailey M R and Xu Z 2011 Cavitation clouds created by shock scattering from bubbles during histotripsy *J. Acoust. Soc. Am.* **130** 1888–98

[67] Goto K, Takagi R, Miyashita T, Jimbo H, Yoshizawa S and Umemura S 2015 Effect of controlled offset of focal position in cavitation-enhanced high-intensity focused ultrasound treatment *Jpn. J. Appl. Phys.* **54** 07HF12

[68] Xu Z, Hall T L, Vlaisavljevich E and Lee F T Jr 2021 Histotripsy: the first noninvasive, non-ionizing, non-thermal ablation technique based on ultrasound *Int. J. Hyperth.* **38** 561–75

[69] Qu S *et al* 2019 Non-thermal histotripsy tumor ablation promotes abscopal immune responses that enhance cancer immunotherapy *J. Immunother. Cancer.* **8** e000200

[70] Lafond M, Yoshizawa S and Umemura S 2019 Sonodynamic therapy: advances and challenges in clinical translation *J. Ultrasound Med.* **38** 567–80

[71] Horise Y *et al* 2019 Sonodynamic therapy with anticancer micelles and high-intensity focused ultrasound in treatment of Canine cancer *Front. Pharmacol.* **10** 545

[72] Lipsman N *et al* 2018 Blood-brain barrier opening in Alzheimer's disease using MR-guided focused ultrasound *Nat. Commun.* **9** 2336

[73] Park *et al* 2020 Safety and feasibility of multiple blood-brain barrier disruptions for the treatment of glioblastoma in patients undergoing standard adjuvant chemotherapy *J. Neurosurg.* **134** 475–83

[74] Simon C, VanBaren P and Ebbini E S 1998 Two-dimensional temperature estimation using diagnostic ultrasound *IEEE Trans. Ultrason. Ferroelectr. Freq. Control.* **45** 1088–99

[75] Pernot M, Tanter M, Bercoff J, Waters K R and Fink M 2004 Temperature estimation using ultrasonic spatial compound imaging *IEEE Trans. Ultrason. Ferroelectr. Freq. Control.* **51** 606–15

[76] Arnal B, Pernot M and Tanter M 2011 Monitoring of thermal therapy based on shear modulus changes: I. Shear wave thermometry *IEEE Trans. Ultrason. Ferroelectr. Freq. Control.* **58** 369–78

[77] Arnal B, Pernot M and Tanter M 2011 Monitoring of thermal therapy based on shear modulus changes: II. Shear wave imaging of thermal lesions *IEEE Trans. Ultrason. Ferroelectr. Freq. Control.* **58** 1603–11

[78] Iwasaki R, Nagaoka R, Takagi R, Goto K, Yoshizawa S, Saijo Y and Umemura S 2015 Effects of cavitation-enhanced heating in high-intensity focused ultrasound treatment on shear wave imaging *Jpn. J. Appl. Phys.* **54** 07HF11

[79] Iwasaki R, Takagi R, Nagaoka R, Jimbo H, Yoshizawa S, Saijo Y and Umemura S 2016 Monitoring of high-intensity focused ultrasound treatment by shear wave elastography induced by two-dimensional-array therapeutic transducer *Jpn. J. Appl. Phys.* **55** 07KF05

[80] Maleke C and Konofagou E E 2008 Harmonic motion imaging for focused ultrasound (HMIFU): a fully integrated technique for sonication and monitoring of thermal ablation in tissues *Phys. Med. Biol.* **53** 1773–93

[81] Sugiyama R *et al* 2015 Real-time feedback control for high-intensity focused ultrasound system using localized motion imaging *Jpn. J. Appl. Phys.* **54** 07HD15

[82] Iwasaki R, Takagi R, Tomiyasu K, Yoshizawa S and Umemura S 2017 Prediction of thermal coagulation from the instantaneous strain distribution induced by high-intensity focused ultrasound *Jpn. J. Appl. Phys.* **56** 07JF23

[83] Yabata H, Umemura S and Yoshizawa S 2020 Effect of shear wave propagation on estimation of heating distribution by high-intensity focused ultrasound using acoustic radiation force imaging *Jpn. J. Appl. Phys.* **59** SKKE19

[84] Yabata H, Umemura S and Yoshizawa S 2021 Effect of difference in shear modulus of biological tissue on heat source distribution of high-intensity focused ultrasound estimated by acoustic radiation force imaging *Jpn. J. Appl. Phys.* **60** SDDE23

[85] Obara N, Umemura S and Yoshizawa S 2021 Comparison between thermal strain and acoustic radiation force imaging methods for estimation of heat source distribution of high-intensity focused ultrasound *Jpn. J. Appl. Phys.* **60** SDDE04

[86] Zheng X and Vaezy S 2010 An acoustic backscatter-based method for localization of lesions induced by high-intensity focused ultrasound *Ultrasound Med. Biol.* **36** 610–22

[87] Mast T D, Pucke D P, Subramanian S E, Bowlus W J, Rudich S M and Buell J F 2008 Ultrasound monitoring of in vitro radio frequency ablation by echo decorrelation imaging *J. Ultrasound Med.* **27** 1685–97

[88] Matsuzawa R, Shishitani T, Yoshizawa S and Umemura S 2012 monitoring of lesion induced by high-intensity focused ultrasound using correlation method based on block matching *Jpn. J. Appl. Phys.* **51** 07GF26

[89] Sasaki S, Takagi R, Matsuura K, Yoshizawa S and Umemura S 2014 Monitoring of high-intensity focused ultrasound lesion formation using decorrelation between high-speed ultrasonic images by parallel beamforming *Jpn. J. Appl. Phys.* **53** 07KF10

[90] Yoshizawa S, Matsuura K, Takagi R, Yamamoto M and Umemura S 2015 Detection of tissue coagulation by decorrelation of ultrasonic echo signals in cavitation-enhanced high-intensity focused ultrasound treatment *J. Ther. Ultrasound* **4** 15

[91] Shishitani T, Matsuzawa R, Yoshizawa S and Umemura S 2013 Changes in backscatter of liver tissue due to thermal coagulation induced by focused ultrasound *J. Acoust. Soc. Am.* **134** 1724–30

[92] Yamamoto M and Yoshizawa S 2021 Analysis of tissue displacement induced by high-intensity focused ultrasound exposure for coagulation monitoring *Jpn. J. Appl. Phys.* **60** 040903

[93] Takeuchi M, Sakai T, Andocs G, Takao K, Nagaoka R and Hasegawa H 2020 Temperature elevation in tissue detected *in vivo* based on statistical analysis of ultrasonic scattered echoes *Sci. Rep.* **10** 9030

[94] Gateau J, Aubry J, Pernot M, Fink and Tanter M 2011 Combined passive detection and ultrafast active imaging of cavitation events induced by short pulses of high-intensity ultrasound *IEEE Trans. Ultrason. Ferroelectr. Freq. Control.* **58** 517–32

[95] Iwasaki R, Nagaoka R, Yoshizawa S and Umemura S 2018 Selective detection of cavitation bubbles by triplet pulse sequence in high-intensity focused ultrasound treatment *Jpn. J. Appl. Phys.* **57** 07LF12

[96] Shiozaki I, Umemura S and Yoshizawa S 2020 Ultrasound imaging of cavitation using triplet pulse sequence in bubble-enhanced ultrasonic heating *Jpn. J. Appl. Phys.* **59** SKKE05

[97] Arnal B, Baranger J, Demene C, Tanter M and Pernot M 2017 *In vivo* real-time cavitation imaging in moving organs *Phys. Med. Biol.* **62** 843–57

[98] Ikeda H, Nagaoka R, Lafond M, Yoshizawa S, Iwasaki R, Maeda M, Umemura S and Saijo Y 2018 Singular value decomposition of received ultrasound signal to separate tissue, blood flow, and cavitation signals *Jpn. J. Appl. Phys.* **57** 07LF04

Milton Keynes UK
Ingram Content Group UK Ltd.
UKHW050219050823
426335UK00002B/23